T0207511

Download Your Included Ebook Today!

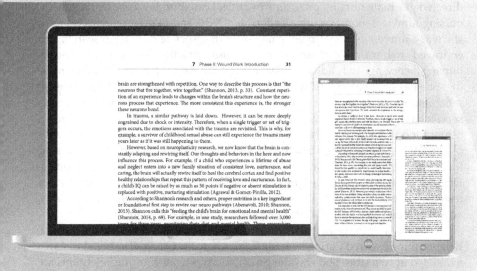

Your print purchase of *Quality Caring In Nursing and Health Systems*, 3e, **includes an ebook download** to the device of your choice—increasing accessibility, portability, and searchability!

Download your ebook today at:
http://spubonline.com/caring
and enter the access code below:

18MP306V1

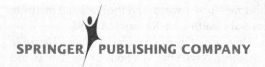

Joanne R. Duffy, PhD, RN, FAAN, is the executive vice president and senior consultant of QualiCare in Winchester, Virginia, and a visiting professor at the Indiana University School of Nursing in Indianapolis, Indiana. Her extensive career encompasses clinical, administrative, and academic roles. Dr. Duffy has directed graduate nursing programs in critical care nursing, care management, nursing administration, executive leadership (DNP), and a PhD program. Formerly, she was a university department chair, interim associate dean for research, and endowed chair for research and evidence-based practice. She currently teaches nursing theory, research, advanced leadership, and data analysis for decision making. She has held various administrative positions in service directing medical, rehabilitation, critical care, emergency, psychiatric, and transplantation nursing services at both community and academic medical centers. She also directed a center for outcomes analysis, a nurse-led department for improving the quality of cardiovascular services. She has published extensively across the nursing literature, but is best known for her work in maximizing patient outcomes. Dr. Duffy was the first to link nurse caring to patient outcomes, designed and tested multiple versions of the Caring Assessment Tool (including the e-CAT), and developed the Quality-Caring Model©, a middle-range theory.

Dr. Duffy was the principal investigator on the national demonstration project, Relationship-Centered Caring in Acute Care, where the Quality-Caring Model was evaluated at two sites. She was the principal investigator for the Telehomecare and Heart Failure Outcomes pilot study that tested a caring-based intervention on readmission and quality of life, and principal investigator for the Improving Safety and Quality in Vulnerable Acute Care Patients Through Interprofessional Collaborative Practice project. She evaluated the feasibility of using the e-CAT on hospitalized older adults, completed a study on nurses' research capacity and use of evidence, assessed the impact of a joint academic–service journal club, and recently completed a study on factors associated with missed nursing care. Dr. Duffy regularly leads research councils and journal clubs, assists staff nurses and nurse leaders in research and practice improvement projects, and provides consultation on professional practice model integration and leadership development.

Dr. Duffy was a consultant to the American Nurses Association in the development and implementation of the National Database of Nursing Quality Indicators and was the former chair of the National League for Nursing's Nursing Educational Research Advisory Council. She is a Commonwealth Fund Executive Nurse Fellow, a Fellow in the American Academy of Nursing, a frequent guest speaker, a former Magnet® appraiser, and a recipient of several awards, including the American Heart Association's Nursing Advisory Council Clinical Article of the Year Award, Virginia's Outstanding Nurse Award, and the National Institute of Health Care Management's Annual Health Care Research Award.

The first edition of this book, *Quality Caring in Nursing: Applying Theory to Clinical Practice, Education, and Leadership,* received the AJN Book of the Year award in 2009 and the model has been embraced by over 54 healthcare organizations, several of which have attained Magnet status.

Quality Caring in Nursing and Health Systems

Implications for Clinicians, Educators, and Leaders

Third Edition

Joanne R. Duffy, PhD, RN, FAAN

SPRINGER PUBLISHING COMPANY

Springer Publishing Company, LLC
11 West 42nd Street
New York, NY 10036
www.springerpub.com

Acquisitions Editor: Joseph Morita
Associate Managing Editor: Kris Parrish
Compositor: S4Carlisle Publishing Services

ISBN: 978-0-8261-8119-0
ebook ISBN: 978-0-8261-8125-1

18 19 20 21 22/5 4 3 2 1

The author and the publisher of this Work have made every effort to use sources believed to be reliable to provide information that is accurate and compatible with the standards generally accepted at the time of publication. Because medical science is continually advancing, our knowledge base continues to expand. Therefore, as new information becomes available, changes in procedures become necessary. We recommend that the reader always consult current research and specific institutional policies before performing any clinical procedure. The author and the publisher shall not be liable for any special, consequential, or exemplary damages resulting, in whole or in part, from the readers' use of, or reliance on, the information contained in this book. The publisher has no responsibility for the persistence or accuracy of URLs for external or third-party Internet websites referred to in this publication and does not guarantee that any content on such websites is, or will remain, accurate or appropriate.

Library of Congress Cataloging-in-Publication Data

Names: Duffy, Joanne R., author.
Title: Quality caring in nursing and health systems: implications for
    clinicians, educators, and leaders / Joanne R. Duffy.
Description: Third edition. | New York: Springer Publishing Company, [2018]
    | Includes bibliographical references and index.
Identifiers: LCCN 2018001649| ISBN 9780826181190 | ISBN 9780826181251 (ebook)
Subjects: | MESH: Nursing Care--standards | Quality Assurance, Health
    Care--standards | Nursing Theory | Nurse-Patient Relations | Nurse's Role
    | Leadership | United States
Classification: LCC RT85.5 | NLM WY 100 AA1 | DDC 610.73--dc23 LC record available at
https://lccn.loc.gov/2018001649

Contact us to receive discount rates on bulk purchases.
We can also customize our books to meet your needs.
For more information please contact: sales@springerpub.com

Printed in the United States of America.

Contents

Preface

While the velocity of societal change in the last 10 years has fueled massive advances in healthcare knowledge and technology, recent healthcare reform efforts have generated confusion and uncertainty among both health professionals and the general public. Within this context, an almost silent revolution is occurring in healthcare today, radically altering how individuals receive care as well as how it is being delivered. Yet, despite our best intentions, patients and families continue to suffer today not only from their illnesses but also from the healthcare system itself.

Notwithstanding the expansive quality improvement programs and dedicated financial resources expended in the past 20 years, the U.S. health system still inflicts unnecessary harms, does not consistently deliver patient-centered care, and does not focus on the fundamental caring processes that undergird healthcare processes. The constant emphasis on procedures, protocols, diagnostic testing, medications, tasks, technology, throughput, and costs has marginalized relationships as the central organizing aspect of professional practice. Evidence of this can be found in numerous professional publications, anecdotal evidence from patients and families, and empirical studies.

Consequently, dedicated time spent with patients and families at the bedside, in health professionals' offices, and at nursing homes, schools, and clinics is limited and often rushed and impersonal. Multiple nameless caregivers, system-created schedules, and distracted clinicians create unnecessary uncertainty, stress, limited opportunities for participation in decisions, incomplete care, and, often, preventable clinical and financial burdens for patients and families. Patients and families, at some of the most vulnerable times of life, are forced into dependency, reluctantly adapting to expectations of the system, and are frequently left to wonder whether they are safe and who will be there for them when they need it most.

This incongruity between the relational core of health services and the needs of patients and families is serious and may be linked to poor health outcomes. Not only has the reduced time spent "in relationship" challenged patients and families but health professionals themselves, leading to work dissatisfaction, diminished personal health, and lack of engagement in the work. The emphasis of today's biotechnical and cost-sensitive health systems often renders professionalism, relationships, and teamwork obscure. And although most health professionals strive to deliver excellent care, many do not regularly incorporate best evidence or timely practice improvement into their workflows. Relationships among health professional students, faculty, and clinical preceptors are, in some cases, considered uncivil, and leadership practices at all levels are not routinely attending to the fundamental relational nature of health system work.

This is particularly difficult for new health professionals who have been educated "to care" and suddenly find themselves working in health systems that do not advance relationships, have little supportive infra-structure, are focused on acquiring the latest gadget while maximizing reimbursement, and offer few incentives for professional development. Nurses, who are the largest group of healthcare professionals and spend the longest time with patients and families, are in a unique position to advance new relationship-centric approaches to healthcare.

This book provides an overview and updates the continuing quality crisis in healthcare, emphasizes the foundational relational aspects of healthcare through an evolving middle-range theory, and offers opportunities for application at several levels. In this updated edition, background literature is updated; the Quality-Caring Model$^©$ is slightly revised to allow for easier comprehension; the previous caring factors have been relabeled; practice analyses appear at the end of most chapters; and an additional appendix has been added.

The intent of the book is to continue the focus on the significance of caring relationships in improving the safety and quality of health systems. Additionally, it is a call to health professionals, particularly nurses, to action. Safe, quality healthcare and meaningful work are at stake. Through exploration of several theoretical concepts drawn from multiple sources, the evolution of the Quality-Caring Model is clarified. The important relationships with self, the community served, patients and families, and the healthcare team are illuminated and updated for current and future practice. Applying the model in clinical, educational, and leadership practice offers possibilities for advancing the value of the nation's health systems. Using the Quality-Caring Model as a foundation for research may point to new evidence regarding the contribution of caring relationships to quality health outcomes.

Part I focuses on the continuing problems inherent in complex health systems, including the continuing, disturbing facts about safety and quality and the state of professional practice, particularly in hospitals. The text continues by describing the evolving Quality-Caring Model, a middle-range theory that emphasizes the value of caring relationships to quality health outcomes. It is a hope-filled approach that is repeatedly emphasized throughout the text with specific exemplars. Part II concentrates on those relationships necessary for quality caring, namely, relationships with self, patients and families, members of the healthcare team, and the community. Concepts in the model are described in depth with case studies and examples. The system characteristics of relational capacity and practice improvement are addressed. Finally, self-advancing systems—those that naturally evolve with attention to caring relationships—end the section. Part III centers on leading and learning in quality-caring health systems, with emphasis on those relational processes that enhance professional practice. To conclude, the future of self-advancing systems—those that add value—is tied to the caring relationships that nurses have always known to be the real foundation for professional practice.

HOW TO USE THIS BOOK

This revised edition is intended for use by nursing students, particularly graduate students, and nursing scholars as well as clinical nurses, nurse educators, nurse researchers, and those in nursing leadership positions. Health professionals in other disciplines may also find it helpful. Each chapter contains an introductory section followed by specific narratives holding new information or applications. Areas of special emphasis are boxed to highlight their importance, and specific "Calls to Action" are included at the end of each chapter. The text offers multiple case examples and includes reflective questions and practice analyses for use in formal education programs, continuing education, workshops and conferences, and general clinical practice. Although these additions are organized for students, nurses in clinical practice, educators, and nurse leaders, they are not mutually exclusive and may be used by health professionals in many different roles. The Appendices provide additional resources for those interested in caring relationships in health systems.

During this confusing period in history where new approaches are drastically needed to meet our social mandate, health professionals at all levels are called to choose caring relationships as the cornerstone of their practice. In particular, professional nurses, the largest group of health professionals, who are educated "to care" and spend the majority of their time with patients and families, are called to lead a more relationship-centric health system by practicing from a quality-caring base, educating and leading health professionals and health systems to create value for vulnerable patients and families.

Acknowledgments

First and foremost, I thank Steve, for steadfastly caring for me as I continue to advance quality caring. His support and tolerance has afforded me the opportunity to pursue this work for many years now, and to him I owe my deepest gratitude.

Secondly, I acknowledge a former professor and colleague, Dr. Lois Hoskins, who passed away last year and who continuously reminds me of the values of discipline, humility, and integrity.

And, finally, I acknowledge the newest nurses—the future of our workforce. These spirited young women and men are transforming nursing at an incredible speed and will no doubt lead the profession to its highest potential as it matures throughout the 21st century. To them, I wish great success and a joy-filled journey.

I

Nursing and Health Systems

1

Quality, Caring, and Health Systems

America's health care system is neither healthy, caring, nor a system.
—Walter Cronkite

PERSISTENT CRISIS OF QUALITY IN HEALTH SYSTEMS

The U.S. healthcare system continues to experience growth in expenditures: expansion of and greater use of technology, data, and personalized treatments; more focus on team-based population health; and unprecedented safety, quality, and security concerns amid a shrinking workforce (Pollack, 2018). Simultaneously, aging baby boomers, increases in lifestyle-induced conditions, emerging global infections, and more engaged consumers present increased demands for services at a time when providers and healthcare organizations are struggling to meet the demanding criteria required for values-based reimbursement (Burd, Brown, Puri, & Sanghavi, 2017). In essence, healthcare is mirroring society as it is transforming right before our eyes! And, it is highly likely that healthcare, as we know it, will be transformed in 10 or 20 years, appearing radically different!

This uncertain state presents many unknowns and resulting concerns, but one thing is certain: patient safety and quality will remain on the radar screen throughout this drastic period of change. In particular, adverse health outcomes, health disparities, and true patient centeredness continue to be problematic today (Cryer, Davis, & Pronovost, 2017; Zuckerman, 2017) and will consume more resources, despite those already expended, in the ever-increasing pursuit of high quality and patient safety. Since the early Institute of Medicine (IOM) safety and quality reports (IOM, 2001a, 2001b; Kohn, Corrigan, & Donaldson, 2000), major efforts and the consumption of massive resources have been expended to measure, improve, and increase access to healthcare. Yet, recent research reveals that, although some progress has been made (e.g., hospital-acquired infections; Centers for Disease Control and Prevention, 2016), improvement in patient safety has been limited and in some cases, huge gaps remain (National Patient Safety Foundation, 2015). In fact, over 200,000 U.S. hospital patients die and countless more are harmed each year as a result of predictable and preventable human errors, costing well over $30 billion annually (Makary & Daniel, 2016). Even worse, the technology meant to improve patient safety may be tied to new, unforeseen types of errors, not anticipated. For example, in the first 6 months of 2016, Pennsylvania hospitals reported 889 medication errors or close calls that were attributed, at least in part, to electronic health records (EHRs) and other technology used to monitor and record patients' treatment (Twedt, 2017). Health disparities linger (Zuckerman, 2017), U.S. life expectancy has dropped (Xu, Murphy, Kochanek, & Arias, 2016), and, despite ample attention to patient centeredness, many healthcare systems and their leaders still do not understand its true meaning (Gunther-Murphy, 2017; Millensen & Berensen, 2015). Of importance is that the actual findings in these data are the same as or worse than those reported in the original IOM report, *To Err is Human: Building a Safer Health System* (Kohn, Corrigan, & Donaldson, 2000), over 19 years ago!

Adverse events, as well as decreased patient functional performance related to hospitalization (not to mention nursing homes, home care, clinics, schools, and outpatient centers), remain a major source of harm, death, and disability for Americans. For example, in one study of hospitalized orthopedic patients, an adverse event rate of 9.5%, of which 56% were preventable, was documented (Rajasekaran, Ravi, & Aiyer, 2016). A systematic review of elderly nursing home residents showed that almost half of them were exposed to potentially inappropriate medications, suggesting an increased prevalence over time (Morin, Laroche, Texier, & Johnell, 2016). Another U. S. Department of Health and Human Services (HHS) report by the Inspector General on Medicare patients revealed that an estimated 22% of Medicare skilled nursing facility (SNF) residents experienced adverse events during their stays and an additional 11% of the residents experienced adverse events that resulted in temporary harm. Worse, physician reviewers determined that 59% of these adverse events and temporary harm events were clearly or likely preventable (Department of Health and Human Services [HHS], 2016).

And in rehabilitation hospitals, an estimated 29% of Medicare beneficiaries experienced adverse or temporary harm events during their stay, resulting in temporary harm, prolonged stay or transfer to other hospitals, permanent harm, life-sustaining intervention, or death. Physician reviewers determined that 46% of these adverse and temporary harm events were clearly or likely preventable and attributed much of the preventable harms to substandard treatment, inadequate patient monitoring, and failure to provide needed treatment. Nearly one-quarter of the patients who experienced adverse or temporary harm events were transferred to an acute care hospital for treatment, with an estimated cost to Medicare of at least $7.7 million in 1 month, or at least $92 million in 1 year (HHS, 2016).

In nursing homes, quality and safety concerns have been long-standing issues. Older adults frequently bounce between nursing homes and hospitals for healthcare. They experience poorer outcomes of care compared to other groups that are not always the result of illness but rather consequences of the hospitalization itself, often resulting in new disabilities, nursing home placements, unanticipated interventions, and significant financial burden (Zisberg, Shadmi, Gur-Yaish, Tonkikh, & Sinoff, 2015). Although the IOM first published *Improving the Quality of Care in Nursing Homes* in 1986, common problems associated with the quality of care in nursing homes, such as pressure ulcers, malnutrition and dehydration, use of physical and chemical restraints, incontinence, pain management, and quality of life, persist. In fact, based on the Centers for Medicare and Medicaid Services (CMS) Star Rating System for nursing homes, 36% of nursing homes certified by Medicare or Medicaid had overall ratings of 1 or 2 stars in 2015, accounting for 39% of all nursing home residents. Furthermore, almost two in five nursing home residents (39%) live in these 1- and 2-star nursing homes (Boccuti, Casellas, & Neuman, 2015). And when elderly patients are admitted to hospitals, they suffer increased prevalence of adverse events compared to their younger counterparts (Gorman, 2016). For example, in one study geriatric syndromes were prevalent in more than 90% of hospitalized adults referred to SNFs and the most prevalent were falls (39%), incontinence (39%), loss of appetite (37%), and weight loss (33%). Most disappointing, treating hospital physicians or registered nurses commonly failed to recognize and document these events in discharge summaries (Bell et al., 2016).

Finally, hospitalization in and of itself may be "the worst place to be when you're sick" (Greider, 2012, p. 1), since infectious organisms, disruption of sleep cycles, inappropriate antibiotics usage, prolonged bedrest, and isolation can lead to unnecessary suffering, needless deaths, and resource waste. And a scorecard of local health performance found access, quality, costs, and health outcomes continue to vary significantly from one local community to another. Despite improved performance in recent years, in many places there was little or no meaningful change on many of the indicators tracked, resulting in improvement on a majority of the scorecard's indicators (17 or more) in only 14 U.S. localities (Radley, McCarthy, & Hayes, 2016). Ghandi, Berwick, and Shojania (2016) suggest that the current focus on measuring and implementing practice changes for specific targets (frequently reimbursable indicators) is not enough to create lasting impact and in fact, patient safety and, therefore, quality, is currently at a crossroads! This is a serious national concern that causes unnecessary harm to patients and families (not to mention increased costs), demanding immediate and systematic attention.

Although the value of the American health system remains stagnant, a large transformation intended to strengthen the system is underway. Since the first edition of this book, the complex Patient Protection and Affordable Care Act (2010), with its emphasis on shared accountability for high-quality care among all providers, disciplines, and associated healthcare organizations, has been implemented. Pay-for-performance programs and value-based purchasing were provisions in the law expected to reimburse and reward health systems that attained certain quality scores and provided better care for five of the most prevalent conditions. One example includes the reimbursement rule for 30-day hospital readmissions for those patients with heart failure (HF), acute myocardial infarction (AMI), or pneumonia. Most hospitals now have initiatives for reducing preventable readmissions of patients with HF or AMI, but the implementation of recommended practices varies widely (Bradley et al., 2012). And, since July 2012, Medicare financially penalized more than 1,621 hospitals—including some with national recognition—in each of the 5 years of the program (Kaiser Health News, 2016). Accountable care organizations (ACOs), another provision in the law intended to promote better integration, coordination, quality and shared costs of ambulatory, inpatient, and post–acute-care services for a defined population of Medicare beneficiaries, have preliminarily shown modest savings (Nyweide et al., 2015).

After 5 years of implementation, according to one study, the availability and affordability of health insurance has improved; nearly 3 million previously uninsured young Americans have gained coverage under their parents' policies, and a slowdown in the rate of healthcare spending to 17% of the gross domestic product (GDP) has occurred. Some reductions in hospital-acquired conditions and Medicare readmissions have also been observed, but the extent to which the ACA influenced these performance trends remains unknown (Blumenthal, Abrams, & Nuzum, 2015). In hospitals, the focus has been on compliance with the law, necessitating multiple changes related to the shifting of reimbursement from volume to value, increased attention to quality, safety, and patient experiences, and added responsibility for population health management. Yet many opposing issues and unforeseen consequences remain, such as an unfriendly website for enrollees, multiple court cases challenging its legality, and endless debates in Washington and the states that consumed national discussion and debate. For example, increased premiums, numerous new regulations, a complicated insurance enrollment system, and a plethora of experiments in payment and delivery system reform have created many hurdles and partisan divide. During the 2016 election cycle, the ACA was the subject of competing political interests and philosophical perspectives that, together with other issues, split the voters. The law continues to be the subject of intense discussions and controversy.

Although several plans have been advanced to repeal and replace key components of the ACA, as of this writing, none has succeeded. It is clear that funding to help stabilize the health insurance marketplace and the children's health insurance program is needed, ensuring high-quality care in rural areas, and limiting hospital cuts for the disadvantaged and drug payments are important. It is also likely that the emphasis on lowering costs, improving healthcare quality (including the patient experience) and safety, will continue to be emphasized. To achieve these aims, health professionals must be ready to lead, understand and implement rigorous practice improvement, have a handle on data and information management, embrace community-based care, and use financial and informed decision-making skills that generate clinical innovations.

During this uncertain period in American history and in the context of a rapidly changing and error-prone healthcare system, advancing patient safety and quality remains a primary responsibility of healthcare professionals. Consistently prioritizing the well-being and safety of patients and families, as well as the healthcare workforce, requires remembering our values and using those, along with improvement science, to remove the emphasis on fragmented performance improvement (PI) projects or indicators and advance a more holistic approach, where patient safety and quality is embedded in clinical workflow, healthcare professionals are held accountable for it, and patients have the power to insist on it. Such is the never-ending battle of pursuing excellence. The role of the professional nurse in such a transformed system is evolving.

QUALITY AND PROFESSIONAL NURSING CARE

The consensus report *The Future of Nursing: Leading Change, Advancing Health* (IOM, 2011) was intended to shape nursing's role in a transformed health system. It recommended four key improvements:

- Nurses should practice to the full extent of their education and training.
- Nurses should achieve higher levels of education and training through an improved education system that promotes seamless academic progression.
- Nurses should be full partners, with physicians and other health-care professionals, in redesigning healthcare in the United States.
- Effective workforce planning and policy making require better data collection and information infrastructure.

The report highlighted nurses' fundamental role in transforming the healthcare system and offered specific recommendations for action, including the key message that strong leadership is necessary to effect significant change in healthcare systems. The report holds that professional nurses must assume accountability for high-quality care, including "taking responsibility for identifying problems and areas of waste, devising and implementing plans for improvement, tracking improvement over time, and making necessary adjustments to realize established goals" (IOM, 2011, p. 8). Furthermore, the report advocated nurses as decision makers who shape health policy while serving on committees, boards, and commissions, and who understand and use data across the health professions to improve patient care. The call for an expanded scope of practice for nurses who regularly collaborate with physicians, other health professionals, and administrators to develop new systems of care delivery and generate performance data has begun, but still has a way to go. In 2015, the IOM released a progress report and suggested several areas where barriers remain (Altman, Butler, & Shern, 2015).

Although many of the recommendations couldn't be quantified due to lack of good data, some progress was seen. For example, a 17% increase in enrollment in pre-licensure BSN programs from 2010 to 2014 and an increase in enrollment in RN-to-BSN programs by 69% from 2010 to 2014 is documented. Overall, BSN-prepared nurses increased from 49% of the workforce in 2010 to 51% of the workforce in 2014 (Altman et al., 2015). Despite the higher levels of education documented, the report cited the need for continued and higher levels of education, starting at the time nurses enter the profession and throughout their careers. Barriers to expanding APRN scope of practice and major gaps in understanding numbers and types of health professionals, where they are employed, and what roles they fill remain were highlighted. And, while many healthcare organizations, academia, and federal and state governments took active steps to increase the diversity of the nursing and health professions workforce, the report recommended continued prioritization of diversity goals with specific actions intended to advance it at all levels. Thus, revised recommendations for consideration included:

- Supporting academic pathways toward the baccalaureate degree
- Exploring ways to create and fund transition-to-practice residency programs
- Promoting doctoral degrees, with an emphasis on the PhD
- Promoting expanded interprofessional and lifelong learning to enhance interprofessional collaboration and leadership development (Altman et al., 2015)

Also recommended were more nurses serving in executive and leadership positions in all types of health systems to encourage involvement in the redesign of healthcare delivery and payment systems. Finally, the report recommended more robust data sets to track the nursing workforce, including how they can be made available to researchers, policy makers, and planners. Thus, while several of the original recommendations showed a little progress, many could not be quantified.

Nursing practice continues to undergo persistent quality difficulties and some indications suggest that, with the impending shortage, it may worsen (Simpson, Lyndon, & Ruhl, 2016). For example, issues such as patient falls (some with injury), pressure injuries, catheter-associated urinary tract infections (CAUTIs), problems related to transitions in care, alarm fatigue, struggles with early mobility, inadequate medication teaching, hand hygiene, infections, workplace violence, and medication errors continue to plague hospitals, nursing homes, schools, and outpatient facilities. Anecdotal evidence of this can be found in newspaper reports and individual stories (Cohen, 2016; Skutch, 2017; Sun, 2016).

Other reports of recent poor quality nursing care can be found in abundance through publicly accessed journals as well as the professional literature: discontinuity of nursing care (Yakusheva, Costa, & Weiss, 2017), loneliness among nursing home residents (Pitkala, 2016), poor quality teamwork between junior doctors and nurses (O'Connor et al., 2016), poor oral hygiene care in hospitalized elders (Coker, Ploeg, Kaasalainen, & Carter, 2017), and inadequate early mobility in hospitalized patients (Manojlovich, Ratz, Miller, & Krein, 2017). A common theme in all of these reports is lacking, limited, or missed basic nursing care.

Missed nursing care is defined as any aspect of required patient care that is omitted (either in part or in whole) or delayed (Kalisch, Landstrom, & Hinshaw, 2009). Missed nursing care is considered an error of omission that potentially leads to negative outcomes, varies across hospitals, and is impacted by several variables (Kalisch, Tschannen, & Lee, 2011). Although missed nursing care is considered a process indicator, it appears to be occurring on a regular basis in hospitals internationally, and is increasingly associated with adverse outcomes. Missed nursing care has been correlated with patient falls (Kalish, Tschannen, & Lee, 2012), poorer patient satisfaction (Lake, Germack, & Viscardi, 2016), 30-day readmissions among patients with HF and AMI (Brooks-Carthon, Lasater, Rearden, Holland, & Sloane, 2016; Carthon, Lasater, Sloane, & Kutney-Lee, 2015), phlebitis in emergency departments (Palese et al., 2015), nosocomial infections and medication errors (Lucero, Lake, & Aiken, 2010), pressure ulcers (Schubert et al., 2008), urinary tract infections (UTI) among nursing home residents (Nelson & Flynn, 2015), new-onset delirium (Karmel, Iqbal, Mogallapu, Maas, & Hoffmann, 2003), pneumonia (Mundy, Leet, Darst, Schnitzler, & Dunagan, 2003), increased length of stay and delayed discharge (Karmel et al., 2003; Mundy et al., 2003; Whitney & Parkman, 2004), increased pain and discomfort (Price & Fowlow, 1994), physical disability (Yohannes & Connolly, 2003), and even mortality (Schubert, Clarke, Aiken, & de Geest, 2012). To date, studies indicate that the volume of missed care is underestimated and that the consequences to patients could be greater than currently understood (Kalisch, 2006; Kalisch et al., 2009; Kalisch & Xie, 2014). According to Kalisch et al. (2011), we have allowed a "culture of missing care" to evolve over time and nurses who have practiced more than 20 years point to a major decline in completeness of nursing care over the last several decades. Built on 10 years of extensive research, Kalisch's (2016) recent text, *Errors of Omission: How Missed Nursing Care Imperils Patients*, highlights research pointing to the correlation between missed nursing care and adverse outcomes in both patients and nurses.

Interestingly, the unmet care needs associated with missed nursing care fall in the categories of patient teaching, discharge planning, comfort, inadequate patient–nurse interactions, ambulation, oral hygiene and skin care, adequate documentation, and updating care plans—all basic responsibilities of nursing. In addition to patient outcomes, nursing job satisfaction, intention to leave, turnover, and perceived quality of care have been linked to missed nursing care (Kalisch et al., 2011). Taken together, the complexity of forces impacting professional nursing and other health professionals has never been greater; in fact, it is revolutionary in nature!

Within this challenging context, RNs continuously monitor and assess patients' illness trajectories, deliver independent and collaborative interventions to a wide variety of patients, delegate and supervise assistive personnel, participate in research, shared governance, and departmental committees, complete continuing education requirements, lead interprofessional teams, and provide services 24 hours/day 7 days/week, creating an intense and unpredictable work environment that may or may not meet patient needs. But while the ACA is awaiting replacement, new nurse turnover and vacancy rates seem to be rising and a major nursing shortage (one-third of the workforce) is occurring (Snavely, 2016). Losing the tacit knowledge of many experienced nurses has never occurred before in this country and will likely leave a huge gap in the workforce. According to Buerhaus, such massive change occurring simultaneously will require savvy new graduates with an understanding of values-based reimbursement models and electronic databases, who are good team players, are flexible, and who can withstand constant change (Buerhaus, 2016). Such recommendations have repercussions for schools of nursing in terms of curricula and faculty competencies. And since the delivery system is changing, more nurses will be in demand in the community where most patients will be cared for. All this is occurring as the state of nursing quality remains problematic. But despite this ongoing evolution, the basics of professional nursing endure—advocating for patients and families, ensuring a holistic perspective and, most importantly, preserving the human-to-human caring connection to patients.

> Because their continuous interactions and intimate relationships with patients and families uniquely position nurses to positively influence experiences of care and other significant health outcomes, nurses are in a position to harness and leverage that power to their full advantage.

In particular, the most fundamental role of all nursing processes—caring relationships with patients, families, and other health professionals—provides the context for all healthcare actions and is tied to important patient and system outcomes (Duffy, 2013). Yet, such relationships seem to be taking a back seat to the seemingly larger and more important concerns, particularly in hospitals. How is it that the largest of all the health professions still cannot claim the value they contribute to patient outcomes and health systems? Is it protective in some way? Is the incessant focus on performance metrics set by others so pervasive that the patient's view is not considered important? Are "smart" systems, EHRs or other new initiatives getting in the way? Do those who assist or support nursing understand and value the connection between basic nursing tasks and health outcomes? Are nurses just plain tired?

IMPROVING QUALITY IN NURSING AND HEALTH SYSTEMS

Nursing-sensitive indicators are used widely today by many organizations, accrediting agencies, and insurers as measures of nursing care quality. This set of performance indicators, first developed by the American Nurses Association (ANA, 1995), provides internal and benchmarking information related to nursing care. Described in detail in the first chapter of *Quality Caring in Nursing* (Duffy, 2009), many organizations have used these indicators to improve their performance and now receive reimbursement on adequate attainment of several of them, for example falls and pressure ulcers.

Another gold standard of nursing excellence and patient quality has been the attainment of Magnet® designation. Some research has demonstrated that Magnet-designated hospitals provide positive work environments for nurses and may improve nurse satisfaction; however, research on *patient* outcomes in Magnet hospitals is unclear. For example, a study in *Health Affairs* found that hospitals recognized for nursing excellence through the Magnet program tended to have better patient outcomes (failure to rescue and mortality rates), but did not continuously improve after gaining recognition, suggesting that the Magnet program recognizes existing excellence but may not lead to sustained excellence (Friese, Xia, Ghaferi, Birkmeyer, & Banerjee, 2015).

Although striving for excellence through the attainment of external designations or certifications and routinely examining internal performance is laudable and oftentimes required, the use of external evidence—such as that found in the professional literature, in the form of practice guidelines and research—provides a more comprehensive evidence base from which to activate practice changes. One example of this is the focus on 30-day hospital readmission rates.

Hospital readmissions are a national concern tied to reimbursement. Variation in these rehospitalizations is well documented (Ramey et al., 2016), and although many organizations are actively working on improving readmission rates, there is limited evidence that guide nurses on how best to do this. Yet, various nursing-led initiatives are occurring across the United States, oftentimes without an evidence base or proper evaluation. Another example is the known link between healthcare worker fatigue and patient safety (Scott, Rogers, Hwang, & Zhang, 2006). The practice of working long shifts contributes to high levels of worker fatigue and reduced productivity, which impacts patient safety, yet nurses and nurse leaders continue to support, hire, and promote 12-hour shifts (that frequently extend to 16-hour or longer shifts). Heeding recent research findings may promote a healthier, safer work environment for both patients and nurses.

To significantly improve safety and quality while better meeting patient needs (and ultimately patient outcomes) in a timely fashion, imagining new approaches to nursing practice and its improvement are needed. Of importance is the recognition that quality and safety are continuously embedded in the daily work of healthcare rather than activities pursued occasionally or as projects. Some examples of approaches to better ingrain quality and safety activities in daily work are active learning communities at the unit/department level, improvement activities included in staffing plans, clinical supervision (yes, on medical–surgical units), multisite improvement collaboratives, academic–service partnerships, authentic simulations, nurse leader focus on patient-centeredness, and a focus on more positive (vs. adverse indicators). Such approaches may provide the performance data and actionable practice changes necessary to accelerate improvements in practice.

For example, using a specific research measure (Q-sort methodology), multiple stakeholders identified and prioritized state measures for child and adolescent health and established a learning agenda for targeted quality improvement (QI) activities (Fifolt, Preskitt, Rucks, Corvey, & Benton, 2017). Importantly, the open dialogue among stakeholders spurred greater organizational buy-in for the collaborative and increased its credibility. Another example is the academic–service partnership to help mentor new advanced practice nurses in the integration of research, QI, and evidence-based activities into their practices (Harbman et al., 2017). Finally, enhancing patient centeredness through nurse leader attention to and role-modeling the patient–nurse relationship may foster better patient experiences.

Assessing the quality of and continuously improving patient–provider relationships are crucial concerns for health systems today as evidence is beginning to mount that the quality of patient–provider relationships is linked to important safety and quality outcomes (Sullivan & Ellner, 2015). A recent study cited the important role nurses play in patient experience and patient safety and showed a significant correlation between the safety culture of an organization and positive patient experiences (Abramson, Hass, Morgan, Fulton, & Ramanujan, 2016). Registered nurses represent a continuous and stabilizing force that engages patients, monitors and validates their progress, provides encouragement, ensures dignity and confidentiality, guarantees safety, coordinates care among multiple health care providers, and performs specialized interventions. Thus, "the patient–nurse relationship provides the context for care as vulnerable patients and families depend on RNs for safe and high-quality services" (Duffy & Brewer, 2011, p. 79). However, little data are routinely collected informing RNs of the quality of the patient–nurse relationship.

> Attending to the regular evaluation and improvement of the patient–RN relationship may demonstrate the significance of the RN's role in the provision of patient-centered care (and the patient experience) and facilitate the attainment of high-reliability health systems, where consistently safe and high-quality services thrive.

SUSTAINING A VALUABLE HEALTH SYSTEM

Because the U.S. health system today performs at a relatively lower level than other countries while simultaneously costing more, the problem of sustaining a high-value system is demanding. Americans still must wait long periods for office visits, diagnostic tests (and their results), and procedures; read about or experience adverse outcomes such as hospital-acquired infections, bedsores, or wrong-site procedures; endure multiple providers who do not talk to one another; receive outrageous charges for services; experience sleeplessness, unnecessary pain, and anxiety during hospitalization; and worst of all, be made to feel as if they don't matter, are unimportant, or are not invited to participate in the decision making about their health.

A sustainable high-value health system will not be realized with EHRs, comparative effectiveness research, or new payment mechanisms alone. All of these will contribute of course, but at its core, delivering high-value healthcare depends on *caring* for patients and families. Nurses, the largest group of health professionals who interact 24/7 with patients and families, are key. The increasing evidence that caring patient–nurse relationships are worthy contributors to safe and quality health systems provides a unique, but brief, opportunity to showcase its potential. Accountability, an important aspect of professional practice, may help nurses to leverage the power that continues to be invisible and underused.

Accountability signifies intent, ownership, commitment, obligation, and willingness (Rachel, 2012), or to use a baseball metaphor, stepping up to the plate. It is no longer *okay* to languish in a job, to *not* engage in lifelong learning, to *not* consider caring relationships essential to professional practice, to *not* partner with professional colleagues, to *not* use data for decision making, or to *not* participate in practice improvement. These behaviors are pertinent to the entire practice of nursing—clinical, educational, and leadership.

Strengthening the nursing workforce through advanced academic progression that is accessible, meaningful, and values based is paramount. Caring relationships, the most often described value associated with nursing, must remain a major thrust of nursing education with appropriate didactic and experiential learning opportunities to understand, cultivate, and appreciate its significance to safe and quality health systems.

> We must hold each other accountable for caring professional practice, including recognizing, listening, observing, and confronting unacceptable caring behaviors and attitudes. Although many nurse educators are working on curricular change as this text is being written, careful attention to the need for "relational capacity" (described in Chapter 6) is necessary to effectively prepare the next generation of nurses. More comprehensive and efficient program evaluation with explicit indicators of learning are needed by nurse educators to assess whether the curricula they design is meeting the needs of creating a valuable health system. Holding each other accountable by attending to the evidence related to valuable health systems, how best to help students learn, and one's own teaching abilities will ensure responsible curricular changes and, we hope, engaged, caring nurse graduates.

Nursing leaders at all levels must hold each other and those they supervise accountable for caring professional practice. This includes consistently modeling accountability, being clear and direct in terms of what defines and is acceptable nursing professional practice, and how caring professional practice will be recognized and rewarded. Increasing time that professional nurses spend in direct patient care, insisting on high-quality patient–nurse relationships as the basis for professional practice, enhancing the work environment, stimulating career development, and demanding that those who assist professional nurses effectively contribute to the team are some approaches that nursing leaders may find advantageous. Of course, using evidence to guide practice is paramount.

As Barbara Resnick recently stated, "I don't think . . . providers truly understand, from the patient perspective, what patient-centered care really is. It seems facilities are rewarded for their patient-centered care approach if they implement certain practices" (Resnick, 2017, p. 7). Unfortunately, the routinization of practices in health systems meant to advance patient centeredness will not work. Rather, capitalizing on the unique, intimate human connections between patients and those delivering services to them is the key. To meet the demand for this foundational aspect of practice, nurse leaders and educators must value, display, educate, and reward the human caring relationships that are central to professional practice, and embrace those theoretical frameworks that honor them. With the patient and family at its core, nurses who practice from a caring professional base will advance the value of the nation's health system.

SUMMARY

In this chapter, the persistent crisis of health system quality has been reviewed. Of particular concern is the continuing slow progress toward its improvement, including cost-reduction efforts, despite the massive resources that have been devoted to it. The value of the U.S. health system lags behind many other countries, and although recent legislation aims to improve it, it remains stagnant. Professional nursing, the largest health system discipline, continues to have quality problems as perceived by patients, families, and nurses themselves. In fact, a "culture of missing care" has evolved over time and now seems rather usual in acute care hospitals. Although routine evaluation of nurse-sensitive indicators and attainment of certifications has stimulated some improvement, speedier translation of external evidence to the bedside will advance the value of nursing care even further. Attending to the routine evaluation, continuous improvement, and scientific investigation of patient–RN relationships may demonstrate the significance of the RN's role in the provision of patient-centered care and facilitate the attainment of high-reliability health systems. Accountable professional practice may help nurses leverage the caring power that continues to be invisible and underused to positively benefit the evolving health system.

Call to Action

The value of the nation's health system is, in part, dependent on the accountability of its professional nurses for delivering caring patient–nurse relationships. **Accept** the responsibility for high-quality patient–nurse relationships.

REFLECTIVE QUESTIONS/APPLICATIONS

. . . for Students

1. What are your perceptions about the value of the health system?
2. Analyze the Patient Protection and Affordable Care Act in terms of its ability to increase the value of the U.S. health system.
3. Reflect on the role of the professional nurse in a reformed health system. How will he or she be spending the majority of time?
4. Outline your plans to acquire the skills necessary for collaboration with other health professionals and generate performance data.
5. How would you go about evaluating and improving the patient–RN relationship? Provide specific examples.

. . . for Professional Nurses in Clinical Practice

1. Discuss the persistent quality problems in your healthcare institution.
2. Is there an accepted "culture of missing care"? If so, who is responsible for its evolution?
3. How or should missed nursing care be corrected?
4. How have collecting and reporting on nursing-sensitive quality indicators improved nursing care in your institution?
5. What new evidence-based nursing interventions or care guidelines have recently been introduced in your unit? Was the evidence from which they were based explicit? How have they been evaluated?
6. How do you hold yourself and fellow nurses accountable for caring relationships?

. . . for Professional Nurses in Educational Practice

1. Has curricular revision taken hold in your institution? If yes, what evidence did you use to shape it? How did you attend to the relational capacity of your graduates?
2. Reflect on the Affordable Care Act. How do you think your educational program will change as a result? What new knowledge and skills will be expected of nursing graduates?
3. How have the learning outcomes specified in your evaluation plan improved over the past 3 years? How does/did this inform curriculum revision?
4. How do you assess caring competence? Is it even necessary?

. . . for Professional Nurses in Leadership Practice

1. How has the value of nursing care improved over the past 3 years at your institution?
2. How have you articulated the role of the professional nurse at your institution?
3. Reflect on the career development activities in place at your institution. Are they working? How do you know?
4. Describe the evidence base that is routinely used to make leadership decisions at your institution.
5. How do you ensure accountability for caring patient–nurse relationships?

PRACTICE ANALYSIS

A large Magnet-accredited academic medical center recently participated in a study of missed nursing care along with six other hospitals, all within the same region of the United States. After receiving their aggregated results, it was apparent that "opportunities for improvement were great." Although the results were reported in aggregate, the principal investigator relayed that individual department results were available and could be obtained in confidence through request by the directors and department managers. Of particular interest was that ambulation, mouth care, delayed feedings, attention to evaluating pain medication effects, turning, hourly rounding, and intake and output recordings were high on the list of missed nursing care. The deficiencies were greatest on medical–surgical units and were tied to "not enough resources and poor physician–nurse communication."

Upon discussion at the practice council, RNs admitted that they were not sure that tasks and responsibilities delegated to nursing assistants (NAs) were being carried out. In fact, the nurses stated they often did not have enough time to assess their patient's psychological status or follow up on NA care. Although the nurses, upon hearing the data, expressed feelings of regret and frustration that they were not able to complete all of the care for their patients, they were not able to come up with specific action plans. Three months after the initial results were reported, no requests from the nursing directors or departmental managers for specific data on their units had been received and the nursing department, in the midst of a major revision to the EHR, had not taken action on the results.

1. What is the urgency associated with these missed nursing care results for this organization?
2. How did the nurses' reaction to the results advance safety and quality for the organization?
3. Describe some approaches that nursing leadership could take to improve safety and quality at this organization.

REFERENCES

Abrahamson, K., Hass, Z., Morgan, K., Fulton, B., & Ramanujan, R. (2016). The relationship between nurse-reported safety culture and the patient experience. *Journal of Nursing Administration, 46*(12), 662–668. doi:10.1097/NNA.0000000000000423

Altman, S. H., Butler, A. S., & Shern, L. (Eds.) (2015). *Assessing progress on the Institute of Medicine report*: The Future of Nursing. Retrieved from https://www.nap.edu/read/21838/chapter/1#ii

American Nurses Association. (1995). *Nursing report card for acute care.* Washington, DC: American Nurses Publishing.

Bell, S. P., Vasilevskis, E. E., Saraf, A. A., Jacobsen, J. J. M., Kripalani, S., Mixon, A. S., . . . Simmons, S. F. (2016). Geriatric syndromes in hospitalized older adults discharged to skilled nursing facilities. *Journal of the American Geriatric Society, 64*(4), 715–22. doi:10.1111/jgs.14035

Beurhaus, P. (2016). The 4 forces that will reshape nursing social and health care changes put pressure on the profession. *Hospitals & Health Networks*. Retrieved from https://www.hhnmag.com/articles/7522-the-4-forces-that-will-reshape-nursing

Blumenthal, D., Abrams, M., & Nuzum, R. (2015). The Affordable Care Act at 5 years. *New England Journal of Medicine, 372*, 2451–2458. doi:10.1056/NEJMhpr1503614

Boccuti, C., Cassallas, G., & Neuman, T. (2015). Reading the stars: Nursing home quality star ratings, nationally and by state. *The Henry J. Kaiser Family Foundation*. Retrieved from http://kff.org/report-section/reading-the-stars-nursing-home-quality-star-ratings-nationally-and-by-state-issue-brief

Bradley, E. H., Curry, L., Horwitz, L. I., Sipsma, H., Thompson, J. W., Elma, M., . . . Krumholz, H. M. (2012). Contemporary evidence about hospital strategies for reducing 30-day readmissions: A national study. *Journal of the American College of Cardiology, 60*(7), 607–614. doi:10.1016/j.jacc.2012.03.067

Brooks-Carthon, J. M., Lasater, K., Rearden, J., Holland, S., & Sloane, D. M. (2016). Unmet nursing care linked to rehospitalizations among older black AMI patients: A cross-sectional study of US hospitals. *Medical Care, 54*(5), 457–465. doi:10.1097/MLR.0000000000000519

Burd, C., Brown, N. C., Puri, P., & Sanghavi, D. (2017). A Centers for Medicare and Medicaid Services lens toward value-based preventive care and population health. *Public Health Reports, 132*(1), 6–10. doi:10.1177/0033354916681508

Carthon, J. M. B., Lasater, K. B., Sloane, D. M., & Kutney-Lee, A. (2015). The quality of hospital work environments and missed nursing care is linked to heart failure readmissions: A cross-sectional study of US hospitals. *BMJ Quality and Safety, 24*(4), 255–263. doi:10.1136/bmjqs-2014-003346

Centers for Disease Control and Prevention. (2016). *Healthcare-associated infections (HAI) progress report*. Retrieved from https://www.cdc.gov/hai/surveillance/progress-report

Cohen, D. (2016). The stories clinicians tell: Achieving high reliability and improving patient safety. *The Permanente Journal, 20*(1), 85–90. doi:10.7812/TPP/15-039

Coker, E., Ploeg, J., Kaasalainen, P., & Carter, N. (2017). Observations of oral hygiene care interventions provided by nurses to hospitalized older people. *Geriatric Nursing, 38*(1), 17–21. doi:10.1016/j.gerinurse.2016.06.018

Cryer, D., Davis, R., & Pronovost, P. (2017). Mutual mentorship: Patient-partnered care starts at the patient-CEO level. *Quality Management in Health Care, 26*(1), 49–50. doi:10.1097/QMH.0000000000000122

Department of Health and Human Services. (2014). Adverse events in skilled nursing facilities: National incidence among Medicare beneficiaries. Retrieved from https://oig.hhs.gov/oei/reports/oei-06-11-00370.pdf

Department of Health and Human Services. (2016). Adverse events in rehabilitation hospitals: National incidence among Medicare beneficiaries. Retrieved from https://oig.hhs.gov/oei/reports/oei-06-14-00110.pdf

Duffy, J. R. (2009). *Quality caring in nursing: Applying theory to clinical practice, education, and leadership.* New York, NY: Springer Publishing.

Duffy, J. R. (2013). *Quality caring in nursing and health systems: Implications for clinicians, educators, and leaders* (2nd ed.). New York, NY: Springer Publishing.

Duffy, J. R., & Brewer, B. B. (2011). Feasibility of a multi-institution collaborative to improve patient-nurse relationship quality. *Journal of Nursing Administration, 41*(2), 78–83. doi:10.1097/NNA.0b013e3182059463

Fifolt, M., Preskitt, J., Rucks, A., Corvey, K., & Benton, E. C. (2017). Promoting continuous quality improvement in the Alabama child health improvement alliance through Q-sort methodology and learning collaboratives. *Quality Management in Health Care, 26*(1), 33–39. doi:10.1097/QMH.0000000000000124

Friese, C. R., Xia, R., Ghaferi, A., Birkmeyer, J. D., & Banerjee, M. (2015). Hospitals in "Magnet" program show better patient outcomes on mortality measures compared to non-"Magnet" hospitals. *Health Affairs, 34*(6), 986–992. doi:10.1377/hlthaff.2014.0793

Ghandi, T. K., Berwick, D. M., & Shojania. K. G. (2016). Patient safety at the crossroads. *Journal of the American Medical Association, 315*(17), 1829–1830. doi:10.1001/jama.2016.1759

Gorman, A. (2016). The older you are, the worse the hospital is for you. *Central News Network.* Retrieved from http://www.cnn.com/2016/08/15/health/elderly-hospital-patients

Greider, K. (2012, March). The worst place to be when you're sick and how to protect yourself. *AARP Bulletin.* Retrieved from https://www.aarp.org/health/doctors-hospitals/info-03-2012/protect-yourself-from-hospital-errors.html

Gunther-Murphy, C. (2017). Why a patient and family advisory council doesn't make you patient-centered? *Institute for Healthcare Improvement.* Retrieved from http://www.ihi.org/communities/blogs/_layouts/ihi/community/blog/itemview.aspx?List=7d1126ec-8f63-4a3b-9926-c44ea3036813&ID=348

Harbman, P., Bryant-Lukosius, D., Martin-Misener, R., Carter, N., Covell, C. L., Donald, F., . . . Valaitis, R. (2017). Partners in research: Building academic-practice partnerships to educate and mentor advanced practice nurses. *Journal of Evaluation in Clinical Practice, 23*(2), 382–390. doi:10.1111/jep.12630

Institute for Healthcare Improvement. (2009). *Improving the patient experience of inpatient care evidence.* Retrieved from http://www.ihi.org/IHI/Topics/PatientCentered Care/PatientCenteredCareGeneral/EmergingContent/Improvingthe PatientExperienceofInpatientCare.htm

Institute of Medicine. (2001a). *Crossing the quality chasm: A new health system for the 21st century.* Washington, DC: National Academies Press.

Institute of Medicine. (2001b). *New health care system for the 21st century: Health care organizations as complex adaptive systems.* Washington, DC: National Academies Press.

Institute of Medicine. (2011). *The future of nursing: Leading change, advancing health.* Retrieved from https://www.nap.edu/read/12956/chapter/1

Kaiser Health News. (2016). Medicare's readmission penalties hit new high. Retrieved from http://khn.org/news/more-than-half-of-hospitals-to-be-penalized-for -excess-readmissions

Kalisch, B. J. (2006). Missed nursing care: A qualitative study. *Journal of Nursing Care Quality, 21*(4), 306–313. Retrieved from https://journals.lww.com/jncqjournal/ Fulltext/2006/10000/Missed_Nursing_Care__A_Qualitative_Study.6.aspx

Kalisch, B. J. (2016). *Errors of omission: How missed nursing care: Imperils patients.* Silver Spring, MD: American Nurses Association.

Kalisch, B. J., Landstrom, G., & Hinshaw, A. S. (2009). Missed nursing care: A concept analysis. *Journal of Advanced Nursing, 65*(7), 1509–1517. doi:10.1111/j.1365-2648.2009.05027.x

Kalisch, B. J., Tschannen, D., & Lee, H. (2011). Does missed nursing care predict job satisfaction? *Journal of Healthcare Management, 56*(2), 117–131. doi:10.1097/00115514-201103000-00007

Kalisch, B. J., Tschannen, D., & Lee, K. H. (2012). Missed nursing care, staffing, and patient falls. *Journal of Nursing Care Quality, 27*(1), 6–12. doi:10.1097/ NCQ.0b013e318225aa23

Kalisch, B. J., & Xie, B. (2014). Errors of omission: Missed nursing care. *Western Journal of Nursing Research, 36*(7), 875–890. doi:10.1177/0193945914531859

Karmel, H. K., Iqbal, M. A., Mogallapu, R., Maas, D., & Hoffmann, R. G. (2003). Time to ambulation after hip fracture surgery: Relation to hospitalization out-comes. *Journal of Gerontology, Series A-Biological Sciences and Medical Sciences, 58*(11), 1042–1045. doi:10.1093/gerona/58.11.M1042

Kohn, L. T., Corrigan, J. M., & Donaldson, M. S. (2000). *To err is human: Building a safer health system.* Washington, DC: National Academies Press.

Lake, E. T., Germack, H., & Viscardi, M. (2016). Missed nursing care is linked to patient satisfaction: A cross-sectional study of US hospitals. *BMJ Quality & Safety, 25*, 535–543. doi:10.1136/bmjqs-2015-003961

Lucero, R. J., Lake, E. T., & Aiken, L. H. (2010). Nursing care quality and adverse events in U.S. hospitals. *Journal of Clinical Nursing, 19*(15–16), 2185–2195. doi:10.1111/j.1365-2702.2010.03250.x

Makary, M. A., & Daniel, M. (2016). Medical error—The third leading cause of death in the US. *British Medical Journal, 353*, i2139. doi:10.1136/bmj.i2139

Manojlovich, M., Ratz, D., Miller, M., & Krein, S. L. (2017). Use of daily inter-ruption of sedation and early mobility in US Hospitals. *Journal of Nursing Care Quality, 32*(1), 71–76. doi:10.1097/NCQ.0000000000000222

Millenson, M. L. & Berenson, R. A. (2015). *The road to making patient-centered care real.* Washington, DC: Urban Institute. Retrieved from https://www.urban .org/sites/default/files/alfresco/publication-pdfs/2015.10.12_Millenson _Berenson.pdf

Morin, L., Laroche, M.-L., Texier, G., & Johnell, K. (2016). Prevalence of potentially inappropriate medication use in older adults living in nursing homes: A systematic review. *Journal of the American Medical Directors Association, 17*(9), 862.e1–862.e9. doi:10.1016/j.jamda.2016.06.011

Mundy, L. M., Leet, T. L., Darst, K., Schnitzler, M. A., & Dunagan, W. C. (2003). Early mobilization of patients hospitalized with community-acquired pneumonia. *Chest, 124*(3), 883–889. doi:10.1378/chest.124.3.883

National Patient Safety Foundation. (2015). *Free from harm: Accelerating patient safety improvement fifteen years after To Err is Human.* Retrieved from http://www.aig.com/content/dam/aig/america-canada/us/documents/brochure/free-from-harm-final-report.pdf

Nelson, S. T., & Flynn, L. (2015). Relationship between missed care and urinary tract infections in nursing homes. *Geriatric Nursing, 36*(2), 126–130. doi:10.1016/j.gerinurse.2014.12.009

Nyweide, D. J., Lee, W., Cuerdon, T. T., Pham, H. H., Cox, M., Rajkumar, R., & Conway, P. H. (2015). Association of pioneer accountable care organizations vs traditional Medicare fee for service with spending, utilization, and patient experience. *Journal of the American Medical Association, 313*(21), 2152–2161. doi:10.1001/jama.2015.4930

O'Connor, P., O'Dea, A., Lydon, A., Offiah, G., Scott, J., Flannery, A., . . . Byrne, D. (2016). A mixed-methods study of the causes and impact of poor teamwork between junior doctors and nurses. *International Journal of Quality Health Care, 28*(3), 339–345. doi:10.1093/intqhc/mzw036

Palese, A., Ambrosi, E., Fabris, F., Guarnier, A., Barelli, P., Zambiasi, P., . . . Saiani, L. (2015). Nursing care as a predictor of phlebitis related to insertion of a peripheral venous cannula in emergency departments: Findings from a prospective study. *Journal of Hospital Infection, 92*(3), 280–286. doi:10.1016/j.jhin.2015.10.021

Patient Protection and Affordable Care Act, 42 U.S.C. § 18001 (2010).

Pitkala, K. H. (2016). Loneliness in nursing homes. *Journal of the American Medical Directors Association, 17*(8), 680–681. doi:10.1016/j.jamda.2016.04.007

Pollack, R. (2018). 2018 environmental scan: Trends that are shaping health care. *Hospitals & Health Networks.* Retrieved from https://www.hhnmag.com/articles/8640-trends-that-are-shaping-health-care

Price, P., & Fowlow, B. (1994). Research-based practice: Early ambulation for PTCA patients. *Canadian Journal of Cardiovascular Nursing, 5*(1), 23–25.

Rachel, M. M. (2012). Accountability: A concept worth revisiting. *American Nurse Today, 7*(3), 36–40. Retrieved from https://www.americannursetoday.com/accountability-a-concept-worth-revisiting

Radley, D. C., McCarthy, D., & Hayes, S. L. (2016). Rising to the challenge: The Commonwealth Fund Scorecard on local health system performance, 2016 edition. *The Commonwealth Fund.* Retrieved from http://www.commonwealthfund.org/interactives/2016/jul/local-scorecard

Rajasekaran, S., Ravi, S., & Aiyer, S. N. (2016). Incidence and preventability of adverse events in an orthopaedic unit: A prospective analysis of four thousand, nine hundred and six admissions. *International Orthopaedics (SICOT)*, 40(11), 2233–2238. doi:10.1007/s00264-016-3282-4

Ramey, L., Goldstein, R., Zafonte, R., Ryan, C., Kazis, L., & Schneider, J. (2016). Variation in 30-day readmission rates among medically complex patients at inpatient rehabilitation facilities and contributing factors. *Journal of the American Medical Directors Association*, 17(8), 730–736. doi:10.1016/j.jamda.2016.03.019

Resnick, B. (2017). Patient centered care: We are definitely not there yet! *Geriatric Nursing*, 38(1), 7–8. doi:10.1016/j.gerinurse.2016.12.011

Schubert, M., Clarke, S. P., Aiken, L. H., & de Geest, S. (2012). Associations between rationing of nursing care and inpatient mortality in Swiss hospitals. *International Journal for Quality in Health Care*, 24(3), 230–238. doi:10.1093/intqhc/mzs009

Schubert, M., Glass, T. R., Clarke, S. P., Aiken, L. H., Schaffert-Witvliet, B., Sloane, D. M., & de Geest, S. (2008). Rationing of nursing care and its relationship to patient outcomes: The Swiss extension of the International Hospital Outcomes Study. *International Journal of Quality Health Care*, 20(4), 227–237. doi:10.1093/intqhc/mzn017

Scott, L., Rogers, A. E., Hwang, T., & Zhang, Y. (2006). Effects of critical care nurses' work hours on vigilance and patients' safety. *American Journal of Critical Care*, 15(1), 30–37. Retrieved from https://pdfs.semanticscholar.org/310e/69eb55 1410b62b176e1e016cf442fce69a45.pdf

Simpson, K. R., Lyndon, A., & Ruhl, C. (2016). Consequences of inadequate staffing include missed care, potential failure to rescue, and job stress and dissatisfaction. *Journal of Obstetric, Gynecologic & Neonatal Nursing*, 45(4), 481–490. doi:10.1016/j.jogn.2016.02.011

Skutch, J. (2017). Savannah's three major hospitals hit with federal penalties for patient-care issues. *Savannah Morning News*. Retrieved from http:// savannahnow.com/news/2017-01-07/savannah-s-three-major-hospitals -hit-federal-penalties-patient-care-issues

Snavely, T. M. (2016). A brief economic analysis of the looming nursing shortage in the United States. *Nursing Economic$*, 34(2), 98–100. Retrieved from https://search.proquest.com/openview/916ab671da5f4a469a15718f4ae854 22/1?pq-origsite=gscholar&cbl=30765

Sullivan, E., & Ellner, A. (2015). Strong patient-provider relationships drive healthier outcomes. *Harvard Business Review*. Retrieved from https://hbr .org/2015/10/strong-patient-provider-relationships-drive-healthier-outcomes

Sun, L. H. (2016, May 10). Exclusive: Patient safety issues prompt leadership shake-up at NIH hospital. *The Washington Post*. Retrieved from https:// www.washingtonpost.com/national/health-science/exclusive-patient-safety -issues-prompt-leadership-shake-up-at-nih-hospital/2016/05/10/ad1f71f6 -0ffb-11e6-8967-7ac733c56f12_story.html?utm_term=.3e3b109b189f

Twedt, S. (2017, April 10). Medication errors in hospitals don't disappear with new technology. *Pittsburgh Post-Gazette*. Retrieved from http://www .post-gazette.com/business/healthcare-business/2017/04/10/medication -error-electronic-health-record-hospitals-patient-safety-authority/stories/ 201704090072

Whitney J. A., & Parkman S. (2004) The effects of early postoperative physical activity on tissue oxygen and wound healing. *Biological Research in Nursing,* 6(2), 79–89. doi:10.1177/1099800404268939

Xu, J., Murphy, S. L., Kochanek, K. D., & Arias, E. (2016). Mortality in the United States, 2015 (NCHS Data Brief No. 267). Retrieved from https://www.cdc .gov/nchs/data/databriefs/db267.pdf

Yakusheva, O., Costa, D., & Weiss, M. (2017). Patients negatively impacted by discontinuity of nursing care during acute hospitalization. *Medical Care, 55*(4), 421–427. doi:10.1097/MLR.0000000000000670

Yohannes, A. M., & Connolly M. J. (2003) Early mobilization with walking aids following hospital admission with acute exacerbation of chronic obstructive pulmonary disease. *Clinical Rehabilitation, 17*(5), 465–471. doi:10.1191/0269215503cr637oa

Zisberg, A., Shadmi, E., Gur-Yaish, N., Tonkikh, O., & Sinoff, G. (2015). Hospital-associated functional decline: The role of hospitalization processes beyond individual risk factors. *Journal of the American Geriatrics Society, 63*(1), 55–62. doi:10.1111/jgs.13193

Zuckerman, D. M. (2017). A major shortcoming in the public health legacy of the Obama administration. *American Journal of Public Health, 107*(1), 29–30. doi:10.2105/AJPH.2016.303559

2

Professionalism in Health Systems

Professionalism is about having the integrity, honesty, and sincere regard
for the personhood of the customer, in the context of always doing what is
best for the business. Those two things do not need to be in conflict.
—Eric Lippert

THE PROFESSION OF NURSING

Professionalism is a fluid concept that is not easy to articulate. However, most definitions of a profession discuss a societal need that is met through the service of individuals who practice from a unique knowledge base, use a code of ethics to guide their behavior, and conform to regulations or legal standards (Cutliffe & Wieck, 2008; Hodson & Sullivan, 2011). Nursing holds a unique set of concepts that are grounded in theory and embedded throughout most formal educational programs. RNs' specialized education and subsequent entry into practice are regulated via the professional licensure process; once nurses are employed in a practice setting, the American Nurses Association's (ANA) *Code of Ethics* (2015) and established practice standards provide overarching principles to guide behavior. Furthermore, Nursing's Social Statement (ANA, 2010) describes the essence of the profession through its definition of nursing, the description of its knowledge base and societal authority for practice, and the scope and standards of practice. Finally, nursing enjoys a body of ongoing research that shapes its growing knowledge base for practice.

Along with the required knowledge, regulations, and ethical conduct associated with professional nursing, several advantages associated with professionalism are routinely observed, among them a certain status in society; a level of autonomy; unique cultural norms with special language, symbols, and dress; and presumed authority over clients (Hodson & Sullivan, 2011). Nurses work autonomously within the scope of their practice by designing and evaluating plans of care, making judgments and clinical decisions, coordinating services among multiple providers, and employing specific nursing interventions. In the context of clinical practice, some would argue that nursing holds special authority over patients and families.

Although the traits and privileges associated with a profession are somewhat characteristic of nursing today, contrary to other professions (e.g., law, medicine), nursing is learned primarily at the undergraduate level even as debates continue over what that entry-level education should be. Furthermore, nursing theory, although learned in some educational programs, is not typically used as the foundation for clinical practice (Hussein & Osuji, 2017) and many nurses are not empowered to base their practice on evidence (Melnyk et al., 2016). On a more practical level, most nurses are still compensated based on a shift or time worked approach, routinely clock in and out, and perform repetitive tasks. Thus, the debate over whether nursing is a profession continues.

The rapidly shifting transformation of healthcare, and consequently the practice of nursing (Chapter 1), however, is demanding increasingly sophisticated nursing behaviors.

Extensive participation of nurses in collaborative models of practice, increased levels of education, including the PhD, acceptance of full accountability for nursing-sensitive and multidisciplinary outcomes, engagement in highest-level leadership, translation of evidence into everyday practice, promotion of workforce diversity, and application of data in decision making are some of those essential behaviors often associated with professionalism that are essential to current and future nursing practice (Altman, Butler, & Shern, 2015). Guidance is needed, however, on effective professional attitudes and behaviors to help nurses manage issues that arise at the societal, organizational, and clinical levels of practice. For example, how do nurses protect patients and families as they navigate the complex health system

(continued)

(*continued*)

> or how do nurses create policy that guides professional behaviors regarding informed consent in an organization? The revised 2015 Code of Ethics for Nurses (ANA, 2015) outlines some significant updates to language, the role of nursing leadership, and emphasis on nurses' more global and societal roles. This code provides the foundation for nursing practice and its corresponding professional behaviors.

PROFESSIONALISM

Professionalism refers to the values and behaviors of those who serve the public and is most likely a multidimensional concept (O'Sullivan, van Mook, Fewtrell, & Wass, 2012). There are numerous definitions and few cohesive interpretations of the word *professionalism*. Thus, professionalism is difficult to teach and even more difficult to assess (Rogers & Ballantyne, 2010). In an effort to evaluate professionalism among physicians, Wilkinson, Wade, and Knock (2009) conducted a systematic review and identified five characteristics that were commonly found in definitions of professionalism. They were adherence to ethical practice principles, effective interactions with patients and with people who are important to the patients, effective interactions with other people working within the health system, reliability, and commitment to autonomous maintenance and continuous improvement of competence. Interestingly, under the theme of effective interactions with patients and others important to them, the authors listed the more specific behaviors of caring, respect for uniqueness, demeanor, and inclusion of patients in decision making. Furthermore, similar behaviors were noted in the theme of effective interactions with other people working within the health system. Taking responsibility, being accountable for lifelong learning, and reflecting on one's own practice, including seeking and using feedback, were listed under the themes of reliability and commitment to autonomous maintenance and continuous improvement of competence.

In nursing, Miller's (1988) model provides a framework for considering professionalism that remains of importance today. In essence, this model includes behaviors such as adherence to the code of ethics, participation in theory development and use, performing community service, engaging in ongoing continuing education, development, evaluation and use of research, being self-regulating, participation in professional organizations, and public dissemination and communication. These behaviors form the basis for nursing autonomy, competence, maintaining public trust, decision making, and nursing's evolving knowledge base.

In essence, professionalism is about relationships—those we have with ourselves, between patients and families, among other healthcare providers, and with the wider community in which we serve. The professional nurse, grounded by a set of ethical values, exhibits professionalism in all of these relationships but upholds the patient–nurse relationship at the center of the practice.

This relationship is primary because it is during this encounter that nurses recognize the unique human person who is suffering and use specialized knowledge and skill to attend to the human experience of health and illness. Thus, it is within this reciprocal relationship that professional nurses demonstrate their commitment to, and contract with, individuals and society. Theoretically, patients and families who interact with healthcare providers who exhibit professionalism are more apt to disclose, engage, and follow recommended treatment guidelines (Duffy & Hoskins, 2003), leading to improved healthcare outcomes.

Unprofessional conduct, on the other hand, refers to behavior that does not conform to the ethical or performance standards set by the profession. Unfortunately, unprofessional behavior among healthcare providers is visible and of concern to regulatory bodies. For instance, improper use of social media sites, lateral violence in hospitals, inappropriate public conversations about patients, organized cheating among undergraduate students enrolled in health professional programs, scientific integrity among health researchers, elder abuse, and even irresponsible use of resources among healthcare leaders have dominated the literature in the last few years. Yet, ethical values and resulting behaviors form the very foundation of healthcare organizations, ultimately influencing patient–clinician encounters. In turn, professionally driven patient–clinician encounters may impact quality and safety of services, reimbursement patterns, regulatory requirements, and mitigate potential conflicts.

In nursing, for example, the integration of electronic health records (EHRs), use of "smart" systems, shortened lengths of stay, and the complexity of the work in the face of limited resources may trigger stress. Under these conditions, unprofessional behaviors versus the obligations to society derived from the ethical codes of conduct may flare up. Those in healthcare leadership and educational practice face similar pressures and may also act unprofessionally at times. When displayed to patients and families, such behavior may lead to diminished communication with health professionals, anxiety, sleeplessness, feelings of insecurity, dissatisfaction, and even safety and quality concerns (Dupree, Anderson, McEvoy, & Brodman, 2011).

The commitment of health professionals to put the needs of patients and families ahead of personal gain, whether that gain is monetary or just being able to complete the tasks of a particular shift, represents the duty to society that undergirds professional practice.

Contrast the professional behavior of nurses in the following health systems:

The first system is a 300-plus-bed community hospital in a major midwestern suburban city. The hospital has a strong heritage and competes with another acute care organization in the same city. Its nurses are undergoing some change as they are transitioning to new leaders and practice models. Recently, a nurse on a particular unit was deemed "unprofessional" for her inappropriate interaction with family members of a patient. The nurse manager evaluated the situation and reported it to her division director. The matter was taken to Human Resources for consultation and it was determined that a suspension pending review was appropriate (per hospital policy). This was a Thursday and as the nurse was scheduled for the weekend, the nurse manager requested that the suspension begin on Monday, so the nurse could work the weekend, keeping the schedule intact.

The second system is a 217-plus-bed community hospital in a major northeastern suburban city. This hospital too has a strong heritage and competes with numerous acute care organizations in nearby towns. Its nurses have been guided by a professional practice model for the last 3 years and are undergoing change as the hospital has recently expanded its services by merging with another acute care system. In this organization, a young nurse was intimidated by a senior nursing assistant and failed to appropriately follow up on a patient's blood sugar. The patient became hypoglycemic and lost consciousness. The nurse's colleague, an experienced nurse who observed the predicament, assessed the situation and immediately corrected it by first treating the patient and then alerting the medical team. Once the patient was stabilized, she initiated a confidential meeting with the young nurse, made her observations known, and labeled the young nurse's actions as unprofessional. In other words, she determined that the young nurse did not appropriately assume accountability for the nursing assistant's behavior or the patient's blood sugar, resulting in an untoward outcome. The senior nurse, knowing that the young nurse was uncomfortable with delegating and following up with senior nursing assistants, helped her through this by first referring her to a hospital class on delegation and then holding her accountable by going to the nurse manager together to discuss what happened and how it was handled.

How would you describe the nursing professionalism in the two health systems? Which health system displayed the most professional behaviors? In which health system would you want your family members admitted?

Although the *Code for Nursing* (ANA, 2015) is most often thought of when considering unprofessional behavior in nursing, nonadherence or violations of state practice acts are also considered unprofessional conduct. This is especially important today as the complex practice environment sometimes blurs health workers' roles and responsibilities. Professional nurses themselves and their leaders, however, are responsible and accountable for adhering to state practice acts, including reporting misconduct, advocating for patients and families, and owning those responsibilities delegated to unlicensed assistive personnel.

Lachman, Murray, Isminger, and Ganske (2012) described the moral courage required of nurses to advocate for the best interests of patients and families, regardless of the perceived or actual risks. Moral courage suggests operating within a certain set of personal and professional beliefs and taking a stand or speaking up when such behaviors are violated or absent. Such behavior requires "accountability for providing the best possible patient care" (p. 28). Pertaining to medical education, moral courage has been defined as "voluntary willingness to stand up and act on one's ethical beliefs despite barriers that prohibit the ability to proceed toward right action" (Martinez, Bell, Etchagaray, & Lehmann, 2016). While it is the individual health professional's responsibility to perform with moral courage, creating an environment that supports it, including enacting clear policies that reinforce openness, multilevel communication, administrative support, and staff empowerment, is a significant role of leadership.

While institutional culture and systems influence the actions and behaviors of health professionals, unprofessional conduct in health professionals may be first observed during the educational process as academic dishonesty, incivility, poor reporting of errors, and even disruptive behaviors in the classroom, online, or during clinical courses. It is precisely during this time of formation that the health profession's educators must prepare students for profession conduct, including the behavioral and dynamic nature of professionalism. In fact, using nontraditional and reflective educational strategies, educators can be instrumental in helping health profession students develop expressions of moral courage (Bickoff, Levett-Jones, & Sinclair, 2016; Krautscheid, 2017).

The Carnegie Study of Nursing Education (Benner, Sutphen, Leonard-Kahn, & Day, 2008) concluded that nurses are unprepared for the complexities of professional practice. Directed at nurse educators, the report noted that "most of the teaching about everyday ethical comportment and formation of the identity, character, and skilled capacities of nurses was confined primarily to clinical practice sites and preclinical and postclinical conferences" (Benner et al., 2008, p. 473). Although formal courses provided the foundational ethical principles and standards, the report advocated for activities that helped healthcare professionals learn what "good practice" means within a particular discipline. During the interviewing of several senior nursing students, the students identified many strong formative nursing experiences that they believed deepened their understanding of good nursing practice. They were:

- Understanding the patient as a person
- Preserving the dignity and personhood of patients
- Responding to substandard practice
- Advocating for patients and families
- Seriously engaging in learning to do "good" nursing
- Learning how to be present with patient and family suffering

These central but everyday concerns of professional nursing must be dealt with during the educational process in order to enhance professionalism, an important societal obligation that many health professionals are struggling to safeguard. As Wolf (2012) so aptly stated, "Nursing programs are the first filters of character for the profession, and modeling good nursing care begins in schools of nursing" (p. 16). Likewise, employers of nurses and nurses themselves have a duty to acknowledge, assess, and address those unprofessional behaviors that some nurses display. Perhaps a behavioral, more dynamic view of professionalism that starts during undergraduate education and continues throughout the workplace with regular assessment and ongoing development provides an alternative approach (Lesser et al., 2010). Linking professionalism to patient outcomes and approaching lapses in professionalism, such as some form of medical error (Lucey & Souba, 2010), may help nurses appreciate their commitment to the values of professionalism, despite the inevitable challenges of the workplace.

PROFESSIONAL NURSING IN A TRANSFORMED HEALTH SYSTEM

Accountability in professional practice is a crucial component of the newly emerging health system. To ensure health professionals are practicing at the highest levels of professionalism, all health professionals must constantly safeguard professional behavior by observing, identifying, and reporting conduct that does not conform to ethical standards. One way to facilitate ethical conduct is to perform values clarification exercises every 3 to 5 years to clearly articulate those values that guide practice and then embed them in pertinent documents such as philosophy and mission statements, professional practice models, and even patient care delivery systems. Some organizations frame and post these core values on clinical units, letterheads, or even web pages as constant reminders of the foundational beliefs of the profession. Using such values for decision framing (all decisions), performance evaluations, recognition programs, and continuing education provides clarity and a focus on action. Similarly, using individual performance data to increase ownership and accountability of nurses' practice or peer review principles provided specific and actionable information (Cline, 2016; Semper, Halvorson, Hersh, Torres, & Lillington, 2016). On a personal level, individual health professionals who routinely reflect on their practice, both individually and in groups, and who maintain a level of awareness about ethical behavior may be able to recognize tendencies toward unethical behaviors early enough to impede their full development.

Leaders and educators can expedite professionalism by creating an open, safe culture for discussion and reporting of unethical behavior, clarifying behavioral expectations, organizing ongoing education, consistently implementing policy, recognizing how their own actions guide the practice of employees or students (living the organization's values), creating peer support groups for themselves and employees/students to help stay grounded on important values and to safely reflect on their conduct, and creating an ongoing professional development program. Measuring the ethical climate in the organization and matching results of procedural audits with established ethical values may provide baseline information from which professional practice can be reframed and improved. Regular review and discussion of revised ethical codes, standards, and state nurse practice acts draws attention to professional behaviors in the context of safe, high-quality services.

In *Nursing's Social Policy Statement*'s (ANA, 2010) definition of professional nursing, the "assurance of safe, quality, and evidence-based practice" (p. 9) is emphasized.

Attending to the "protection, promotion, and optimization of health and abilities, prevention of illness and injury, alleviation of suffering through the diagnosis and treatment of human response, and advocacy in the care of individuals, families, communities, and populations" (ANA, 2010, p. 10) with knowledge-based nursing actions that produce beneficial outcomes for patients, families, and communities is a social responsibility that requires professional nurses to practice with a spirit of inquiry, always mindful of how health outcomes are tied to organizational and process aspects of care.

Professional nursing is accountable to society for its performance; consequently, routine measuring, monitoring, reporting, and using outcomes to improve nursing care are social responsibilities. However, the complexity associated with measuring and interpreting outcomes of care can be overwhelming to healthcare professionals who do not routinely discuss methodological issues associated with interpreting data on outcomes. Lack of sufficient awareness about the methodologies associated with measurement of outcomes, however, contributes to errors in interpretation, oftentimes generating unnecessary remediations and wasting resources. For example, in a recent discussion of the annual results of nursing-sensitive quality indicators, a nursing leadership team was presented with raw data that was highlighted with red (poor), yellow (average), and green (good) marks. At first glance, certain units were considered better or worse and the expectation was that the poorer quality units would explain and develop recommendations for improvement. However, after more in-depth analysis with a nurse researcher, it was learned that confounding factors (such as patients' age, severity of illness, or comorbidities and RNs' experience and credentials) were not accounted for, giving the data a somewhat false meaning. The interface between measurement of indicators and accountability for quality outcomes calls for creative thinking with attention to methods used. This particular strength is important for ongoing performance improvement and is essential for professional practice.

> In the developing future healthcare system, nurses already are participating with other health professionals in publicly documenting the results of care, and workplaces are reimbursed accordingly. Nurses, therefore, must recognize that ongoing performance improvement is nonnegotiable evidence of their work and an obligation of professionalism that translates into beneficial outcomes for patients and health systems.

THE GROUNDING BENEFITS OF THEORY-GUIDED PROFESSIONAL PRACTICE

Because disciplinary values and beliefs (philosophies) undergird nursing theory, professional nursing practice that is based on theory, often referred to as theory-guided practice, directs nurses in their thinking, provides a frame of reference for assessments and interventions, specifies a structure for ongoing development and evaluation, and promotes nursing autonomy and accountability. Theory provides nurses with a framework for practice (or rationale) that includes the specific parameters of the discipline and suggests what data to collect, specific actions to use, and how to evaluate services (Kenney, 2002). However, there is relatively little evidence in the professional literature related to the application of theory to contemporary professional practice.

Despite the potential value of nursing theory to professional practice, especially the more recent middle range theories, many nurses anecdotally report that nursing theory is not routinely applied in the daily care of patients or practice improvement efforts. In reality, most health systems tend to address practice improvement by progressing straight from recommendations to implementation, limiting the critical benefits of considering theory. More importantly, specific improvement interventions are commonly launched without a theory of change to guide needed practice revisions, and oftentimes outcomes measurement plans, or baseline data required for meaningful analyses, are not considered. Furthermore, without theory, any contextual consideration that might impact the improvement intervention or how the intervention will be evaluated is often forgotten. In fact, this last point is often quite costly to organizations and is an explanation for why many nursing contributions are left unknown (Duffy, 2016). Without a good grasp of an underlying theory and its critical components (concepts, assumptions, and propositions), it is difficult to articulate the components of an intervention or demonstrate a particular intervention's impact. Alternatively, including theory in practice continually informs and guides practice and practice improvement, while simultaneously assisting in the advancement of nursing knowledge.

To meet the challenge of professionalism in a transformed health system, middle range theory may be a more practical approach for attending to human responses to actual and potential health problems. It tends to be less abstract than grand theory and helps nurses to focus on more specific phenomena in different care settings. Middle range theory in particular adds meaning to practice as it is applied in daily care, in research studies, and in practice changes. To be most useful, however, theories should be realistic and provide some evidence of benefit (to patients and families). Of note, many middle range theories are amenable to empirical testing, making evaluation of outcomes easier and actionable practice changes faster. However, selecting theories for application are decisions that require evaluation, including analysis of a theory's value, worth, and significance (Smith & Parker, 2015) and its alignment with nurses' values and beliefs, the organization's mission, and its feasibility for implementation and evaluation.

The Quality-Caring Model© (QCM) is a middle range theory that is congruent with nursing's disciplinary beliefs and values, the Social Policy Statement standards (ANA, 2010), and offers language and concepts consistent with professional nursing practice. It has literature support, empirical measures for evaluation, and has been implemented in multiple sites, several of which have successfully attained Magnet® designation. This model can be used as a basis for nursing assessment, to guide job descriptions and advancement programs, as a basis for nursing interventions, and as a foundation for research and improvement. And, most importantly, as the model is integrated into practice and used to routinely evaluate and improve quality, professionalism is advanced.

In a qualitative study of caring theories, the author notes that certain theories play a role in confirming and verifying nurses' practice by putting into words their professional experience (Ranheim, Kärner, & Berterö, 2011). It is especially crucial in this global and evolving health system that healthcare professionals maintain their focus on the human experience of individuals in need of health services, keeping in mind the holistic and contextual nature of humans and health systems. The need for a grounding framework for practice could never be greater.

SUMMARY

Characteristics of professionalism are described and examined in relation to nursing and healthcare. Relationships form the basis of professionalism, guided by ethical codes of conduct, standards, and regulatory mechanisms. Unprofessional behaviors in nursing and healthcare are exposed and linked to patient outcomes. The accountability of health professionals, educators, and leadership for professional conduct is highlighted in light of the transitioning health system. Finally, the value of a grounding framework for practice is presented.

Call to Action

Professionalism is a social mandate based on advanced knowledge and a strong ethical foundation. Professional nursing validates the nature of humans as they exist in union with the universe. **Consider** how nursing serves society. **Assume** accountability for placing the needs of patients and families first.

REFLECTIVE QUESTIONS/APPLICATIONS

. . . for Students

1. What are your beliefs about nursing and the health system?
2. Analyze the *Code for Nurses* and the *Social Policy Statement* for their ability to enhance professionalism of health professionals.
3. Reflect on the role of the professional nurse. Based on your clinical experience, how do professional nurses display professionalism?
4. Outline your plans to develop professional behaviors consistent with your discipline. How will you know you have achieved professionalism?
5. How would you go about evaluating nursing professionalism? Provide specific examples.

. . . for Professional Nurses in Clinical Practice

1. Discuss professionalism in your healthcare institution.
2. Is there an accepted code of behavior? If so, who is responsible for its application and evaluation?
3. How or should unprofessional nursing care be corrected?
4. How are health outcomes reported in your institution? Are nurses held accountable for nursing-sensitive health outcomes? How do you know?
5. What nursing theory is used on your unit? How was it chosen? How has it been evaluated?
6. How do you hold yourself and fellow nurses accountable for professional conduct?

. . . for Professional Nurses in Educational Practice

1. What specific curricular revisions have you developed that addressed ethical comportment among nursing students? What evidence did you use to shape them? What teaching strategies will you use to help undergraduate and graduate students learn ethical comportment?
2. Reflect on today's nursing practice environment. How do you think your educational program helps graduates stay focused on the patient–nurse relationship as the central component of practice? What new knowledge and skills will be required to meet the societal obligations associated with professionalism?

3. Have the learning outcomes specified in your evaluation plan informed curricular revision regarding professionalism over the last 3 years?
4. How do you assess professionalism in students? Is it even necessary?

. . . for Professional Nurses in Leadership Practice

1. How has professionalism in nursing improved/worsened over the last 3 years at your institution?
2. How have you articulated the specific professional conduct required of professional nurses at your institution?
3. Reflect on the developmental activities in place at your institution. Do they include aspects of professionalism? Are they working? How do you know?
4. How are data on patient outcomes used to advance professionalism at your institution?
5. How do you ensure accountability for professional behavior?

PRACTICE ANALYSIS

A day shift nursing director in a large tertiary hospital was reporting off to the night nursing director when an RN called in sick. The RN was scheduled to work on a busy medical–surgical unit. Since there were no other available RNs, the day shift nursing director communicated this via telephone to the unit charge nurse suggesting that she rearrange assignments to accommodate for the absent RN. (The unit was originally intended to be staffed with five RNs [two with <6 months of experience] and two NAs for 36 patients, leaving them with four RNs and two NAs. Furthermore, there were four empty beds and several admitted patients in the emergency department.) Specifically, the nursing director asked the charge nurse to assign some extra duties to the two NAs to lighten the remaining RNs' workloads and maybe assign herself to a couple of patients. About 15 minutes later, the charge nurse called the day shift director to express that one of her scheduled night RNs was distraught about having to work short. She threatened to leave if another RN was not assigned to care for the 36 patients on the unit. Furthermore, the charge nurse communicated that the nurse stated, "I will not continue to put up with this constant shortage of help. It is the number 1 reason everyone quits around here. We are overworked, underpaid, and hospital management does nothing about it. Patients deserve better. This place needs to be investigated." A senior baccalaureate student who was completing a clinical assignment on the unit and overheard the charge nurse asked her instructor, "Does this happen often? Doesn't the nursing director have some responsibility for providing the unit with more RNs?" The day shift director, who has just worked the last 12 hours, asks the charge nurse to do the best she can to calm down the employee and suggests that the night nursing director will come and check on them as soon as she is able.

1. What behaviors did the day nursing director and the distraught staff RN display that were professional and/or unprofessional?
2. What about the nursing student?
3. Was moral courage displayed in this situation? If so, by whom?
4. Were any ethical codes, practice acts, or professional responsibilities violated? If so, what were they?
5. How did the relational aspects of the situation demonstrate and/ or not demonstrate professionalism?
6. If you were the nursing instructor, what would you have communicated to the student?
7. What advice do you have for the nurses in this situation?

REFERENCES

Altman, S. H., Butler, A. S., & Shern, L. (Eds.). (2015). *Assessing progress on the Institute of Medicine report*: The Future of Nursing. Retrieved from https://www.nap.edu/read/21838/chapter/1#ii

American Nurses Association. (2010). *Nursing's social policy statement: The essence of the profession*. Silver Spring, MD: Author.

American Nurses Association. (2015). *Code of ethics for nurses with interpretive statements*. Silver Spring, MD: Author.

Benner, P., Sutphen, M., Leonard-Kahn, V., & Day, L. (2008). Formation and everyday ethical comportment. *American Journal of Critical Care, 17*(5), 473–476. Retrieved from http://ajcc.aacnjournals.org/content/17/5/473.full

Bickoff, L., Levett-Jones, T., & Sinclair, P. M. (2016). Rocking the boat—Nursing students' stories of moral courage: A qualitative descriptive study. *Nurse Education Today, 42,* 35–40. doi:10.1016/j.nedt.2016.03.030

Cline, M. (2016). Increasing RN accountability in professional practice: Development of a pain reassessment documentation scorecard. *Journal of Nursing Administration, 46*(3), 128–131. doi:10.1097/NNA.0000000000000311

Cutliffe, J. R., & Wieck, K. L. (2008). Salvation or damnation: Deconstructing nursing's aspirations to professional status. *Journal of Nursing Management, 16*(5), 499–507. doi:10.1111/j.1365-2834.2008.00894.x

Duffy, J. (2016). *Professional practice models in nursing: Successful health system integration*. New York, NY: Springer Publishing.

Duffy, J., & Hoskins, L. (2003). The Quality-Caring Model©: Blending dual paradigms. *Advances in Nursing Science, 26*(1), 77–88. doi:10.1097/00012272-200301000-00010

Dupree, E., Anderson, R., McEvoy, M. D., & Brodman, M. (2011). Professionalism: A necessary ingredient in a culture of safety. *The Joint Commission Journal on Quality and Patient Safety, 37*(10), 446–454. doi:10.1016/S1553-7250(11)37057-2

Hodson, R., & Sullivan, T. A. (2011). *The social organization of work* (5th ed.). Belmont, CA: Cengage-Wadsworth.

Hussein, M. T., & Osuji, J. (2017). Bridging the theory-practice dichotomy in nursing: The role of nurse educators. *Journal of Education and Practice, 7*(3), 20–25. doi:10.5430/jnep.v7n3p20

Kenney, J. W. (2002). *Philosophical and theoretical perspectives for advanced nursing practice* (3rd ed.). Sudbury, MA: Jones & Bartlett.

Krautscheid, L. C. (2017). Embedding microethical dilemmas in high-fidelity simulation scenarios: Preparing nursing students for ethical practice. *Journal of Nursing Education, 56*(1), 55–58. doi:10.3928/01484834-20161219-11

Lachman, V. D., Murray, J. S., Isminger, K., & Ganske, K. M. (2012). Doing the right thing: Pathways to moral courage. *American Nurse Today, 7*(5), 24–29. Retrieved from https://www.americannursetoday.com/doing-the-right-thing-pathways-to-moral-courage

Lesser, C. S., Lucey, C., Egener, B., Braddock, C. H., Linas, S. L., & Levinson, W. (2010). Behavioral and systems view of professionalism. *Journal of the American Medical Association, 304*(24), 2732–2737. doi:10.1001/jama.2010.1864

Lucey, C., & Souba, W. (2010). Perspective: The problem with the problem of professionalism. *Academic Medicine, 85*(6), 1018–1024. doi:10.1097/ACM.0b013e3181dbe51f

Martinez, W., Bell, S. K., Etchagaray, J. M., & Lehmann, L. S. (2016). Measuring moral courage for interns and residents: Scale development and initial psychometrics. *Academic Medicine, 91*(10), 1431–1438. doi:10.1097/ACM.0000000000001288

Melnyk, B. M., Gallagher-Ford, L., Thomas, B. K., Troseth, M., Wyngarden, K., & Szalacha, L. (2016). A study of chief nurse executives indicates low prioritization of evidence-based practice and shortcomings in Hospital performance metrics Across the United States. *Worldviews on Evidence-Based Nursing, 13*(1), 6–14. doi:10.1111/wvn.12133

Miller, B. K. (1988). A model for professionalism in nursing. *Today's OR Nurse, 10*(9), 18–23.

O'Sullivan, H., van Mook, W., Fewtrell, R., & Wass, V. (2012). Integrating professionalism into the curriculum: AMEE guide No. 61. *Medical Teacher, 34*(2), e64–e77. doi:10.3109/0142159X.2012.655610

Ranheim, A., Kärner, A., & Berterö, C. (2011). Eliciting reflections on caring theory in elderly caring practice. *International Journal of Qualitative Studies on Health and Well-Being, 6*, 14–18. doi:10.3402/qhw.v6i3.7296

Rogers, W., & Ballantyne, A. (2010). Towards a practical definition of professional behaviour. *Journal of Medical Ethics, 36*(4), 250–254. doi:10.1136/jme.2009.035121

Semper, J., Halvorson, B., Hersh, M., Torres, C., & Lillington, L. (2016). Clinical nurse specialists guide staff nurses to promote practice accountability through peer review. *Clinical Nurse Specialist, 30*(1), 19–27. doi:10.1097/NUR.0000000000000157

Smith, M., & Parker, M. E. (2015). *Nursing theories and nursing practice.* Philadelphia, PA: F. A. Davis.

Wilkinson, T., Wade, W., & Knock, L. D. (2009). A blueprint to assess professionalism: Results of a systematic review. *Academic Medicine, 84,* 551–558. doi:10.1097/ACM.0b013e31819fbaa2

Wolf, Z. R. (2012). Nursing practice breakdown: Good and bad nursing. *MedSurg Nursing, 21*(1), 16–36.

3

Evolution of the Quality-Caring Model©

Caring can be learned by all human beings, can be worked into the design of every life, meeting an individual's need as well as a pervasive need in society.

—Mary Catherine Bateson

COMPLEX HEALTH SYSTEMS

A complex system is one that comprises a large number of parts that continuously interact (Simon, 1996), much like health systems. Complexity in this sense refers to the valuable interconnectivity among the many parts that often transforms them in unexpected and irreversible ways (Uhl-Bien & Arena, 2017). Health systems, in particular, are composed of multiple systems—individuals, groups, departmental (or unit-based), organizational, and larger community or societal systems. The delivery of health services includes all of these systems; it follows, then, that the delivery of healthcare is not a linear process, but rather a complex, dynamic process that allows for continual interaction, contextual influences, relationship forming, feedback among the many parts, relationship remodeling, and adaptation. Complex adaptive systems (CAS) refer to the application of Complex Systems Theory (a.k.a. complexity science) to living, dynamic systems (e.g., health and health systems; Engebretson & Hickey, 2011).

In such systems, individual diverse agents (e.g., human beings, a hospital department, a single cell) continually and dynamically interact and connect, and over time develop patterns that inform behaviors. These accumulated experiences and resultant behaviors enable adaptations that shape the evolution of the system, oftentimes generating unexpected behaviors that emerge in ways that can neither be predicted nor controlled. Over time, these dynamics allow for the process of self-organization, or new patterns of behavior, labeled *emergence or co-emergence* (Institute of Medicine, 2001; Mahajan, Islam, Schwartz, & Cannesson, 2017; Rickles, Hawe, & Shiell, 2007). For example, typically nurses on one hospital unit befriend those on their same unit (they have shared interests). However, through meeting and working with other nurses on different units in shared governance committees (interaction and connection), relationships and interdependencies form. Over time, nurses who work in the ICU might be observed interacting comfortably with other nurses from the postanesthesia care unit (PACU) sharing lunch in the cafeteria. Through continuous interaction, a new pattern of behavior forms (emergence) in which the two groups of nurses transition to a more tightly knit group of "critical care" nurses (self-organization). Interestingly, these diverse agents interact in a manner that allows for creative adaptations and do so in an unpredictable manner that does not require centralized control. The nursing profession has long emphasized and valued connections and interactions within a systems paradigm and has a long, rich tradition of appreciating patterns. And healthcare in general is recognized as a CAS because of the dynamic network of interactions needed to execute complex plans of care both for individuals and for groups (i.e., patient populations).

In fact, in the larger health system context, connections and relationships continuously occur in a complex, dynamically changing environment, much like a spinning cyclone or tornado. Over time, the interaction of multiple individuals fosters collective learning from that context and re-influences the context to better prepare for future advancement. But because a health system is embedded within its context, when one part of the health system changes, so does the context in a constant interplay of coexisting correction or revision. This intricacy of interdependent related parts, together with the constant flux of the external environment, creates a natural cycle of coevolution such that the system and the agents within it evolve (or coevolve) together over time (Lindberg, Nash, & Lindberg, 2008; Marshall & Broome, 2016). For example, in a health system where a new service is introduced, operationalization of the new service (including the involved patients and employees) together with the context will coevolve over time as each interacts with the other and learns to advance.

In the social systems of healthcare, interactions among various team members affect the processes and outcomes of work. Sociologists have labeled this phenomenon Social Network Theory and use this as a framework for analysis (Freeman, 2004; Knoke & Yang, 2008; Scott, 2000; Valente & Pitts, 2017; Wasserman & Faust, 1994). In social networks, individuals (nodes) and their relationships/connections (ties) influence how information is relayed, the performance of professionals, and improved quality and safety outcomes (Cunningham et al., 2012). In fact, in the systematic review by Cunningham et al. (2012), evidence for cohesive and collaborative health professional networks facilitating the coordination of care and contributing to improved quality and safety of care was apparent.

Because of the many connections among nursing (and other health professions) within the complex nature and social structures of health systems, the Quality-Caring Model© (QCM) has evolved from its initiation in 2003. Once depicted in a linear manner between patients and care providers, it is now situated within several relationships. These relationships form the complex "system within a system" echelons of healthcare, much like nesting doll toys, absent the boundaries among them. The level of relationships that characterize health systems (see Figure 3.1)

FIGURE 3.1   Levels of relationships in health systems.

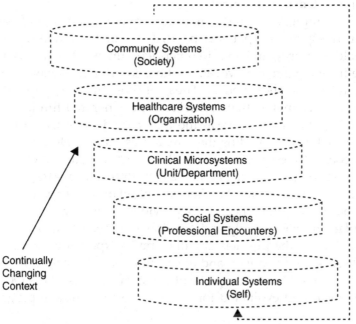
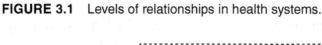

influences the application of the QCM, enabling adaptations that shape the evolution of both the system and the model.

Healthcare providers and patients serve as individual systems (or agents) who cocreate social systems during healthcare encounters. Healthcare encounters typically occur within departments or units, medical offices, or homes/schools (microsystems) that coexist in larger organizations that are embedded within a community. Nursing units in a hospital, for example, exist within a larger health system that serves a particular community that is part of still larger societal systems (state and federal). These multiple systems continually interact, form relationships, and generate feedback that informs the development of new ways of being.

Interestingly, the more emphasis placed on interaction, relationships, and continuous learning among the levels, the more interdependent (robust) they become, facilitating progress or advancement of the larger system. Thus, the relationships between and among systems are paramount. This is not complicated, but rather a straightforward tenet that affirms the significant influence that relationships and connections play in systems' progress. It also demonstrates the lack of outside control that is necessary to evolve or advance. This is a particularly difficult concept for health professionals and their leaders, who are used to continually anticipating and controlling. The continual interaction, reshaping, feedback, and adaptation common to relationships in complex systems actually creates the energy (or flow) required to sustain the system and expedite system advancement.

For example, seemingly small improvements in a unit (such as improved responses to patients' pain), if attended to and nurtured, may take hold, multiply, and shift to other departments. For this to happen in an efficient manner, however, reactions to this new behavior must be quick, direct, and show benefit. Thus, for those in leadership positions, feedback mechanisms that are delayed or generated through a third party will not be as effective as those that are disseminated directly to clinicians who are providing the care. In this example, leadership effort is best concentrated at the local level (vs. upper organizational levels), supporting health professionals in their efforts to improve response times to patients' reports of pain. Another example of the power of relationships is that observed among healthcare providers. Over time, as nurses in a particular unit consistently and genuinely collaborate with physicians during rounds, the physicians will come to expect this behavior and actively seek out the nurses and their opinions at the start of rounds.

At each level in the larger health system, aspects of the QCM can be employed and evaluated for effects on overall system progress or advancement. Developed as an approach to the professional practice of nursing, the QCM has also been used at the organizational level with all health professionals attuned to its concepts. In one large organization that uses the model to guide overall professional practice, board members who greatly believed in the QCM model devoted an entire annual meeting to its integration in the system.

THE EVOLVING QUALITY-CARING MODEL

The philosophical and theoretical underpinnings of the QCM remain rooted in earlier theories of healthcare quality (Donabedian, 1966) and relational aspects of nursing (Irvine, Sidani, & McGillis Hall, 1998; King, 1981; Peplau, 1988; Swanson, 1993; Watson, 1979) but more recently are influenced by the complexity and systems theories associated with the continuously evolving health system. In essence, the relationships and interactions among the agents in the healthcare system are viewed as fundamental and central to its operations and require different approaches to clinical practice, leadership, change, and ongoing professional development. And although the term *quality* was originally defined as excellence or worthiness of a service (Duffy, 2009), it is now seen as a broad construct that incorporates the concepts of safety and value and includes advanced practice (Duffy, 2013).

In this perspective, quality is not an endpoint per se, but a relational *process* of continuous learning and improvement. Such a broad view connotes a dynamic system of practice improvement that treats patients as full partners, is operationalized through educated, multidisciplinary teams that find meaning in their work, transparently serves its community (Leape et al., 2009), and is fully integrated into the work of health professionals.

Through continuous improvement processes, individual healthcare providers and systems attend to revising their practice using internal and external evidence as guides, generating practice changes that are ongoing and innovative, and allowing for natural self-advancement. Collectively, these individual agents facilitate continuous learning organizations or organizational learning.

Continuous learning organizations create the infrastructure and capacity (behavioral, social, information, computing, mathematical, and engineering sciences) for iterative, rapid improvements that generate value for patients and families through shared knowledge and team-based approaches (Friedman et al., 2017). The American Heart Association recently issued a scientific statement on learning health systems that calls for the development and activation of science and informatics, patient–clinician partnerships, incentives, and culture in health systems as a roadmap to continuous learning and by extension, value creation and possibly new evidence generation (Maddox et al., 2017). From an individual healthcare professional basis, continuous learning and resultant practice change is a professional responsibility that, when integrated into practice, fulfills our social obligation while also adding meaning to the work.

Today's technological advances enable patients, individual health professionals, departments, and whole health systems to gather, analyze, and disseminate internal data. Furthermore, regular external benchmarking and access to current research are regular features of health systems that are available to guide practice improvement. From the individual health professional's perspective, this implies that all are actively involved in improving their practice, including those parts that interact with other health professionals. Using knowledge to advance practice helps one learn about himself or herself and ensures patients and families are provided the highest value.

An open and safe environment for inquiry and regular reflection facilitates such practice. Such an environment engages health professionals in discussions, allows for education and development of new ideas, and encourages pilot studies that test feasibility of new approaches. Of course, leadership is key to promoting a learning culture, including the design and sustainment of the infrastructure required to support learning.

> Caring, on the other hand, is implicitly tied to the relational aspect of human beings, who are multidimensional beings worthy of our ongoing consideration. Caring relationships, when attended to and sustained, facilitate advancement of individual, social, micro, organizational, and community systems, ultimately influencing self-advancement.

Make no mistake, caring is work, nursing's primary work. Other health professionals also establish caring relationships and must be recognized for this; however, nursing, in many healthcare environments, is the only health profession that maintains a 24/7 presence, has the most direct contact with patients and families, is a stabilizing force in a fragmented health system, and remains very influential in the prevention of adverse outcomes (Hughes, 2008; Needleman & Hassmiller, 2009; Rosenkoetter,

2016). Since caring is the foundation for nurses' work, it remains a crucial phenomenon that is expressed daily in the attitudes, behaviors, and skills of professional nurses.

Caring is a process that involves the human person of the nurse relating to the human person of the patient. This reciprocal relationship forms the foundation for all nursing practice and generates "feeling cared for," a positive emotion experienced by both the patient and the nurse. It is this feeling of being "cared for" that gives rise to patients' sentiments that they matter in the complex health system and is an important performance indicator of high-quality nursing care.

Caring relationships many times are viewed as soft, intangible, and unworthy by some. Caring relationships are not often measured as an indicator of professional performance (Duffy, Kooken, Wolverton, & Weaver, 2012), but patients and families know when it is lacking (Baird, Rehm, Hinds, Baggott, & Davies, 2016). It is most often associated with "basic nursing care" or those seemingly inconsequential routine activities that professional nurses often delegate to unlicensed assistive personnel. Yet, caring relationships honor the dignity of persons and provide the foundation for future interactions (required for patient-centered care), create a spirit of transparency (necessary ingredient for safety cultures), and enable the conditions for advancement (may help patients better participate in care and attain health goals while engaging employees in meaningful practice). These are beneficial, progressive consequences that contribute to health system value.

But, because the health system is so focused on disease, cures, and technology, we often fail to notice the advantages associated with its more routine (or buried) human caring aspects. A more optimistic and broad-minded view may help nursing appreciate its strengths, including specifically how we contribute to the larger whole. Furthermore, acknowledging strengths (vs. limitations) may stimulate more innovative approaches to practice change. To reinforce and intensify human caring in health systems, this essential relational process of nursing must be valued, consistently applied, tied to outcomes, and rewarded.

In summary then, the term *quality* in the evolving QCM is viewed as a dynamic process of learning that is fully embedded in practice. It uses qualitative and quantitative evaluative techniques to provide the data required for actionable practice changes. *Caring* is a seminal attribute of nursing practice that, together with continuous learning (and resultant practice improvement), facilitates *feeling cared for* and, ultimately, *self-advancing* individuals, communities, and health systems.

ASSUMPTIONS, MAJOR CONCEPTS, AND PROPOSITIONS OF THE QUALITY-CARING MODEL

Assumptions

Assumptions of a model include the theorist's underlying values and beliefs that are used as premises for its development. In the QCM, they are the following:

- Humans are multidimensional beings capable of growth and change.
- Humans exist in relationship to themselves, others, communities or groups, the environment (including the workplace), and the larger universe.
- Humans evolve in a dynamic, interconnected continuum.
- Humans are inherently worthy.
- Caring consists of interpersonal processes that are used individually or in combination and often concurrently.
- Caring is a social process that is done "in relationship."
- Caring for self enhances caring for others.
- Caring relationships are protective.
- Caring is embedded in the daily work of professional nursing.
- Professional nursing work is done in the context of human relationships.
- The display of caring relationships varies.
- Caring is a tangible concept that can be measured.
- Caring relationships benefit both the carer and the one being cared for.
- Caring relationships benefit society.
- Caring relationships generate feeling "cared for."
- Feeling "cared for" is a positive emotion.
- Feeling "cared for" is adaptive for individuals, groups, and systems.
- Caring relationships influence advancement.
- Feeling "cared for" positively influences self-advancing systems.
- Self-advancing systems evolve over time and in context.

Major Model Concepts

Major concepts are those ideas or components that form the essence of the model. In the QCM, the major concepts are humans in relationship, relationship-centered professional encounters, feeling "cared for," and self-advancing systems (see Figure 3.2). Humans, with their unique beliefs, attitudes, behaviors, physical attributes, and life experiences, are

FIGURE 3.2 Quality-Caring Model©.

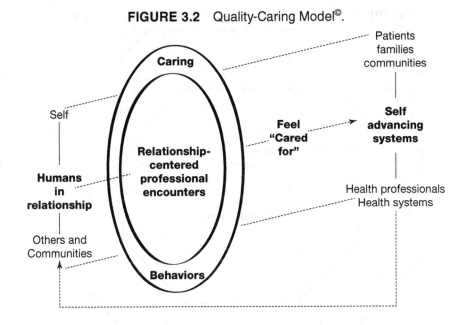

holistic in nature and relate throughout their lives to others, including their families and communities, and the larger universe.

During illness or suffering, specific health characteristics (such as severity of illness, years living with a disease, number of comorbidities) and the aforementioned unique individual characteristics become important considerations since they may impact processes and outcomes of care. Through their many relationships, individuals live, work, and die, and if caring in nature, relationships enable individuals to progress, evolve, achieve healthy states, and advance. If, however, those relationships are uncaring, individuals may respond by withdrawing or falling behind, or even becoming ill.

In healthcare professional encounters, persons with health needs relate to healthcare providers who function independently and collaboratively with them (see Figure 3.3). Independent relationships are those between patients and families and a healthcare provider. Collaborative relationships are those among healthcare providers and patients that occur as three-way encounters and are necessary to cohesively deliver needed services. When healthcare providers work in harmony and mutually partner with patients and families, such collaborative relationships can be instrumental in attaining specific health goals.

Furthermore, when relationships are grounded in caring behaviors, human connections occur that are transpersonal (extending beyond the individuals alone) and have the potential to be transformative for all

FIGURE 3.3   Relationship-centered professional encounters.

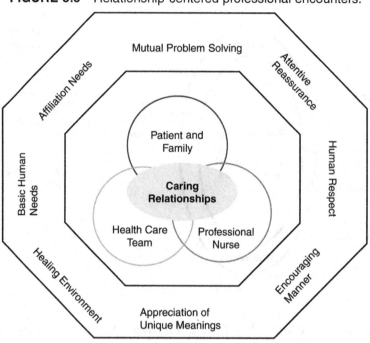

involved. Specific behaviors or processes, namely, *mutual problem solving, attentive reassurance, human respect, encouraging manner, healing environment, appreciation of unique meanings, affiliation needs,* and *basic human needs,* have been used as guides for understanding and practicing the QCM (see Table 3.1 for definitions of the caring behaviors). Although derived from theory, these actions and demeanors coexist in relationships (Duffy, Brewer, & Weaver, 2014; Wolverton, 2016) and are often delivered concurrently based on the particular clinical situation. When delivered expertly and over time, however, they lead to "feeling cared for" in the recipient. This reaction is a positive emotion generated as a result of the caring processes (Duffy, 2013) that leads to feelings of ease, worth, comfort, hope, security, and confidence to name a few (see Figure 3.4). These positive emotions, necessary antecedents to risk-taking, learning, following-through, disclosure, and future interactions have been reported to facilitate very specific intermediate outcomes such as timely discharge and the patient experience in the stroke population (Baggett et al., 2016). Although depicted as a linear process in Figure 3.2, caring relationships and their immediate and longer term consequences are dynamic processes influenced by individual and contextual processes that can "speed up" or "slow down" responses.

TABLE 3.1 Definitions of the Caring Behaviors

Caring Factors	Definitions
Mutual problem solving	Behaviors that help patients and caregivers understand how to confront, learn, and think about their health and illness. Providing information, reframing, facilitating learning, exploring alternatives, brainstorming together, deciding questions to ask, validating, accepting feedback from patients, and experimenting with different approaches all involve mutual input and participation from *both* patients and health professionals. This factor implies that health professionals are informed, actively listen, are continuously learning, and engaged.
Attentive reassurance	Behaviors that assure health professionals are reliable. They include availability, hopeful outlook, confidence, conveying possibilities, presence, paying attention. This factor implies that health professionals postpone action long enough to be authentically accessible to notice, actively listen, focus, and to concentrate fully on the patient at that moment.
Human respect	Refers to honoring the worth of humans through unconditional acceptance, kind and careful handling of the human body, recognition of rights and responsibilities, and appreciation of the *whole* human person (body–mind–spirit).
Encouraging manner	An affective factor consisting of the demeanor or attitude of the health professional and expressed through verbal and nonverbal messages of support, positive thoughts and feelings, openness to others, belief in the health system, tolerance for positive and negative feelings, creation of "safe space," and encouragement.
Appreciation of unique meanings	Concerned with a person's context or worldview. Knowing what is important to patients, including their distinctive sociocultural connections; avoidance of assumptions; acknowledging the subjective value placed on persons, situations, or events; recognizing the significance of the patient's frame of reference and using that in the provision of care.
Healing environment	Refers to the setting where care is taking place, including the surroundings, spaces, stressors (noise, lighting), culture, workflow, and structures for maintaining privacy, safety, aesthetics, confidentiality, and quality.
Basic human needs	Recognizing and responding to the primacy of those needs identified by Maslow—physical needs, safety and security needs, social and relational needs, self-esteem, and self-actualization.
Affiliation needs	Persons' needs for belonging and membership in families or other social contexts. Includes appreciation and engagement of the family/caregivers in the healthcare situation, including decision making.

Source: Maslow, A. (1954). *Motivation and personality.* New York, NY: Harper.

FIGURE 3.4   Feeling "cared for."

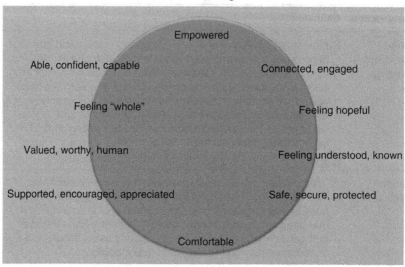

Feeling "cared for" is a significant concept for nurses because it is tied to the fundamental relational aspect of our work. Caring relationships engender this reaction and arouse persons', groups', and systems' capabilities to change, learn and develop, or self-advance. In other words, new, unique attitudes and behaviors gradually emerge through these multiple complex interactions, fueled by the relational energy shared among the participants. Whether they are individual behaviors, groups of persons' behaviors (microsystem performance), or organizational performance, they manifest as progression or advancement. And, because they were allowed to emerge on their own, they are naturally self-advancing.

Self-advancing systems reflect dynamic positive progress that enhances well-being and evolves naturally without external control. This process is not linear, but has peaks and troughs, and emerges gradually over time and space, and is influenced by the context. Self-advancing systems can be evaluated through empirical indicators that are used to provide ongoing evidence for practice changes. Crucial to self-advancing systems are those relationship-centered professional encounters that are grounded in caring and enable attainment of feeling "cared for."

Propositions of the Quality-Caring Model

Propositions are those relational statements that tie model concepts to each other and in some instances can be the basis for hypothesis testing. Propositions of the QCM include the following:

- Human caring capacity can be improved.
- Caring relationships are composed of processes or behaviors that can be observed.
- Caring relationships require intent, specialized knowledge, and time.
- Engagement in communities through caring relationships enhances self-caring.
- Independent caring relationships between patients and healthcare providers influence feeling "cared for."
- Collaborative caring relationships among nurses and members of the healthcare team enhance team cohesiveness.
- Caring relationships influence health behaviors.
- Caring relationships influence feeling "cared for" in the recipient.
- Caring relationships facilitate change.
- Feeling "cared for" facilitates cooperation, engagement, and disclosure in recipients.
- Feeling "cared for" is an antecedent to self-advancing systems.
- Self-advancing systems are naturally self-caring or self-healing.
- Feeling "cared for" contributes to individual, group, and system self-advancement.

ROLE OF THE NURSE

The overall role of the professional nurse in this model is to engage in expert caring relationships with self and others, enabling feelings of being "cared for" in recipients. Such actions are theorized to positively influence intermediate and terminal health outcomes (advancement), including those that are nursing sensitive.

Some specific responsibilities of the professional nurse include the following:

- Attain and continuously advance knowledge and expertise in caring processes
- Initiate, cultivate, and sustain caring relationships with patients and families
- Initiate, cultivate, and sustain caring relationships with other nurses and all members of the healthcare team
- Maintain an ongoing awareness of the patient's and family's point of view
- Carry on self-caring activities, including personal and professional development

- Integrate caring relationships with specific evidence-based nursing interventions to positively influence health outcomes
- Engage in continuous learning and practice improvement
- Use caring relationships to enhance the professional work environment
- Use the expertise of caring relationships embedded in nursing, to actively participate in community groups
- Contribute to the knowledge of caring and, ultimately, to health systems using all forms of knowing, including research
- Maintain an open, flexible perspective
- Use measures of caring to evaluate professional practice

HOPEFUL INSIGHTS FOR A MORE CARING FUTURE

The complexity and uncertainty that hangs over the U.S. health system at the time of this writing appear ominous. With so many unstable and unpredictable concerns, many questions are evident, such as:

- How will the replacement of the Affordable Care Act affect health system reimbursement?
- What will happen to the healthcare workforce in the face of massive retirements?
- Speaking of retirement, what will our own retirement portfolios look like?
- How will nursing be situated in a reformed health system?
- How will we educate future nurses with less nursing faculty?
- How can we best optimize patients' experiences and reduce adverse events?

These unanswered questions impact the unique cultures of health systems and pose an uneasiness that is palpable in the workplace. Health professionals are tired, many are disengaged, leaders come and go, new gimmicks are tried each week in an effort to boost system outcomes, and there is a deep sense that future, as yet unnamed, challenges are on the horizon. Professional nurses report that time spent with patients and families has decreased relative to other demands, and this presents a source of concern that many find is tied to less meaningful work. Patients and families are not consistently receiving the care they need and often report less than desirable hospital experiences (see Chapter 1). Sometimes it seems as if health systems of today are losing ground.

I t is precisely at these times of doubt that deeply held beliefs or philosophical values can provide direction. Rather than reacting, being alert to and intentionally engaging in learning about and practicing nursing's (or other health professions') most deeply held values may in fact facilitate adaptations in behavior that lead to the development of new and generative patterns of behavior (self-organization).

Many nursing pioneers have espoused the relational aspect of nursing as the core or central most fundamental component of the discipline (King, 1981; Peplau, 1988; Travelbee, 1966; Watson, 1979, 1985, 2012), and patients consistently point out that it is important to them (Theis, Stanford, Goodman, Duke, & Shenkman, 2017). The QCM is derived from those early pioneers in nursing who believed that while nursing draws on other disciplines, it is, by its very nature, an assistive, compassionate discipline that provides services in the context of relationships. The model is now 15 years old and has been used as the theoretical framework in many PhD dissertations and Doctor of Nursing Practice (DNP) scholarly projects, master's theory classes, as a guide for undergraduate students' honors projects, as the framework for the development of nursing interventions, and to guide research studies. It has been used to develop measures of caring from the patients' perspective, nurses' views, and students' views; and some of these measures have been translated into Spanish and Japanese. Most notably, the model has been adopted at over 54 U.S. hospitals to guide professional practice. Several of these organizations have gone on to achieve Magnet® designation and some have now changed their professional practice model to incorporate the QCM *after* initial Magnet designation. The QCM has undergone some expected revisions and much more work needs to be done relative to its validation, but promising signs of nursing's adoption of this way of being are occurring.

Many organizations (community hospitals, academic medical centers, educational institutions) and countless health professionals (chief nurse executives, chief operating officers, chief executive officers, directors of professional practice, deans, physicians, and faculty members) who have been or are in the process of adopting a more relationship-centric approach to practice have expressed their experiences with this author. Common to all was that through systematic integration of the QCM added benefit to patients and families, health professionals, and health systems was evidenced!

For example, in one mid-Atlantic academic medical center that has adopted the model, integration of model components into nurses' clinical workflow is beginning to show positive improvements in patients' experiences of care (HCAHPS scores; Centers for Medicare and Medicaid Services, 2014). In another hospital, nurse researchers are using the model to evaluate "feeling cared for" in the workplace. Specifically, they are evaluating staff nurses' perceptions of their leaders' use of caring behaviors before and after a QCM immersion experience; analysis is forthcoming.

At the Miriam Hospital in Providence, Rhode Island, annual readings of nursing exemplars using the professional practice model as a guide is used to share the work of nursing and highlight the particular caring behaviors applied. At this same health system, the QCM model components, caring for self and caring for others, are applied to stress management, compassion fatigue, lateral violence, and conflict resolution among nurses. The charge nurses have also integrated the QCM into their workshops. Another organization has instituted real-time medication teaching (rather than at discharge) using caring behaviors to "ground" the learning (mutual problem solving). And, in one outstanding Magnet-designated organization, reviewers were astonished at the re-designation review to learn how the nursing staff detailed the revision and implementation of a revised professional practice model (using the QCM as the theoretical foundation). In fact, the thoughtfulness behind each step in the process was highlighted by the staff nurses in a timeline as they reported to the reviewers that if other hospitals did it quicker, they were probably doing it wrong!

At the MD Anderson Cancer Center in Houston, Texas, the QCM is prominently described as a seminal content area in the *Academic Online Orientation Packet* and is operationalized through a primary-team patient care delivery system that focuses on outcomes of "feeling cared for." Finally, two large nursing organizations, namely the Association of Women's Health, Obstetric and Neonatal Nurses (AWHONN) and the International Association of Forensic Nurses Sexual Assault Nurse Examiner (SANE) Program have adopted the QCM to guide practice and evaluation of care (AWHONN, 2014; United States Office of Justice Programs, 2017).

Many organizations using the QCM as the foundation for practice have health professionals who are leading members of their communities serving on local boards and nonprofit agencies. Furthermore, professional nurses at these organizations have been engaged in leading the dissemination of results of their work with the model and creatively designing programs and interventions that promote relationship-centered practice. Daisy awards (Daisy Foundation, 2012) abound in organizations that use the QCM, with nurses who relate to patients and families in a caring manner being most often recognized. One medical center so embraces the model that it has become the basis for all health professionals' practice. Another academic medical center has provided funding to create an endowed professorship to advance the use of the QCM, including its contributions to research and evidence-based practice.

Health systems use the caring assessment tool (CAT; Duffy et al., 2014) to evaluate feeling "cared for" at patient discharge and are using these results to improve nursing practice. Some even use the tool in nursing portfolios designed for clinical advancement. And one large well-known academic medical center has consistently used the CAT—Admin Version (CAT-adm; Duffy, 2008) annually for the last 7 years to evaluate the caring behaviors of the leadership team.

These successful health systems are only a few of the many that are leading the way to a more caring future, one that is optimistic and offers promising practice revisions that might take hold, show favorable results, and reshape the larger health system. Interestingly, the example organizations have engaged professional nurses, many of whom are leading governance committees, continuing their education, and taking action in their communities.

SUMMARY

The QCM has evolved as expected since its introduction over 15 years ago, more recently influenced by complexity science and sociological structures. The terms *quality* and *caring* are redefined as dynamic *processes*, with caring remaining the central, organizing component of nursing work. Relationship-centered professional encounters are situated within large health systems and are influenced by this ever-changing context. Model assumptions, major concepts, and propositional statements are revised and the concept, feeling "cared for," and its consequences are explained. The roles of nursing are highlighted and examples from health systems using the QCM as the foundation for professional practice are revealed.

Call to Action

Complex health systems demand caring relationships. **Notice** what you are doing and what you are **not doing**. Caring for patients and families is a complex, social process that remains the foundation of nursing work. Appreciating the impact of health and illness on patients' holistic nature is an underlying premise of caring relationships. **Observe** how illness is affecting the physical, emotional, social, cultural, and spiritual dimensions of your next patient. Reliably implementing caring interpersonal relationships with members of the health team is a nursing responsibility according to the QCM. Practicing this way upholds each health team member's unique contribution and enhances the meaning of professional nurse work. **Appraise** the consistency of your own interprofessional behavior. **Attend** to caring relationships by making them the central, organizing aspect of your practice.

REFLECTIVE QUESTIONS/APPLICATIONS

... for Students

1. Explain how complexity science impacts health systems.
2. What are the philosophical underpinnings of the QCM?
3. Reflect on the role of the professional nurse. Explain how caring is the central, organizing aspect.
4. Define the model component "self-advancing systems."
5. List some intermediate outcomes that result from feeling "cared for." How important are these to a patient's health outcomes?
6. What are propositional statements in a theory?

... for Professional Nurses in Clinical Practice

1. Discuss whether aspects of the QCM are visible in your healthcare institution.
2. Are nurses' relationship oriented or task oriented? Does it matter?
3. What avenues exist at your institution for nurses to adopt a professional practice model?
4. What specific health outcomes may be advanced as a result of implementing a more relational approach to care?
5. What is your assessment of the examples provided in this chapter that many nursing departments have implemented? Do they seem feasible?
6. How do you envision the future of nursing?

... for Professional Nurses in Educational Practice

1. Is middle range theory presented to students at your institution? If so, how and at what levels of education? What learning strategies are used to help students translate them into practice?
2. Reflect on the QCM—its foundation, evolution, major concepts, and propositional statements. How do students best learn these phenomena? What new knowledge and skills are required to help students learn the value of nursing theory?
3. How can you bring real-life examples of quality caring into the classroom?
4. What avenues exist to help students realize the power of relationships between patients and nurses? Among healthcare professionals? Is this a necessary aspect of undergraduate learning? Of graduate learning?

... for Professional Nurses in Leadership Practice

1. Describe how complexity science has influenced leadership practice.
2. How is professional nursing organized at your institution? Is it based on nursing theory? Should it be?
3. Reflect on the levels of relationships at your institution. Are processes and outcomes assessed at each of these levels? If so, how are they observed as a system?
4. Are you leading a continuous learning organization? How do you know?
5. In what innovative ways do nurses at your facility demonstrate caring relationships? How often are these disseminated to the larger nursing community?

PRACTICE ANALYSIS

XYZ Health is a nonprofit community-based healthcare system located in a rural, semi-mountainous area of the mid-Atlantic region of the United States. Its mission is to improve the health of the communities it serves with a special focus on wellness and preventative care. XYZ Health has 604 licensed inpatient beds, 166 long-term care beds, 5,300 employees, and a medical staff exceeding 500 professionals. There are over 500,000 residents in its primary service area; 7% are >65 years old, with a projected growth in older adults and non-White populations. A high percentage of individuals are uninsured and mental and behavioral health issues were recently cited as the second most frequent health condition, with access to primary care cited as first. Chronic disease and substance abuse are ongoing health challenges.

Often individuals in outlying counties who need acute care services are transported via ambulance to the flagship hospital. Due to the rural nature of the community, it sometimes takes 2 hours for an ambulance to get from the originating site to the larger hospital. Emergency department nurses in the large hospital are complaining that patients often arrive in unstable condition with little information about their past and present health conditions. At least six times in the last month, a patient transported from an outlying hospital presented to the ED unstable and either needed resuscitation in the ED or was admitted to the ICU. In one instance, after admission to a medical–surgical unit, a 49-year-old transferred male experienced cardiac arrest, could not be resuscitated, and died.

The Director of Performance Improvement has directed his team to create a database that will track all transfers so that analysis could be performed to better understand and prevent further such experiences. However, defining what should be included in the database, identifying specific sources of data, and how to capture them among system hospitals has become a nightmare. Some of the hospitals say they have no data, others are reluctant to share, and still others, while willing to comply, do not have competent staff to facilitate the process. Eight months later, the project has stalled and relationships among personnel at the various hospitals are tense.

1. What aspects of the above scenario reflect a CAS?
2. How do the relationships among the agents in this CAS contribute to the natural cycle of coevolution in this health system? How is the system coevolving over time?
3. How can knowledge of complexity science inform ongoing behavioral adaptations in this large health system?
4. What suggestions do you have for helping the system move toward a more continuous learning environment?

REFERENCES

Association of Women's Health, Obstetric and Neonatal Nurses. (2014). AWHONN position statement: Nursing care quality measurement. *Journal of Obstetric, Gynecologic, and Neonatal Nursing, 43*(1), 132–133. doi:10.1111/1552-6909.12276

Baggett, M., Giambattista, L., Lobbestael, L., Pfeiffer, J., Madani, C., Modir, R., . . . Davidson, J. E. (2016). Exploring the human emotion of feeling cared for in the workplace. *Journal of Nursing Management, 24*(6), 816–824. doi:10.1111/jonm.12388

Baird, J., Rehm, R. S., Hinds, P. S., Baggott, C., & Davies, B. (2016). Do you know my child? Continuity of nursing care in the pediatric intensive care unit. *Nursing Research, 65*(2), 142–150. doi:10.1097/NNR.0000000000000135

Centers for Medicare and Medicaid Services. (2014). HCAHPS: Patients' perspectives of care survey. Retrieved from https://www.cms.gov/medicare/quality-initiatives-patient-assessment-instruments/hospitalqualityinits/hospitalhcahps.html

Cunningham, F. C., Ranmuthugala, G., Plumb, J., Georgiou, A., Westbrook, J. I., & Braithwaite, J. (2012). Health professional networks as a vector for improving health quality and safety: A systematic review. *BMJ Quality and Safety, 21,* 239–249. doi:10.1136/bmjqs-2011-000187

The Daisy Foundation. (2012). Daisy Award. Retrieved from http://daisyfoundation.org/daisy-award

Donabedian, A. (1966). Evaluating the quality of medical care. *Milbank Memorial Fund Quarterly, 44,* 166–206. doi:10.1111/j.1468-0009.2005.00397.x

Duffy, J. (2008). The caring assessment tools—Administrative version. In J. Watson (Ed.), *Assessing and measuring caring in nursing* (2nd ed.). New York, NY: Springer Publishing.

Duffy, J. (2009). *Quality caring in nursing and health systems: Applying theory to clinical practice, education, and leadership.* New York, NY: Springer Publishing.

Duffy, J. (2013). *Quality caring in nursing and health systems: Implications for clinicians, educators, and leaders.* New York, NY: Springer Publishing.

Duffy, J., Brewer, B., & Weaver, M. (2014). Revision and psychometric properties of the Caring Assessment Tool. *Clinical Nursing Research, 23*(1), 80–93. doi:10.1177/1054773810369827

Duffy, J., Kooken, W., Wolverton, C., & Weaver, M. (2012). Evaluating patient-centered care: Feasibility of electronic data collection in hospitalized older adults. *Journal of Nursing Care Quality, 27*(4), 307–315. doi:10.1097/NCQ.0b013e31825ba9d4

Engebretson, J. C., & Hickey, J. V. (2011). Complexity science and complex adaptive systems. In J. B. Butts & K. L. Rich (Eds.), *Philosophies and theories for advanced nursing practice.* Boston, MA: Jones & Bartlett.

Freeman, L. C. (2004). *The development of social network analysis: A study in the sociology of science.* Vancouver, BC, Canada: Empirical Press.

Friedman, C. P., Allee, N. J., Delaney, B. C., Flynn, A. J., Silverstein, J. C., Sullivan, K., & Young, K. A. (2017). The science of Learning Health Systems: Foundations for a new journal. *Learning Health Systems, 1*(1), e10020. doi:10.1002/lrh2.10020

Hughes, R. (2008). *Patient safety and quality: An evidence-based handbook for nurses.* AHRQ Publication # 08-0043. Rockville, MD: Agency for Healthcare Research and Quality. Retrieved from http://www.ahrq.gov/qual/nurseshdbk

Institute of Medicine. (2001). *Crossing the quality chasm: A new health system for the 21st century.* Washington, DC: National Academies Press.

Irvine, D. M., Sidani, S., & McGillis Hall, L. (1998). Linking outcomes to nurses' roles in health care. *Nursing Economic$, 16*(2), 58–64.

King, I. M. (1981). *A theory for nursing: Systems, concepts, process.* New York, NY: Wiley.

Knoke, D., & Yang, S. (2008). *Social network analysis* (2nd ed.). Los Angeles, CA: Sage.

Leape, L., Berwick, D., Clancy, C., Conway, J., Gluck, P., Guest, J., . . . Isaac, T. (2009). Transforming healthcare: A safety imperative. *Quality and Safety in Health Care, 18*(6), 424–428. doi:10.1136/qshc.2009.036954

Lindberg, C., Nash, S., & Lindberg, C. (2008). *On the edge: Nursing in the age of complexity.* Bordentown, NJ: Plexus Press.

Maddox, T. M., Albert, N. M., Borden, W. B., Curtis, L. H., Ferguson, T. B., Kao, D. P., . . . Tcheng, J. E. (2017). The learning healthcare system and cardiovascular care: A scientific statement from the American Heart Association. *Circulation, 135*(14), e826–e857. doi:10.1161/CIR.0000000000000480

Mahajan, A., Islam, S. D., Schwartz, M. J., & Cannesson, M. (2017). A hospital is not just a factory, but a complex adaptive system—Implications for perioperative care. *Anesthesia & Analgesia, 125*(1), 333–341. doi:10.1213/ANE.0000000000002144

Marshall, E. S., & Broome, M. E. (2016). Understanding contexts for transformational leadership: Complexity, change, and strategic planning. In *Transformational leadership in nursing: From expert clinician to influential leader* (2nd ed.). New York, NY: Springer Publishing.

Maslow, A. (1954). *Motivation and personality.* New York, NY: Harper.

Needleman, J., & Hassmiller, S. (2009). The role of nurses in improving hospital quality and efficiency: Real-world results. *Health Affairs, 28*(4), w625–w633. doi:10.1377/hlthaff.28.4.w625

Peplau, H. (1988). *Interpersonal relations in nursing: A conceptual frame of reference for psychodynamic nursing.* New York, NY: Springer Publishing.

Rickles D., Hawe P., & Shiell A. (2007). A simple guide to chaos and complexity. *Journal of Epidemiology in Community Health, 61*(11), 933–937. doi:10.1136/jech.2006.054254

Rosenkoetter, M. (2016). Overview and summary: Organizational outcomes for providers and patients. *OJIN: The Online Journal of Issues in Nursing, 21*(2), 1. doi:10.3912/OJIN.Vol21No02ManOS.

Scott, J. (2000). *Social network analysis: A handbook* (2nd ed.). Newbury Park, CA: Sage.

Simon, H. A. (1996). *The sciences of the artificial* (3rd ed.). Cambridge, MA: MIT Press.

Swanson, K. M. (1993). Nursing as informed caring for the well-being of others. *Image, 25*(4), 352–357. doi:10.1111/j.1547-5069.1993.tb00271.x

Theis, R. P., Stanford, J. C., Goodman, J. R., Duke, L. L., & Shenkman, E. A. (2017). Defining "quality" from the patient's perspective: Findings from focus groups with Medicaid beneficiaries and implications for public reporting. *Health Expectations, 20*(3), 395–406. doi:10.1111/hex.12466

Travelbee, J. (1966). *Interpersonal aspects of nursing.* Philadelphia, PA: F. A. Davis.

3 EVOLUTION OF THE QUALITY-CARING MODEL©   **63**

Uhl-Bien, M., & Arena, M. (2017). Complexity leadership: Enabling people and organizations for adaptability. *Organizational Dynamics, 46*(1), 9–20. doi:10.1016/j.orgdyn.2016.12.001

United States Office of Justice Programs. (2017). SANE program development and operational guide. Retrieved from https://www.ovcttac.gov/saneguide/introduction

Valente, T. W., & Pitts, S. R. (2017). An appraisal of social network theory and analysis as applied to public health: Challenges and opportunities. *Annual Review of Public Health, 38,* 103–118. doi:10.1146/annurev-publhealth-031816-044528

Wasserman, S., & Faust, K. (1994). *Social network analysis: Methods and applications.* New York, NY: Cambridge University Press.

Watson, J. (1979). *Nursing: The philosophy and science of caring.* Boston, MA: Little, Brown and Company.

Watson, J. (1985). *Nursing: Human science and human care.* Norwalk, CT: Appleton-Century-Crofts.

Watson, J. (2012). *Human caring science.* Sudbury, MA: Jones & Bartlett.

Wolverton, C.L. (2016). Staff nurse perceptions' of nurse manager caring behaviors: Psychometric testing of the Caring Assessment Tool-Administration (CAT-adm©). Retrieved from https://scholarworks.iupui.edu/handle/1805/10462

II

Practicing in Quality-Caring Health Systems

Humans in Relationship

Human relationships help us to carry on because they always presuppose
further developments, a future . . .
—Albert Camus

THE RELATIONAL CONTEXT OF BEING HUMAN

Relationships are the context for human birth, living, working, growing, learning, advancing, and dying. As multidimensional beings, humans exist in relationship to others and their environment and, to a larger extent, the universe. Humans also exist as individuals, separate from other people, with unique characteristics and life experiences. Philosophically, human beings are differentiated from other forms of life by features such as consciousness, the ability to reason and move autonomously, and the capacity to use language. From most formal religious perspectives, such uniqueness confers respect, dignity, and value for human life.

Through relational life experiences and ordinary growth processes, humans develop throughout the life span biologically, cognitively (Piaget, 1972, 1990), psychologically (Buhler & Allen, 1972; Buhler & Marschak, 1967; Erikson, 1964, 1968; Gould, 1978; Havighurst, 1953; Jung, 1933; Levinson, 1966; Levinson, Darrow, & Klein, 1978; Sheehy, 1976), morally (Kohlberg, 1986), and some would say spiritually, all influenced by specific sociocultural dimensions, such as gender, race, and societal status combined with the social interactions that dominate human behavior.

This relational context associated with *being human* suggests a mutual connectedness among individuals that may facilitate individual and group behavior, including creativity (Dong, Bartol, Zhang, & Li, 2016), well-being (Graham, Powell, & Truscott, 2016), and human development (Grusec, 2011). Such a perspective is known as relationship science (Reis, Collins, & Berscheid, 2000).

Relationship science is an "interdisciplinary field that employs empirical methods to understand the initiation, development, maintenance, and dissolution of interpersonal relationships" (Finkel, Simpson, & Eastwich, 2017, p. 4.2) and is undergirded by several social and psychological theories. According to this way of thinking, relationships among humans are characterized by:

- Interdependence
- Uniqueness
- Integration
- Trajectory
- Evaluation
- Responsiveness
- Resolution
- Maintenance
- Predisposition
- Instrumentality
- Standards
- Diagnosticity
- Alternatives
- Stress
- Culture

(Finkel et al., 2017)

Such characteristics address what relationships are, how they operate, the unique features that people bring to relationships, and the contextual factors that affect relational processes and outcomes. Relationship science is emerging as a powerful approach to understanding how humans behave and advance in society.

The characteristics of relationships are varied—romantic, parental, employee, boss, neighbor, friend, business partner/s, and in the case of healthcare, helping relationships. At the core of relationships, however, are the interactions that take place between the partners—these interactions are influential to all and take place in a context that is ever-changing. Importantly, the quality of relationships impacts health

(Allen et al, 2017; Feeney & Collins, 2015; L. H. Hall, Johnson, Watt, Tsipa, & O'Connor, 2016). The complex blend of relational life experiences (including those experienced in healthcare) shapes the *whole* person (Serlin & DiCowden, 2007). When relationships are good, persons feel reassured, safe, and are likely to advance. When, however, relationships are flawed or conflicted, individuals feel isolated, distressed, or even sick. Thus, relationships have a profound influence on human behavior, interpersonal interactions, health, longevity, and overall development.

Early transpersonal psychologists were concerned with understanding the unity and connectedness of persons as well as the benefits of higher levels of consciousness (Jung, 1977; Maslow, 1966; Rogers, 1961). Some of these views understand human persons, psychological concepts, theories, and methods integrated with the spiritual disciplines, taking on a holistic view of persons as connected to the larger universe. Relationships that use this approach are nonjudgmental and oftentimes transformative for all participants. Humans are viewed as capable of cognitive and psychological growth through all phases of life, which has implications for learning, advancement, and optimum health. A key to such human progression is self-awareness or clarity about one's relationship to the environment and other people.

The process of being aware of the present moment is a contrast to much of what health professionals experience in their daily lives. In fact, unintentional wandering of the mind (being on automatic pilot) or pushing away negative thoughts is common. In such a state, individuals tend to function more habitually or mechanistically. Mindless experiences or inactive states of mind use past experiences to define the present, leading to rigidity, insensitivity, and application of old behaviors even though the context has changed. How many of us have witnessed health professionals walk into a patient's room or enter an elevator and mindlessly ask, "How are you?" never really expecting to get a real answer? Likewise, how often do we observe some health professionals stuck in their old ways or driving home from work and missing their exit on the freeway? Unfortunately, without paying attention to what is observed and experienced, decreases in competence, focus, health, mood, and creativity can occur leading to burnout and even ineffective patient care. Thus, maintaining awareness is crucial for busy health professionals.

This awareness of *both* subjective and objective phenomena in life is not static; rather, it occurs on a continuum from being fully awake and aware of oneself to being asleep or unaware (Morin, 2011). Subjective or internally focused self-awareness grounds the self to see with clarity how life experiences (including those faced at work) shape thoughts and behaviors. Concepts such as the perception of the physical body or body image, self-concept, agency (one's capacity to act), or social identity are understood and refined as self-awareness or consciousness is heightened. Such a view of humans suggests that a depth of understanding is possible that may empower one to self-monitor and regulate behaviors, advance his or her full potential, have meaningful relationships, heal, and achieve some form of contentment or peace (Crane et al, 2017; Kabat-Zinn, 2012).

Regrettably, as humans go about relating, working, and caring for each other, the self is often forgotten or lost along the way. Disappointments, insecurities, losses, physical ailments, and the everyday fast-paced demands of life build up over time leaving many individuals stressed and exhausted. Furthermore, many aspects of workplace performance, such as attention, cognition, emotions, behavior, and even physiology, can be interrupted or limited by the unnecessary demands and approaches to the work, ultimately impacting key workplace outcomes, individual and group performance, relationships, and well-being (Good et al., 2015). The 24/7 connectivity that has consumed humans' lives in the last few years has added to the inability to be in touch with ourselves. To make matters worse, learned ways of knowing (externally derived), such as formal education and religious training, may limit or constrain the view of oneself. In this restricted view of the world, individuals tend to be more reactive, feel separated or disjointed, and function under an individualistic or misplaced perspective.

Nurses and other health professionals, in particular, tend to get accustomed to multiple work demands and "run on adrenalin" to accomplish them; in fact, many nurses are proud of their multitasking abilities! But, balancing highly acute patient needs with limited resources, the physical demands of nurse work, and making life-and-death decisions according to the latest evidence, along with family responsibilities, annoyances like traffic, and information overload leaves many nurses feeling drained and worn out. Experiencing such pressures generates intense emotion; without awareness of them, human energy is squandered and general dissatisfaction and even the development of physical symptoms may occur.

> Balancing internal authentic awareness of self along with external worldly stimuli may strengthen one such that an integrated, more resilient, and healthy self is more available for patients and families.

The empirical evidence beginning to emerge demonstrating connections between emotions and physiological processes is noteworthy (Cross &

Pressman, 2017; Norman, Necka, & Berntson, 2016; Pivetti, Camodeca, & Rapino, 2016). The relatively new field of interpersonal neurobiology integrates findings from recent brain research with human interactions and emphasizes the brain as a social organ developed over time and through experiences with others. Many in this field would argue that human relationships actually shape neural connections and modify how the brain develops (Siegel, 2015).

Professional nurses and other health professionals interact and relate to others with ease; yet, most have not traditionally been taught how to do this for themselves (see Figure 4.1).

Learning how to stop "doing" and just "being" for a while permits one to slow down enough to actually focus on one's inner thoughts and feelings and access new ways of seeing the whole. Once accessed, this attention to self helps one see his or her situation more clearly. In turn, such actions may help health professionals appreciate and honor the work they do.

This interaction is believed to be so necessary to therapeutic relationships and positive health outcomes that many centers have led efforts to help patients and health professionals learn better self-awareness practices. For example, at the University of Massachusetts Center for

FIGURE 4.1   Balancing "being" and "doing."

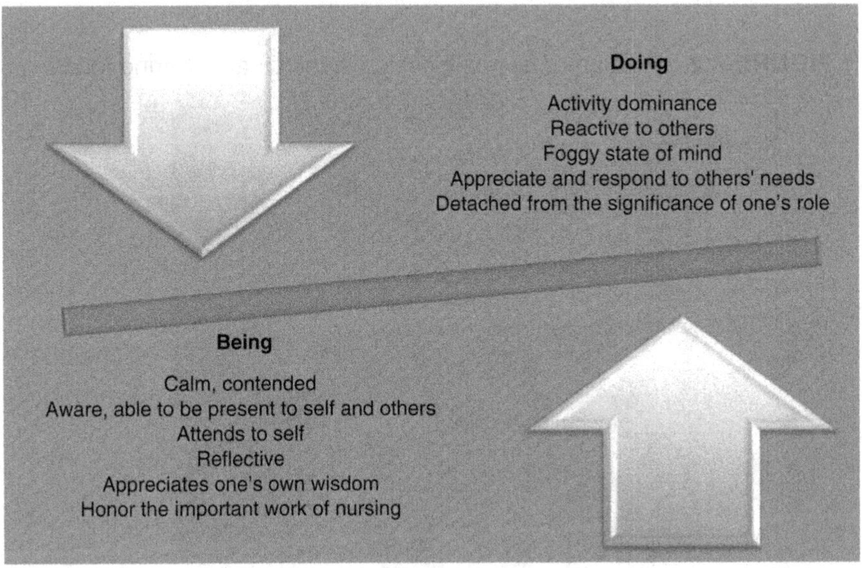

Doing
Activity dominance
Reactive to others
Foggy state of mind
Appreciate and respond to others' needs
Detached from the significance of one's role

Being
Calm, contended
Aware, able to be present to self and others
Attends to self
Reflective
Appreciates one's own wisdom
Honor the important work of nursing

Mindfulness, attention to the self is taught to health professionals and patients to reduce stress and enhance leadership and educational effectiveness. In these programs, Kabat-Zinn and others have spent decades in regular efforts to increase conscious awareness while demonstrating important results (including increases in regional gray matter) through research. Similarly, at the University of California at Los Angeles (UCLA) Mindful Awareness Research Center, programs of research are conducted and classes on mindful awareness are available in person and online for the general public and health professionals.

THE FUNDAMENTAL RELATIONSHIPS OF THE QUALITY-CARING MODEL©

Because of the interpersonal nature of humans as the primary focus of healthcare, the Quality-Caring Model (QCM) relies on relationships to position itself. Four relationships (Figure 4.2), in particular, are considered foundational to the QCM and must be attended to in order to practice from this relationship-centered stance. Each will be described in the next few pages.

Relating to Self

Most nurses have been taught "to do," to assist others, to teach, and to provide answers. In fact, task or activity dominance (being observed as

FIGURE 4.2   Fundamental relationships in the Quality-Caring Model.

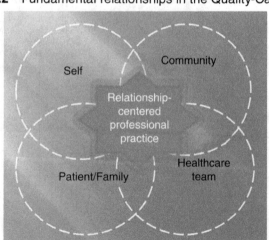

busy) is considered proper behavior for nurses. Together with the incessant background noise, competing priorities, interruptions, and nonstop automatic doing common to health systems, this endless acting is stressful, error promoting, and even unhealthy to health professionals. It is easy in this environment to remain in a persistent fog or oblivious state of mind where mechanistic routines and practices dominate the work. This lack of awareness, however, does not contribute to one's own personal development, attention to the quality of performance, or generate meaningful relationships with patients and families.

Being more aware (or mindful) is a particularly healthy way to work and deepens one's ability to be present to patients and families. Mindfulness has drawn the attention of health educators and health professionals, and is the focus of current research. Systematic cultivation of mindfulness begins during the educational process and is nurtured in the work environment. The willingness to look deeply at one's practice—reflectively—regardless of what it holds and in a spirit of acceptance and caring toward oneself helps us see possibilities and value in what we do. In the work environment, regular efforts to increase conscious awareness may help health professionals focus more attentively on the human person of the patient, holistically assess patients' needs, make better clinical judgments, and use best evidence to improve the quality of care. Short pauses between patient rooms, taking brief time-outs to sit and reflect, and using routine tasks such as handwashing, documenting, or walking from room to room as opportunities to feel one's body and emotions may, in fact, be therapeutic to both the patient and the health professional.

More formal reflective activities such as regularly soliciting feedback from patients, families, and coworkers, or reflective analyses where thoughts and feelings are actually written out or spoken into a recorder, are revealing. In such activities, nurses learn from their own practice by examining who they are as nurses, questioning their place in or their view of the discipline, encouraging deep thoughts about certain encounters to come to the surface, and using these experiences to clarify and enhance the practice. To do this, one must be disciplined and willing to make the effort. Although somewhat threatening (to self), if taught to honor themselves this way early on, nurses may come to view such behaviors as less risky and be able to uncover the hidden meanings and learning opportunities embedded during clinical work and integrate them into future practice. In some organizations, nurses are provided "safe space" whether on a computer or in groups to place written reflections for other nurses to view and comment on. Others are using the annual evaluation time to consider reflective questions and use the interaction between supervisor and employee to discuss how practice has evolved during the past year.

Practicing Self-Caring

Regular attention to the self helps one see situations more clearly and, over time, generates self-wisdom. Taking the time to look back (reflect), clarify, and become aware of where one is (in relation to one's practice) is liberating and helps to remind us of the important work we do.

Making time to "be with" oneself, gaining insight into emotions, thoughts, bodily sensations, and other feelings, contributes to well-being (Kushlev et al., 2017; Siegel, 2015). Health professionals need to acknowledge and allow themselves to feel the meanings associated with their work, including suffering. In essence, this is a form of self-caring that may be a necessary antecedent to caring for others.

Some researchers have been able to demonstrate the benefits of self-caring for nurses and other health professionals. For example, Kravits, McAllister-Black, Grant, and Kirk (2010) were able to show improved scores related to emotional exhaustion and depersonalization after a 6-hour psychoeducational program (including stress and relaxation responses, coping patterns, guided imagery, and a wellness plan) was offered twice a month to nurses. Proposed implications for practice suggested that regular, systematic efforts to support positive self-care behaviors of nurses may be beneficial to help resolve the organizational challenges related to patient workload, conflict, and professional empowerment. Durkin, Beaumont, Hollins Martin, and Carson (2016) showed that high levels of self-compassion in community nurses were linked with lower levels of burnout. Furthermore, when the nurses reported greater compassion and satisfaction, they also reported more compassion for others, increased well-being, and less burnout. Dyess, Prestia, Marquit, and Newman (2018) demonstrated a statistically significant drop in perceived stress among nurse leaders at 6 weeks and again at 12 weeks after a simple meditation practice. Other nursing researchers have studied mindfulness practices in nursing students, nurses, and nurse leaders and reported improved caring (Hunter, 2016), decreased stress (Pipe & Bortz, 2009), promotion of self-care (Shields, 2011), and improving sleep patterns (Gross et al., 2011).

Making time for true relaxation—not just time off from work, but authentic quiet time by oneself—is essential. Nursing is so people oriented and other-focused that time alone is often not seen as valuable. Yet, alone time can become a practice that enhances self-caring. In the nursing culture of self-sacrifice and adrenalin-induced nervous energy, creating balance through regular private time is therapeutic. For example, a few minutes alone practicing deep breathing or taking a leisurely walk by oneself can promote insight and help one reframe a situation or experience, not to mention the physiologic benefits!

Likewise, committing to private time each day is a requisite for quality nursing care. Similar to physical exercise, obligating oneself to quiet time requires altering of daily habits. Waking up 15 minutes early or creating an evening ritual of quiet time, or just sitting quietly with oneself, is essential to nurses' well-being. These kinds of experiences help one become attuned to the larger whole, allowing connections to surface that might otherwise remain buried. The key word here is *practice*; a verb, practice requires *action*. Although the exact nature of what constitutes mindfulness is still being pursued, mindfulness practices usually encompass several elements (Schlitz, Vieten, & Amorok, 2007).

First is *intention* or making the choice to stay open and aware. Second is *directing attention inward*; in other words, being present to the self. Third, committing to a more conscious way of living requires *repetition*. Repeating components of a mindfulness practice reinforces the habit. Finally, *guidance* in the form of both external learning and/or accessing internal wisdom can increase the value of mindfulness practices.

Several methods are available to practice mindful awareness. Deep relaxation and meditation practices, yoga and tai chi, contemplative prayer, walking, rehearsing a song, even service itself—when performed in a conscious manner—can be transpersonal experiences. The key to such practice is found in the four essential elements (Schlitz et al., 2007).

> In the personal practice of deep relaxation, for example, making the commitment (intent) to devote the necessary time as well as focused attention to breathing or other bodily functions (directed attention inward), repeating the practice in the same way and at the same time each day (repetition), and reading about or taking a class on relaxation techniques (receiving guidance) are all reinforcers that enable positive self-care behaviors.

Expression of oneself through artistic or creative pursuits, such as music, painting, sewing, quilting, gardening, woodworking, or noncompetitive sports, when consciously pursued, can be awareness-raising. These activities keep us "in the moment" and, although considered recreation, with the right intent, attention, repetition, and guidance, they can provide the same accessibility to the self as more traditional practices (Schlitz et al., 2007). In the case of music, there is some evidence that it may even be physically and emotionally therapeutic (Bilgiç & Acaroğlu, 2017; Gallagher, Lagman, & Rybicki, 2017; Mofredj, Alaya, Tassaioust, Bahloul, & Mrabet, 2016; Sachs, 2007).

Another way to access the inner self is to spend time in nature. Professional nurses are most often found working in drab, enclosed environments with artificial lighting and limited temperature controls. Often, there are no windows or opportunities to even see the outside surroundings. Being in the natural environment, however, and using the experience to appreciate its mystery provides a reflective way to ponder and even dream. In this way, one can learn to quiet the self and see the sacred in everyday life. Taking a walk around the building at lunchtime or sitting near a window while eating in the cafeteria may help assist nurses recharge during their working hours.

Taking care of the body through regular exercise and healthy eating are self-caring acts that many nurses forget to do for themselves as they take care of others. Yet, caring for the physical body is crucial to quality nursing practice and promotes effective modeling for patients and families. And, the particularly serious nature of healthcare often diminishes opportunities to see some of the lighter sides of human nature. The use of humor, particularly in the workplace, can be a source of joy even in the most difficult of circumstances (Mesmer-Magnus, Glew, & Viswesvaran, 2012). Establishing a support network or taking classes that reinforce and help perfect awareness practices enhances one's performance. Monitoring oneself during working hours by regularly observing one's behavior and asking, "Am I stressed or at ease?" or "Am I busy doing or am I present to myself, my coworkers, and my patients?" keeps one alert and in the moment. Regular reminders to practice mindfulness, such as listening to relaxation techniques in the car, and pictures or other symbols in the workplace, may assist health professionals to practice mindfulness daily.

Caring for self by allowing oneself to feel physical as well as emotional sensations, reflecting on them slowly, making meaning of them, and using this introspection to relate to others in a continual pattern of action and inaction keeps one balanced and more "in tune" to the world's energy. The regular performance of personal and professional self-caring practices sets up the conditions for self-knowing, a prerequisite for helping others.

As humans have the capacity to continuously learn and grow, it follows that caring for self both personally and professionally may have the potential to positively influence lives—both our own and those we care for. According to Siegel (2010), "Creating well-being—in our mental life, in our close relationships, and even in our bodies—is a learnable skill" (p. xv). Connecting work experiences with those at home, in the classroom, at church, and elsewhere helps unite body, mind, and soul—enabling integration essential to health, flexibility, and creativity (Siegel, 2010).

Caring for oneself holistically leads to improved positive states and creates the possibility for greater well-being. Compelling research findings from the field of integrative medicine (whole person [body–mind–spirit] health) show decreased cardiovascular risk factors, decreased negative reactions, improved insulin resistance, decreased back pain, and improved quality of life after more holistic self-caring activities (Edelman et al., 2006; Feldman, Greeson, & Senville, 2010; Goebel-Fabbri et al., 2011; Greeson, Krucoff, Moon, Moon, & Shaffer, 2010; Greeson et al., 2011; Smith & Gettings, 2016). If the emerging evidence is accurate, caring for the whole self may lead to better overall health, enabling the other three foundational relationships.

Valuing the self enough to care for oneself, including appreciating the internal meanings of our experiences, may change our perceptions, build confidence, optimize our ability to care for others, and create more positive workplaces. Just as nurses do with patients, creating and implementing a plan for self-caring is an essential aspect for attaining and maintaining one's health and performing optimally in practice.

Relating to Vulnerable Patients and Families

Before engaging in relationships with patients and families, health professionals must be sensitive to and appreciate the illness experience, including the enormous uncertainty and vulnerabilities that accompany illness and suffering. As complex beings that are constantly changing and relating, humans have objective (physical), subjective (emotional, cultural, spiritual), and social (family, role functions) characteristics. During an illness, these characteristics are all affected and the results can be profound. First, there is the emotional reaction and necessary adjustment to the illness itself. Illness represents a fundamental threat to one's basic sense of wholeness. Persons may form certain meanings about their illnesses based on the knowledge they have about their own bodies, what they have heard or read about others in similar situations, individual psychological traits, and societal/cultural points of view. Physiological changes can create feelings of discomfort, vulnerability, and dependence that generate loss of self-confidence and create doubt. Ambitions or plans must be suspended, and communication patterns change. Fulfilling one's role as parent, grandparent, spouse, worker, or friend is often disrupted and the psychological impact of being ill presents threats to one's sense of wholeness.

Oftentimes, persons experience shock, anger, or fear as the initial emotional response to a new diagnosis or the need for care from others. Over time, these emotions may change and can be viewed on a continuum from courageous acceptance on the one hand to specific self-destructive behaviors that can lead to personal and family turmoil on the other. With this awareness of the illness experience, consider the additional burden of residing (temporarily) in a cold, rushed hospital environment where others have created the conditions under which one will live for a few days.

Early in the hospital admission process, emphasis is placed on payment and consent to treatment versus the transition to a new living space. Once admitted, individuals must conform to the work habits of the employees, including their shift changes, their unique norms and behaviors (the culture of the department), and their disciplinary traditions; the environment, including the noise, lights, facilities, and conversations; and the organization, including its leadership practices, protocols/procedures, and resources. The sudden dependency placed on formerly independent individuals is an uneasy, tenuous state that may interfere with normal human needs such as rest and sleep, mood, feelings of safety and security, dignity, mobility, nourishment and elimination, affiliation needs, and sociocultural–spiritual practices, and it places individuals at high risk for adverse outcomes of their illness.

> Hospitalization unintentionally introduces nonstop invasion of patients' personal spaces by complete strangers, impersonalizes the care experience by labeling patients according to diagnoses, and allows little autonomy in terms of patients' personal routines. Thus, hospitalization itself poses significant risks that are not the result of the illness; in fact, many persons leave the hospital in worse conditions than when they entered.

Hospital-acquired infections and pressure ulcers, deconditioned limbs, development of delirium, falls, and errors, not to mention frustration, unnecessary anxiety, and embarrassment, are examples of this inadvertent consequence of hospitalization.

Websites and magazine articles warn prospective patients about hospital dangers and offer advice about how to safeguard themselves during hospitalization. For example, WebMD offers six tips for patients to protect themselves during hospitalization (www.webmd.com/healthy-aging/hospital-risks-7/default.htm) and the AARP magazine regularly publishes articles providing advice and warnings to older adults regarding healthcare.

Central to providing quality caring is the ability of healthcare professionals to "experience the other person's private world and feelings and to communicate to the other person some significant degree of that understanding" (Watson, 1979, p. 28).

Consider this example:

Recently, a 33-year-old White female who was 10 weeks pregnant had her first prenatal visit at the OB/GYN office. She was a healthy female, worked full time as a human resources benefits analyst, was married for 6 years, and had a 4-year-old son. She recently had a miscarriage (spontaneous) at 10 weeks and was very anxious about the health of this developing child. During the visit, a nurse practitioner (NP), who was new to her, drew blood (several vials) and conducted an ultrasound. She stated that she "could not find the baby" and further announced "there must be something wrong with this machine." She left the room to get another machine and was gone for 15 minutes during which time the young mother imagined the worst had occurred all over again. The NP returned and repeated the procedure with the new machine and still "could not find the baby." She then called the physician, who ordered a vaginal ultrasound. At first, the baby was not visible, but finally the physician was able to locate the fetus. The physician said, "According to your dates, it looks okay but come back in 4 weeks for another ultrasound just to be sure." The mom drove home all the while questioning whether she was being told the truth and whether her baby would develop normally. That evening, she called a family member (who was a nurse) to verify that "they wouldn't lie to me, would they?"

Obviously, the NP failed to appreciate the patient's private world (she had already lost one pregnancy and was extremely anxious about this one). What could/should the NP have done to reassure this anxious mom? What about the physician?

Or, consider this new grandmother's experience whose one-year-old grandson was transferred from a rural hospital to a specialized children's hospital with a high fever and no urine output:

The first few days that he was in the hospital, it was my observation that he wasn't a priority or that he was receiving substandard care. I envisioned he would be transported quickly and received by a team of experts who were ready to treat him immediately. Rather, after the 5 hours it took for the transport service to coordinate and drive through traffic, he was finally admitted. Although a young doctor saw him in the first few hours after admission, his parents were left alone for the next 7 hours with no feedback on a plan of care. After a myriad of interviews with various doctors, a flurry of activity ensued to place a dialysis catheter. No further communication occurred during the first 2 days, so the mother called a hotline number she saw on a hospital pamphlet and finally a hospital administrator appeared to play the role of mediator between the parents, doctors, and nurses. The baby was moved to the PICU where he got better attention but his fever climbed and complicated treatment. Both sets of grandparents and the parents lost confidence in the care provided and began to feel "he wouldn't make it." As the paternal grandmother stated, "I didn't want to insert myself between the parents and the staff—I felt terribly helpless—it was so hard to watch it all unfold. In observing the staff work, there were tremendous delays from when a decision was made to delivering the care—for example, 6 hours from the ordering of an important antibiotic medication to administration. In this case, although there were a whole slew of people involved in decision making and checking and rechecking—the patient paid a high price in delayed care. And yet, mistakes were made . . . several. The excuses we received several times were that there were more patients than usual. Don't they routinely plan for higher volumes of patients? However, sometimes I'd go out to the nurses' station and see nurses sitting at the station clearly not talking about work! Watching this play out and assuming most hospitals run this way, I have to say they are much worse than any environment I have ever worked in—so I would NEVER want to work in a hospital. It's too bad the cost of this hospital stay will be the same whether the care was excellent or not. I don't know of another industry or service where this is the case.

"One positive note—a male nurse in the PICU was exceptional—he went out of his way to coordinate with the doctor to advocate for the baby to have more feedings while being held by his parents since that was the only thing that comforted him. This particular nurse went to the trouble to analyze his treatment plan and spent time with me explaining in detail the rationale for how much and what kinds of fluids the baby could have."

The child received multiple dialysis treatments and eventually got well enough to go home. But six family members (two parents and four grandparents) were anxious, fearful, and received inadequate communication. The child experienced multiple delays in treatment that contributed to a longer length of stay. Why was only one nurse attuned to the needs of the patient and family? What could have been done differently?

A s patients and families present to the health system for needed care, they are already compromised from their illness or situation, but they are further burdened by well-intentioned health professionals and health systems that are not designed to relate. In fact, this ability to relate in a manner that conveys understanding of the other's situation is essential to caring.

The patient experience is increasingly being recognized as an important factor in developing and providing excellence in healthcare. Interestingly, when many patients are asked about their hospital experiences, most discuss their interaction with staff members and talk about issues such as communication patterns, how safe they felt, whether they were treated with respect and included in decision making, and whether "people knew what they were doing" (personal experience). Just as relationships are an important aspect of human living, they are just as important during illness and hospitalization (maybe more so). In fact, relationships with health professionals play an important role in shaping patient experiences.

Practicing Caring for Patients and Families

Therapeutic relationships are considered a cornerstone of all health professionals' practice; yet they are often incomplete, not valued in the overall scheme of healthcare, or simply overlooked. The term *therapeutic* connotes healing, whereas the term *relationship* connotes some sort of interaction with a resulting connection, bond, or partnership. More recently, the operative term has been *therapeutic alliance* or *healing relationships*. Evidence reveals that the therapeutic alliance positively influences treatment outcomes (A. M. Hall, Ferreira, Maher, Latiner, & Ferreira, 2010; Hojat, 2016; Kornhaber, Walsh, Duff, & Walker, 2016). Several healthcare providers have documented certain factors as necessary for therapeutic relationships (Rogers, 1961; Yalom, 1975). Nursing theorists such as King (1981) discussed "perceptual accuracy;" Watson (1979, 1985) identified 10 factors, more recently labeled *clinical caritas processes* (Watson, 2008a, 2008b); Peplau (1952) described orientation, identification, development, and conclusion of patient–nurse relationships; and Travelbee (1966) discussed the humanistic processes of original encounter, emerging identities, empathy, and sympathy. In general, these authors refer to the demeanor, communication style (verbal and nonverbal), along with the specific behaviors of health professionals that are engaging, assistive, and supportive. This relationship is considered therapeutic, healing, or caring when both recipients benefit in terms of the shared process and the attainment of something valuable. Cultivating relational aspects of professional practice requires interaction, knowledge, skills, and presence (time). Experienced health professionals know this and are able to integrate this relational component with the more instrumental activities associated with health services.

A key aspect of therapeutic relating is the recognition that patients' experiences and concerns, versus their diagnosis or procedure, are primary and then responding in a timely and caring manner. Recognizing patient problems, anticipating patient experiences, being (relating) and doing (acting) together, monitoring how patients change in response to clinical practice, and appropriately revising care represent the practice of caring.

Working in this manner is somewhat countercultural in this day of fast-paced, highly intense health systems. As such, it requires the ability to tolerate some uncertainty or ambiguity and remain attentive and open minded. Use of oneself in this way honors the individual patient and the health professional as a life-giving energy source. Specific processes of relating during relationship-centered professional encounters will be described in the next chapter.

Relating to Each Other

Health professionals today are a multigenerational, diverse working group with individual psychosociocultural, spiritual, and life experience characteristics that shape their performance. In addition, many are caring for the most complex, diverse, acute, and chronically ill population this nation has ever seen. Professional nurses supervise unlicensed personnel, provide care 24/7, chase down equipment and supplies, coordinate healthcare teams, participate in shared governance councils and performance improvement meetings, assist in the implementation and evaluation of electronic health records, and many are pursuing advanced education. Meanwhile, the economic constraints of the last few years have forced hospitals and other healthcare agencies to concentrate on cost containment and restructuring efforts, many of which have not been evaluated in terms of their consequences to patients and employees. Health professionals today are frequently working at the interface between the efficiency needs of the health system and the human caring needs of patients and families.

In this environment, there is enormous responsibility, high intensity, and workplace tension. Complicating these system difficulties are future unknowns concerning the workforce, long-term employment, reimbursement, and retirement, all contributing to perceived insensitivities in the workplace. Horizontal violence among peers is sadly prevalent and interprofessional collaboration has not been optimized. Yet, creating a therapeutic context in which healing can occur relies not just on the caring dispositions of individual clinicians but also on the collective relational capacities of interprofessional healthcare teams (Agreli, Peduzzi, & Bailey, 2017; Konrad & Browning, 2012).

Although colleagues typically are associated through common work, *being collaborative* has a stronger meaning. It denotes a commitment to working together—sharing knowledge and power, appreciating each other as role models, making decisions together, relying on each other, rooting for one another—these are all ways that health professionals demonstrate a collaborative nature. *Being collaborative* suggests a higher form of relating to another that assumes sharing followed by collective action so that mutual goals are attained (in this case, what is in the best interest of the patient and family). Furthermore, collaboration is a dynamic process that is interpersonal and interdependent (e.g., two or more disciplines interacting in a trusting manner) and is characterized as a partnership (Rose, 2011; Ward et al., 2017). Although collaboration among health professionals has been studied before, a recent report suggested that nurses and physicians think differently about collaboration (House & Havens, 2017).

Lately, the term *interprofessional practice* has dominated the literature with respect to groups of health professionals working "in relationship." The World Health Organization (WHO, 2010) has published a framework for action on collaboration and interprofessional education (IPE) and practice, core competencies have been established (American Association of Colleges of Nursing, 2011), programs for interprofessional development have been introduced (e.g., Program for Interprofessional Practice, Education and Research [PIPER] at McMaster University's Faculty of Health Sciences), and the National Center for Interprofessional Practice and Education (nexusipe.org) has been established at the University of Minnesota in the hopes of accelerating such practice through research and education.

Interprofessional research has gained momentum nationally in the last few years as recommendations for promoting such research have been mandated. For example, the National Institutes of Health (NIH) Roadmap for Medical Research and NIH Exploratory Centers for Interdisciplinary Research have established interprofessional components. The concept of

FIGURE 4.3   Interprofessional collaborative practice.

"Being" Collaborative	**Interprofessional Collaborative Practice**	**Mutual Goals**
Sharing power Collective action (making decisions *together*) Relational capacity of health professionals	"Team Caring" with patient as functioning member of the team	(What's in the best interest of patients and families)?

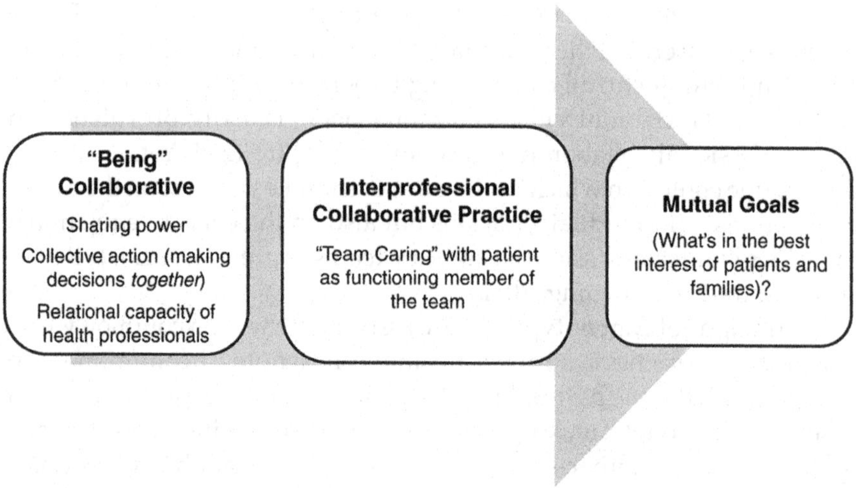

team science as a dimension of interprofessional collaborative practice has evolved (Little et al., 2016) and the National Institute of Nursing Research (NINR) supports strong multidisciplinary research. Such federal directives and funding mechanisms demonstrate the importance of interprofessional collaboration to advancing knowledge related to health. Key to all these initiatives is the collaborative relationships established and cultivated among two or more health disciplines that respect each other's contributions to patient care (see Figure 4.3).

Such collaborative relationships, when optimized, become transpersonal—beyond disciplinary boundaries—with the patient as a functioning participant. Thus, true collaborative relationships are often referred to as team-based care or team care; in the QCM, a more appropriate term may be *team caring*, as the qualities of caring relationships (next chapter) apply.

Teams of healthcare professionals are integral to modern-day professional practice. But teams are easily broken by poor leadership or role models, inadequate training, and cultural barriers. Caring for each other is crucial to high-quality patient care.

Practicing Caring for Each Other

In health systems where interprofessional collaborative practice is optimized, the following characteristics are generally seen: (a) increased communication and shared decision making among practitioners, (b) mutual respect and effective dialogue among all members of the care team in care planning and problem solving, and (c) more efficient and integrated practices that lead to high-quality patient and population-centered outcomes (Health Resources and Services Administration, 2013). Furthermore, organizational leadership is crucial to the success of team caring as is initial and ongoing education. IPE competencies (i.e., values/ethics for IPE, roles and responsibilities, interprofessional communication, and teams and teamwork) are foundational for interprofessional collaborative practice program (IPCP) teams. Caring for each other, nurse to nurse and interprofessionally, is essential to quality health outcomes. It is depicted in the QCM as an integral relationship and has benefits not only for the patient and family but for healthcare providers as well.

As a group of like-minded professionals seeking to care for patients in need, well-balanced nurses (those who integrate self-knowledge together with worldly knowledge and who use caring processes or behaviors) *enable* collaborative relationships to flourish. The QCM advances the notion that intra- and interprofessional collaboration positively impacts healthcare outcomes and is a nursing responsibility. Interprofessionality, however, requires a paradigm shift, since it encompasses unique values, codes of conduct, and ways of working. For example, working collaboratively highlights the patient/client as central to the process with health professionals and patients/families relating interdependently. Patients in this case are simultaneously active members of the team and recipients of the care provided by the team, with their needs determining the interactions between professionals. Interprofessional collaborative practice recognizes and honors the diverse interests and uneven power among the care team as well as the bonds that develop between team members. Finally, taking the time to "know" team members in terms of understanding, at least conceptually, each other's frame of reference, roles and responsibilities helps to move the team from individual exclusive professional "turfs" to sharing a common professional space. Using caring relationships in day-to-day interactions with colleagues fosters this common professional space (aka healthy work environments) that may contribute to improved quality of work life, engaged employees, more opportunities for shared clinical research, and improved and more efficient patient outcomes.

Relating to the Community We Serve

Today's traditional communities are facing tremendous pressures. Diverse members of society are residing in changing neighborhoods often without supportive extended families; many commute long distances to work and often in unpleasant traffic. Others are unemployed, with some receiving needed assistance, while other unfortunate individuals and families remain at the mercy of community organizations. Places are evolving—earlier rural environments have become almost cosmopolitan, while services have not kept pace. Environmental issues such as poor quality air, water and sewage, climate change, and consequences of accessing new energy sources are cropping up, without real solutions. Functions of communities are different as workplaces change or are deleted, sometimes resulting in lower tax revenues, school problems, crime and violence, and even mental health problems. The forces of globalization and Internet communication have disconnected local economies and fractured face-to-face contact. These stressors often lead to less engagement in community service and eventual frustration, apathy, and stagnation as community members begin to feel powerless over their changing circumstances.

For example, the rise in opiate use and its effects have had grave consequences on American communities. Opiate addiction affects marriages and may lead to child abuse and even criminal charges related to theft or violence. Furthermore, implications for schools and universities, local police departments, and hospital emergency rooms have driven some communities to despair. Others have been mobilized—some communities and even entire states have generated new policies and educational programs (Penm et al., 2017). Such community challenges often give rise to new health problems, many of which were unforeseen, but nevertheless instigate serious consequences.

Nurses and other health professionals can augment services to communities simply by using their relationship-centric approach. Healthy communities are dependent on individuals who are committed to healthy environments and who can communicate and drive needed change. For example, health professionals can help drive agendas for community group meetings, share their knowledge of more healthful approaches, help disseminate research, and most importantly, participate through caring relationships in decision making and implementation of local projects. In this way, communities can regain health and enable a shared identity.

Many have suggested that community involvement benefits the health professional as well. For example, Butterfoss, LaChance, and Orians (2006) suggested that opportunities for networking, access to information and resources, personal recognition, learning, and improved relationships among stakeholders may be enhanced. The Centers for Disease Control and Prevention (CDC) views community engagement as necessary for healthy communities (CDC, 2017) and offers grants and programs to enable such participation. Thus, commitment of time and energy in true community partnership is a form of caring that is beneficial for healthcare professionals who often use their unique strengths only in the work environment. It is important to remember that the workplace is a part of the larger community and often is supported financially by it. By actively participating in the larger community, healthcare professionals are contributing to the health of the local population as well as their own personal growth.

Practicing Caring for Communities

Caring communities can take many forms. A fundamental principle of caring is *enabling members* through information and education, establishing linkages, and organizing and procuring resources. The key to creating caring communities is building the network of relationships among members and the informal day-to-day exchanges that occur among them. When individual relationships among members are of a caring nature, individuals feel safe and dignified, resulting in richer public events. Because most community involvement is voluntary, it is important that members see the value of their participation so that continued advancement is possible.

Many initiatives in healthcare are ongoing to increase participation by providers in larger community groups. For example, an organization in the northeast has collaborated with a community group to develop and obtain funding to increase breastfeeding rates among the diverse community they serve. A hospital in Florida that uses the QCM as the basis for practice recognizes departments that are best at "living the model" by bestowing monetary awards that can be used to make charitable contributions to the community, as directed by the employees in the department—this example is publicized as one way to "care for the community served." Nurses lead breast cancer awareness groups; support follow-up community clinics for many chronic diseases; are participants in regional disaster teams and respond to natural disasters; regularly provide education to community groups, including schools; facilitate wellness clinics; and raise money for research and other community health initiatives.

Health educators use service-learning concepts as strategies to bridge the gap between classroom and community. Most universities have formal service-learning curricula that generate genuine linkages among the university, its students, and the community that positively affect student learning and overall community health. Engaging members of the local community by offering information and education assists students in expanding their knowledge of healthcare and appreciation of cultural diversity by participating directly in the community in which they live.

At the graduate level, examples of community-based health professions programs are plentiful. Many health researchers routinely partner with community agencies to consider interventions that may enhance the health of the community. Connecting to the larger community in which one lives provides unique experiences that promote meaning in one's life.

Assisting communities to improve their capacity for ongoing change in specific geographic areas is necessary to tackle their problems and to preserve their unique lifestyle while improving their lives. Without regular interaction among citizens, communities are unable to move forward, ensure social justice, build collective resilience (needed in times of disasters or great change), and promote the common good; in other words, they become unhealthy. Healthy communities, on the other hand, demonstrate authentic citizen participation in which old and new ideas are included. Building community capacity is a civic duty to which healthcare providers can greatly contribute. Healthy communities are fundamental to the health and safety of their citizens and allow citizens to have a voice, promote quality of life and economic opportunity, and raise hope for the future. In healthy communities, there is noticeable collaboration between private and governmental services and attractive, clean surroundings. These outcomes are of special interest to health professionals who are advocates for good health. Actively engaged health professionals will not only realize great personal benefits but will ensure the ongoing vitality of the communities they serve.

IMPORTANCE OF RELATIONSHIPS IN HEALTH SYSTEMS

Although not the primary aim of this book, relationships among personnel and levels within organizations and their surrounding communities must not be overlooked. In fact, Gittell (2003, 2009, 2016) and Carmeli and Gittell (2009) have developed a theory of relational coordination that focuses on the interdependency of health systems and the high-quality relationships that are necessary for quality outcomes. The focus on communication, building shared goals and knowledge, and mutual respect across boundaries (e.g., among departments) aligns well with the QCM and reinforces the power of relationships to effectively coordinate the work. The importance of relationships cannot be underestimated, with increasing evidence that building and maintaining strong caring relationships can be an agent for change in itself, which leads to positive health outcomes.

SUMMARY

The focus of this chapter centered on the four relationships foundational to the QCM—relating to self, relating to patients and families, relating to each other, and relating to the community served. These four relationships form the basic underpinnings for quality caring practice; some evidence links them to improved patient and health professional outcomes. Relationships that are therapeutic (healing or caring) are empowering and foster a sense of belonging and well-being. Furthermore, they may generate positive energy that fuels new or sustained healthy behavior.

Additionally, relationships within and among health systems are explored vis-à-vis the patient experience and its significance to health outcomes.

Call to Action

Relationships are central to the human condition; they **reflect** on the beauty of the human person as he or she lives in relation to the universe. Slowing down enough to contact one's inner world—thoughts, desires, feelings—permits one to gain access to his or her own realty. Linking to this valuable resource of self helps one remember what he or she already knows—the powerful impact of one's work. **Recognize** nursing's power. Balancing external and internal energy requires regularly disengaging oneself from the complex culture of health systems and acquiescing to one of quiet aloneness—such action is renewing. **Sit** in silent reflection for 15 minutes this week. Human persons who are ill are mothers, fathers, sons, daughters, and/or grandparents; they hold societal roles and are members of their unique communities. **Appreciate** the totality of patients and families, including their significance to others. Taking pleasure in patients' roles and responsibilities when they are not ill preserves their honor. **Obtain** information about your patients' roles and responsibilities in society, their families, and their communities. Already vulnerable patients and families are subject to risks, namely, adverse outcomes, merely by virtue of their admission to health systems. **Eliminate** one condition at your institution that could reduce adverse outcomes for patients, families, employees, or students. The duality of doing (actions) and being (authentic use of self in the moment) simultaneously is crucial to quality patient care. Nurses who integrate the two create meaning, are comforting, and affirm human

(continued)

(*continued*)

dignity. **Practice** being and doing together. To attain superior patient and system outcomes, "being collaborative" with members of the health team is essential. This way of being suggests a shared, reciprocal relationship that is focused on the common goal of "what's best for patients and families." **Share** your true self with the health team. Reaching out to health team members to actively listen, being accessible to energetically dialogue about clinical issues, providing encouragement and enthusiasm, reinforcing his or her importance to the health team, respecting privacy and safety, and acknowledging the team member's human and affiliation needs set the tone for future interactions and generate ease in the workplace. **Choose** to be caring with the health team. Commitment to community activities is enhanced by caring relationships and builds community capacity. **Join** a community group today. Caring relationships are essential for safe and quality health systems. **Practice** caring for self, for patients and families, for each other, and for communities served.

REFLECTIVE QUESTIONS/APPLICATIONS

. . . for Students

1. Explain how relationships facilitate human growth and development.
2. Discuss the relationship between authentic self-awareness and neurobiology.
3. How do you specifically practice self-caring?
4. List specific ways health systems can interfere with health. How important are these to a patient's experience?
5. Develop a plan for holistic self-caring.
6. Define interprofessional collaborative practice.
7. Investigate the competencies for effective interprofessional collaborative practice.
8. Cite some personal benefits of caring for communities.

. . . for Professional Nurses in Clinical Practice

1. Are self-caring practices visible in your institution? What are they? Are they routinely used?
2. What is relational coordination? How do you see it working in your institution?

3. What avenues exist at your institution for nurses to integrate mindful practice into the workflow?
4. What specific health outcomes may be at risk as a consequence of hospitalization itself?
5. What is your assessment of the examples provided in this chapter that many nursing departments have implemented? Do they seem feasible?
6. How do you envision interprofessional collaboration in the future?

. . . for Professional Nurses in Educational Practice

1. How would you assist students to learn the four foundational relationships? How would it differ by program or level?
2. Reflect on interprofessional collaborative practice, including the competencies. How do undergraduate students best learn these phenomena? What new knowledge and skills are required to help students learn the value of interprofessional collaborative practice? How do you evaluate attainment of interprofessional collaborative practice at graduation?
3. How do you practice holistic self-caring? Are your students aware of it? Why or why not?
4. What avenues exist to help students realize the personal benefits of caring for communities? What about understanding the vulnerabilities of hospitalization?

. . . for Professional Nurses in Leadership Practice

1. How might relationship science inform your leadership?
2. What environmental reminders could you create to prompt professional nurses at your institution to be mindful of the important work they do?
3. Reflect on the four relationships discussed in this chapter. At what level are they being performed at your institution? How could they be strengthened?
4. Are you leading a relationship-centered organization? How do you know?
5. What innovative ways do nurses at your facility care for the community they serve? How often are these disseminated?
6. How do you specifically care for yourself?
7. In what ways does the organizational culture at your institution demonstrate support for interprofessional collaboration? Be specific.

PRACTICE ANALYSIS

Outside the door of a patient's room on an inpatient unit at a prominent academic health center, 5 individuals were observed shouting, one was crying and two more were sitting on the ground. As it turns out, all were family members of a woman in her 40s who had been healthy prior to admission. Apparently, she had a partial colectomy for a benign mass and was post-op for 2 days when she starting spiking fevers up to 103°–104°F. Over several days, it was determined that she had a widespread abdominal infection and needed IV antibiotics. The nurses asked her to call them when she needed to use the bathroom because she had been unstable on her feet. But early the day before, she got up by herself and fell. A head CT scan and vital signs were negative.

But over the course of the last 24 hours, the nurses observed that she seemed a little lethargic and she didn't seem able to do her own activities of daily living (ADLs). Nevertheless, she was recovering from the infection nicely and the patient's surgeon (who did not see the patient in person) informed the family of this via telephone prior to their arrival. They expected to see a woman well on her way to recovery. In fact, many of them had skipped work that day to be with her. What they saw when they arrived was a huge surprise and not a positive one! They immediately acted out and demanded to see the "head nurse" who came to the bedside and explained that her slight change in status had not yet been communicated to the surgeon who had been in the OR all morning. She assured them that the patient was being well monitored and asked them to please "quiet down" so other patients could rest. This only enraged the family more and they continued to use loud noises, demanding to speak to the doctor and hospital administration. The patient died 2 days later from a cerebral hemorrhage due to the fall.

1. How attuned were the health professionals in this case to the family's experience of hospitalization?
2. What could have helped them better appreciate the family's view?
3. How did the "head nurse" relate to the family members? What would you have done differently?
4. Were the surgeon and nurses collaborating on this patient's care? Why or why not? What would you have done differently, if anything?

REFERENCES

Agreli, H. F., Peduzzi, M., & Bailey, C. (2017). The relationship between team climate and interprofessional collaboration: Preliminary results of a mixed methods study. *Journal of Interprofessional Care, 31*(2), 184–186. doi:10.1080/13561820.2016.1261098

Allen, M. L., Lê Cook, B., Carson, N., Interian, A., La Roche, M., & Alegría, M. (2017). Patient-provider therapeutic alliance contributes to patient activation in community mental health clinics. *Administration and Policy in Mental Health and Mental Health Services Research, 44*(4), 431–440. doi:10.1007/s10488-015-0655-8

American Association of Colleges of Nursing. (2011). *Core competencies for interprofessional collaborative practice.* Washington, DC: Author.

Bilgiç, Ş., & Acaroğlu, R. (2017). Effects of listening to music on the comfort of chemotherapy patients. *Western Journal of Nursing Research, 39*(6), 745–762. doi:10.1177/0193945916660527

Buhler, C., & Allen, M. (1972). *Introduction to humanistic psychology.* Monterey, CA: Brooks/Cole.

Buhler, C., & Marschak, M. (1967). Basic tendencies of human life. In C. Buhler & F. Massarik (Eds.), *The course of human life.* New York, NY: Springer Publishing.

Butterfoss, F. D., LaChance, L. L., & Orians, C. E. (2006). Building allies coalitions: Why formation matters. *Health Promotion Practice, 7*(2 Suppl), 23S–33S. doi:10.1177/1524839906287062

Carmeli, A., & Gittell, J. (2009). High-quality relationships, psychological safety, and learning from failures in work organizations. *Journal of Organizational Behavior, 30*, 709–729. doi:10.1002/job.565

Centers for Disease Control and Prevention. (2017). The community guide. Retrieved from https://www.thecommunityguide.org/sites/default/files/assets/CG_flyer.pdf

Crane, R. S., Brewer, J., Feldman, C., Kabat-Zinn, J., Santorelli, S., Williams, J. M. G., & Kuyken, W. (2017). What defines mindfulness-based programs? The warp and the weft. *Psychological Medicine, 47*(6), 990–999. doi:10.1017/S0033291716003317

Cross, M. P., & Pressman, S. D. (2017). Understanding the connections between positive affect and health. In C. L. Cooper & J. C. Quick (Eds.), *The handbook of stress and health: A guide to research and practice* (pp. 75–95). Chichester, UK: John Wiley & Sons.

Dong, Y., Bartol, K. M., Zhang, Z.-X., & Li, C. (2016). Enhancing employee creativity via individual skill development and team knowledge sharing: Influences of dual-focused transformational leadership. *Journal of Organizational Behavior, 38*(3), 439–458. doi:10.1002/job.2134

Durkin, M., Beaumont, E., Hollins Martin, C. J., & Carson, J. (2016). A pilot study exploring the relationship between self-compassion, self-judgement, self-kindness, compassion, professional quality of life and wellbeing among UK community nurses. *Nurse Education Today, 46*, 109–114. doi:10.1016/j.nedt.2016.08.030

Dyess, S. M. L., Prestia, A. S., Marquit, D. E., & Newman, D. (2018). Self-care for nurse leaders in acute care environment reduces perceived stress: A mixed-methods pilot study merits further investigation. *Journal of Holistic Nursing, 36*(1), 79–90. doi:10.1177/0898010116685655

Edelman, D., Oddone, E., Liebowitz, R., Yancy, W., Olsen, M., Jeffreys, A., . . . Gaudet, T. W. (2006). A multidimensional integrative medicine intervention to improve cardiovascular risk. *Journal of General Internal Medicine, 21*(7), 728–734. doi:10.1111/j.1525-1497.2006.00495.x

Erikson, E. H. (1964). *Insight and responsibility.* New York, NY: Norton.

Erikson, E. H. (1968). *Identity: Youth and crisis.* New York, NY: Norton.

Feeney, B. C., & Collins, N. L. (2015). A new look at social support: A theoretical perspective on thriving through relationships. *Personality and Social Psychology Review, 19*(2), 113–147. doi:10.1177/1088868314544222

Feldman, G., Greeson, J., & Senville, J. (2010). Differential effects of mindful breathing, progressive muscle relaxation, and loving kindness meditation on decentering and negative reactions to repetitive thoughts. *Behaviour Research and Therapy, 48*, 1002–1011. doi:10.1016/j.brat.2010.06.006

Finkel, E. J., Simpson, J. A., & Eastwick, P. W. (2017). The psychology of close relationships: Fourteen core principles. *Annual Review of Psychology, 68*, 383–411. doi:10.1146/annurev-psych-010416-044038

Gallagher, L. M., Lagman, R., & Rybicki, L. (2017). Outcomes of music therapy interventions on symptom management in palliative medicine patients. *American Journal of Hospice and Palliative Medicine, 35*(2), 250–257. doi:10.1177/1049909117696723

Gittell, J. H. (2003). A theory of relational coordination. In K. Cameron, J. Dutton, & R.Quinn (Eds.), *Positive organizational scholarship: Foundations of a new discipline* (pp. 279–295). San Francisco, CA: Berrett-Kohler.

Gittell, J. H. (2009). *High performance healthcare: Using the power of relationships to achieve quality, efficiency and resilience.* New York, NY: McGraw-Hill.

Gittell, J. H. (2016). *Transforming relationships for high performance: The power of relational coordination.* Stanford, CA: Stanford University Press.

Goebel-Fabbri, A. E., Anderson, B. J., Fikkan, J., Franko, D. L., Pearson, K., & Weinger, K. (2011). Improvement and emergence of insulin resistance in woman with type 1 diabetes. *Diabetes Care, 34*, 545–555. doi:10.2337/dc10-1547

Good, D. J., Lyddy, C. J., Glomb, T. M., Bono, J. E., Brown, K. W., Duffy, M. K., . . . Lazar, S. W. (2015). Contemplating mindfulness at work. *Journal of Management, 42*(1), 114–142. doi:10.1177/0149206315617003

Gould, R. (1978). *Transformations: Growth and change in adult life.* New York, NY: Simon & Schuster.

Graham, A., Powell, M. S., & Truscott, J. (2016). Facilitating student well-being: Relationships do matter. *Educational Research, 58*(4), 366–383. doi:10.1080/00131881.2016.1228841

Greeson, J. M., Krucoff, C., Moon, S., Moon, T., & Shaffer, J. (2010). A "whole-person" approach. *Alternative and Complementary Therapies, 16,* 359. Retrieved from https://www.academia.edu/696402/A_whole-person_approach_to_back_pain_

Greeson, J. M., Webber, D. M., Smoski, M. J., Brantley, J. G., Ekblad, A. G., Suarez, E. C., & Wolever, R. Q. (2011). Changes in spirituality partly explain health-related quality of life outcomes after Mindfulness-Based Stress Reduction. *Journal of Behavioral Medicine, 34*(6), 508–518. doi:10.1007/s10865-011-9332-x

Gross, C. R., Krietzer, M. J., Reilly-Spong, M., Wall, M., Winbush, N. Y., Patterson, R., . . . Cramer-Bornemann, M. (2011). Mindfulness-based stress reduction versus pharmacotherapy for chronic primary insomnia: A randomized controlled clinical trial. *Explore: The Journal of Science and Healing, 7*(2), 76–87. doi:10.1016/j.explore.2010.12.003

Grusec, J. E. (2011). Socialization processes in the family: Social and emotional development. *Annual Review of Psychology, 62,* 243–269. doi:10.1146/annurev.psych.121208.131650

Hall, A. M., Ferreira, P. H., Maher, C. G., Latiner, J., & Ferreira, M. L. (2010). The influence of the therapist-patient relationship on treatment outcome in physical rehabilitation: A systematic review. *Physical Therapy, 90*(8), 1099–1110. doi:10.2522/ptj.20090245

Hall, L. H., Johnson, J., Watt, I., Tsipa, A., O'Connor, D. B. (2016). Healthcare staff wellbeing, burnout, and patient safety: A systematic review. *PLoS ONE, 11*(7), e0159015. doi:10.1371/journal.pone.0159015

Havighurst, R. (1953). *Human development and education.* New York, NY: McKay.

Health Resources and Services Administration. (2013). Nurse Education, Practice, Quality, and Retention (NEPQR) program—Interprofessional collaborative practice. Retrieved from http://bhpr.hrsa.gov/nursing/grants/nepqr.html

Hojat, M. (2016). Empathy and patient outcomes. In M. Hojat (Ed.), *Empathy in health professions education and patient care* (pp. 189–201). Cham, Switzerland: Springer.

House, S., & Havens, D. J. (2017). Nurses' and physicians' perceptions of nurse-physician collaboration: A systematic review. *Journal of Nursing Administration, 47*(3), 165–171. doi:10.1097/NNA.0000000000000460

Hunter, L. (2016). Making time and space: The impact of mindfulness training on nursing and midwifery practice. A critical interpretative synthesis. *Journal of Clinical Nursing, 25*(7–8), 918–929. doi:10.1111/jocn.13164

Jung, C. (1933). *Modern man in search of a soul.* New York, NY: Harcourt, Brace.

Jung, C. (1977). *The archetypes and the collective unconscious* (5th ed.). Princeton, NJ: Princeton University Press.

Kabat-Zinn, J. (2012). *Mindfulness for beginners: Reclaiming the present moment—And your life.* Boulder, CO: Sounds True.

King, I. M. (1981). *A theory for nursing: Systems, concepts, process.* New York, NY: Wiley.

Kohlberg, L. (1986). *The philosophy of moral development.* San Francisco, CA: Harper and Row.

Konrad, S. C., & Browning, D. M. (2012). Relational learning and interprofessional practice: Transforming health education for the 21st century. *Work: A Journal of Prevention, Assessment and Rehabilitation, 41*(3), 247–251. doi:10.3233/WOR-2012-1295

Kornhaber, R., Walsh, K., Duff, J., & Walker, K. (2016). Enhancing adult therapeutic interpersonal relationships in the acute health care setting: An integrative review. *Journal of Multidisciplinary Healthcare, 9*, 537. doi:10.2147/JMDH.S116957

Kravits, K., McAllister-Black, R., Grant, M., & Kirk, C. (2010). Self-care strategies for nurses: A psycho-educational intervention for stress reduction and the prevention of burnout. *Applied Nursing Research, 23*, 130–138. doi:10.1016/j.apnr.2008.08.002

Kushlev, K., Heintzelman, S. J., Lutes, L. D., Wirtz, D., Oishi, S., & Diener, E. (2017). ENHANCE: Design and rationale of a randomized controlled trial for promoting enduring happiness & well-being. *Contemporary Clinical Trials, 52*, 62–74. doi:10.1016/j.cct.2016.11.003

Levinson, D. J. (1966). *Seasons of a woman's life.* New York, NY: Alfred A. Knopf.

Levinson, D. J., Darrow, C. N., & Klein, E. B. (1978). *Seasons of a man's life.* New York, NY: Random House.

Little, M. M., St Hill, C. A., Ware, K. B., Swanoski, M. T., Chapman, S. A., Lutfiyya, M. N., & Cerra, F. B. (2016). Team science as interprofessional collaborative research practice: A systematic review of the science of team science literature. *Journal of Investigative Medicine, 65*(1), 15–22. doi:10.1136/jim-2016-000216

Maslow, A. (1966). *Psychology of science.* Chapel Hill, NC: Maurice Bassett.

Mesmer-Magnus, J., Glew, D. J., & Viswesvaran, C. (2012). A meta-analysis of positive humor in the workplace. *Journal of Managerial Psychology, 27*(2), 155–190. doi:10.1108/02683941211199554

Mofredj, A., Alaya, S., Tassaioust, K., Bahloul, H., & Mrabet, A. (2016). Music therapy, a review of the potential therapeutic benefits for the critically ill. *Journal of Critical Care, 35*, 195–199. doi:10.1016/j.jcrc.2016.05.021

Morin, A. (2011). Self-awareness Part 1: Definition, measures, effects, functions, and antecedents. *Social and Personality Psychology Compass, 5*(10), 807–823. doi:10.1111/j.1751-9004.2011.00387.x

Norman, G. J., Necka, E., & Berntson, G. G. (2016). The psychophysiology of emotions. In G. Norman (Ed.), *Emotion measurement* (pp. 83–98). Cambridge, MA: Elsevier. doi:10.1016/B978-0-08-100508-8.00029-1

Penm, J., MacKinnon, N. J., Boone, J. M., Ciaccia, A., McNamee, C., & Winstanley, E. L. (2017). Strategies and policies to address the opioid epidemic: A case study of Ohio. *Journal of the American Pharmacists Association, 57*(2S), S148–S153. doi:10.1016/j.japh.2017.01.001

Peplau, H. E. (1952). Interpersonal relations in nursing. *American Journal of Nursing, 52*(6), 765. doi:10.1097/00000446-195206000-00062

Piaget, J. (1972). *The psychology of the child.* New York, NY: Basic Books.

Piaget, J. (1990). *The child's conception of the world.* New York, NY: Littlefield Adams.

Pipe, T. B., & Bortz, J. J. (2009). A randomized controlled trial evaluating the effects of an intensive mindfulness meditation course for stress symptom management in nurse leaders. *Journal of Nursing Administration, 39*(3), 130–137. doi:10.1097/NNA.0b013e31819894a0

Pivetti, M., Camodeca, M., & Rapino, M. (2016). Shame, guilt, and anger: Their cognitive, physiological, and behavioral correlates. *Current Psychology, 35*(4), 690–699. doi:10.1007/s12144-015-9339-5

Reis, H. T., Collins, W. A., & Berscheid, E. (2000). The relationship context of human behavior and development. *Psychological Bulletin, 126*(6), 844–872. doi:10.1037/0033-2909.126.6.844

Rogers, C. (1961). On becoming a person: A therapist's view of psychotherapy. *Archives of General Psychiatry, 62,* 1377–1384. doi:10.1002/jpoc.20072.95

Rose, L. (2011). Interprofessional collaboration in the ICU: How to define? *Nursing Critical Care, 16*(1), 5–10. doi:10.1111/j.1478-5153.2010.00398.x

Sachs, O. (2007). *Musicophilia: Tales of music and the brain.* New York, NY: Alfred A. Knopf.

Schlitz, M. M., Vieten, C., & Amorok, T. (2007). *Living deeply: The art and science of transformation in everyday life.* Oakland, CA: New Harbinger.

Serlin, I. A., & DiCowden, M. A. (Eds.). (2007). *Whole person healthcare Vol. 1: Humanizing healthcare.* Westport, CT: Praeger.

Sheehy, G. (1976). *Passages: Predictable crises of adult life.* New York, NY: E. P. Dutton.

Shields, L. R. (2011). *Teaching mindfulness techniques to nursing students for stress reduction and self-care* (Doctor of Nursing Practice System Change Projects Paper 18). Retrieved from https://sophia.stkate.edu/cgi/viewcontent.cgi?referer=https://www.google.com/&httpsredir=1&article=1019&context=dnp_projects

Siegel, D. J. (2010). *Mindsight: The new science of personal transformation.* New York, NY: Bantam Books.

Siegel, D. J. (2015). *The developing mind: How relationships and the brain interact to shape who we are.* New York, NY: Guilford.

Smith, C., & Gettings, S. (2016). Reshaping policy to deliver holistic care for adolescents with Crohn's disease. *Nursing Children and Young People, 28*(10), 19–24. doi:10.7748/ncyp.2016.e723

Travelbee, J. (1966). *Interpersonal aspects of nursing.* Philadelphia, PA: F. A. Davis.

Ward, H., Gum, L., Attrill, S., Bramwell, D., Lindemann, I., Lawn, S., & Sweet, L. (2017). Educating for interprofessional practice: Moving from knowing to being, is it the final piece of the puzzle? *BMC Medical Education, 17*(1), 5. doi:10.1186/s12909-016-0844-5

Watson, J. (1979). *Nursing: The philosophy and science of caring.* Boston, MA: Little, Brown and Company.

Watson, J. (1985). *Nursing: Human science and human care.* Norwalk, CT: Appleton-Century-Crofts.

Watson, J. (2008a). *Assessing and measuring caring in nursing and health sciences* (2nd ed.). New York, NY: Springer Publishing.

Watson, J. (2008b). *The philosophy and science of caring* (Rev. ed.). Boulder: University of Colorado Press.

World Health Organization. (2010). *Framework for action on interprofessional education and collaborative practice.* Geneva, Switzerland: Author.

Yalom, I. D. (1975). *The theory and practice of group psychotherapy.* New York, NY: Basic Books.

5

Relationship-Centered Professional Encounters

Never forget that it is not a pneumonia, but a pneumonic person who is your patient.
—William Withey Gull

WHAT PATIENTS AND FAMILIES WANT FROM HEALTH PROFESSIONALS

As vulnerable, sick persons in oftentimes strange places (doctors' offices, outpatient clinics, nursing homes, or hospitals), patients, and their families, assume that health professionals "know what they are doing" (personal conversations with countless patients). What they expect, however, is another story.

In 1993, the Picker Institute, in partnership with patients and families, conducted a multiyear research project and ultimately identified eight characteristics of care, from the patients' perspective, as the most important indicators of quality and safety. They were (a) respect for the patient's values, preferences, and expressed needs; (b) coordinated and integrated care; (c) clear, high-quality information and education for the patient and family; (d) physical comfort, including pain management; (e) emotional support and alleviation of fear and anxiety; (f) involvement of family, including significant others and friends, as appropriate;

(g) continuity, including thorough care site transitions; and (h) access to care (Gerteis, 1993). Success in addressing these dimensions seems to require partnering with patients and families in designing, implementing, and evaluating care systems. In turn, they labeled such care "patient centered."

This concept was reintroduced and specifically recommended in five of the 10 "rules for redesigning and improving care" that were part of the Institute of Medicine's (IOM, 2001) report *Crossing the Quality Chasm.* The associated rules were:

- Care should be based on continuous healing relationships that are available to patients and families wherever they are 24/7.
- Care should be customized based on the patient's needs and values (e.g., designed to respond to patients' needs).
- The patient should be in control.
- The system should encourage shared knowledge and free flow of information, including patients' access to their respective records.
- The system should anticipate patients' needs.

Aspects of patient-centered care (PCC) were seen in several of the other five rules as well. For example, the rule "the system should constantly strive to decrease waste" included not wasting patients' time (IOM, 2001, p. 3). The IOM defined PCC as "care that is respectful of and responsive to individual patient preferences, needs, and values" and ensures "that patients' values guide all clinical decisions" (p. 3).

Ten years later and in response to recent healthcare reform initiatives, Detsky (2011) used his years of experience as a physician to outline, in order of priority, what patients want from health services:

First priorities:

1. A response to and restoration of a good state of health (as defined by them)
2. Access to services in a timely manner
3. Kindness, empathy, and respect for privacy
4. Hope (even when cure is unlikely) and a sense of certainty about the process
5. Continuity, choice, and coordination (with a health professional or team with whom they have an ongoing, secure relationship)
6. A private room when hospitalized
7. No out-of-pocket costs
8. The best (highly qualified clinicians)
9. Medications and surgery (easy fixes) versus behavioral changes

Second order priorities were:

10. Efficiency (so that *their* time is not wasted), including rapid sched-
    uling and reporting of test results—*excessive wait time matters*
11. Aggregate-level statistics about treatments unless it can be tied to
    them personally
12. Equity of services
13. Conflicts of interest (treatments recommended by certain health
    professionals that stand to gain) *if* it makes them feel better

Lowest priority:

14. The real cost of services
15. Percentage gross national product (GNP) devoted to healthcare
    (Detsky, 2011, pp. 2500–2501)

In other words, from an illness perspective, patients and families were
concerned about themselves and the care they received (versus the larger
health system and its costs). To illustrate this further, participants in one
qualitative study reported that during hospitalization, expectations for
basic human needs, respect for time, food delivery, sleep, emotional and
spiritual needs, and knowing clinicians' plans for their care were fundamental needs that demonstrated dignity and respect (Gazarian et al., 2017).

Most of this work on patient needs was done with hospitalized patients,
but interestingly, when community-dwelling persons were asked what they
wanted from health services they overwhelmingly brought up the subject
of interactions with their doctors, consistent with past reports (Wen &
Tucker, 2015). Most people commented on the importance of a clinician who
listens, cares, and explains issues to patients versus their technical expertise.
In summary, individual patients are less likely to be interested in the technological and cost aspects of healthcare and seem to be more affected by
their unique perceptions and experiences as they encounter the healthcare
system and its providers—thus the term *patient-centered care*. What does
this suggest about ongoing caring relationships with health professionals?

Fueled by the ongoing and pervasive safety and quality problems
in health systems, feverish efforts have been undertaken by accrediting
organizations, payers, and health systems to embrace PCC as a means of
improving safety and quality, while meeting the needs of a diverse patient
population. Stakeholders in all health systems—professional organizations,
public policy groups, hospital administration, health professional school
leadership, insurance carriers, and health professionals themselves—have
welcomed the focus on PCC. And while the IOM asserted over 17 years ago
that PCC is a central aim for improving healthcare (Entwistle & Watt, 2013;

IOM, 2001), argued that little improvement had been made. Thus, although the healthcare community universally endorses the ideal of PCC, many organizations are struggling to understand what PCC truly means, how it is displayed, the obligations it entails, and how it is best evaluated. These issues have only just begun to be explored in a health system that is typically centered on health professionals or organizational needs (Fights, 2012).

For example, confusion about what PCC really means has shaped recent costly efforts by health systems to create hotel-like environments, such as the use of greeters and valet parking, indoor gardens and waterfalls, unique coffee kiosks, expensive customer-service consultations, artwork, and fashionable lighting. Others have now implemented the use of electronic tablets as a means to enhance communication and education about health needs. Yet, "hospital patients today are bombarded with surveys, post-discharge calls, opportunities to share 'compliments and concerns,' and requests to 'speak up' . . . . In actuality, patients' perceptions of care are often ignored and rarely translate into improvements" (Mazor et al., 2016, p. 618).

Customer services approaches such as installing beautiful surroundings, having a few classes on customer-service principles, hiring a patient experience specialist, and implementing electronic means of communication are superficial fixes that are not necessarily patient centered, *unless* they strengthen how patients and providers relate. Even the patient-centered medical home is suffering from lack of focus on what matters to patients (Wasson, 2017).

In addition, health systems have unknowingly created barriers to PCC that challenge its consistent delivery; these have been organized into three categories: organizational, professional, and data related (Audet, Davies, & Schoenbaum, 2006). Organizational characteristics such as poor leadership (West, Barron, & Reeves, 2005), clinician relational challenges (Dunn, 2003; Gillespie, Florin, & Gillam, 2004), insufficient attention paid to the specific competencies providers need to optimize PCC (Bernabeo & Holmboe, 2013), competing professional priorities, lack of focus on PCC as a quality issue, and resistance to change have been cited as obstacles. Lack of systematic and timely quality improvement (QI) processes to drive practice changes (Davies & Cleary, 2005; Shaller, 2007), including long delays from data collection to reporting results, measures that do not capture patient perspectives of care *during* hospitalization thus subjecting them to potential recall bias, and irregular dissemination of data to clinicians who actually deliver the care, have been challenging to PCC application (Davies & Cleary, 2005). More recently, lapses in being treated with dignity and respect (or emotional harm) have been reported as barriers to PCC and are considered preventable harms (Gazarian et al., 2017; Sokol-Hessner, Folcarelli, & Sands, 2015). With all the focus on PCC, such continuing system challenges beg the question: Why has there been so little improvement? Furthermore, what does PCC really mean (in terms of delivery)?

WHAT DOES "PATIENT CENTERED" REALLY MEAN?

Patient-centered care is a dynamic, multidimensional construct comprised of characteristics and behaviors that shift the focus of healthcare from a clinical or disease-driven process to one that is patient driven. PCC is a characteristic of individual practitioners, the healthcare system, and relationship quality (Epstein et al., 2005). Definitions of PCC have varied over the years, complicating its theoretical clarity. From the clinical perspective, PCC has been defined as understanding the patient as a unique human being (Balint, 1969; Shaller, 2007) and promoting the trust, confidence, and clarification of patients' concerns by clinicians who have specific knowledge, attitudes, and skills (Lipkin, Quill, & Napodano, 1984). A literature review in 2000 revealed five domains of PCC: a biopsychosocial perspective, understanding the *patient* as person, sharing power and responsibility, building a therapeutic alliance (relationship), and understanding the *clinician* as a person (Kaba & Sooriakumaran, 2007). The terms family-centered care and relationship-centered care have expanded and deepened the meaning of PCC to include families, caring patient–clinician relationships, teamwork and community relationships, and the importance of reflective practice, the clinician's responsibility for ongoing emotional engagement and reflection (Conway et al., 2006; Tresolini and the Pew-Fetzer Task Force, 1994).

The hospitalized patient's perspective of PCC emerged as a unique and important view, and now embraces understanding and responding to "what matters" to patients and families (Schall, Sevin, & Wasson, 2009). In fact, the patient's perspective, particularly at the point of care, is now considered crucial in the evaluation of PCC (Wasson & Baker, 2009). Radwin (2003) heavily drew on the IOM definition of PCC in her evaluation research and Hobbs (2009) conducted a dimensional analysis to identify components of PCC. She reported alleviating vulnerabilities, therapeutic engagement, carrying out information practices, knowing the other, and the constancy of relationship as important components of PCC.

More recently, PCC has been defined as "healing relationships between providers and patients" (Epstein, Fiscella, Lesser, & Stange, 2010, p. 1489) and "a quality of personal, professional, and organizational relationships" (Epstein & Street, 2011, p. 100). The Quality and Safety Education for Nurses (QSEN) initiative has defined PCC as recognition of "the patient or designee as the source of control and full partner in providing compassionate and coordinated care based on respect for patient's preferences, values, and needs" (QSEN, 2012, "Patient-centered Care"). And based on a literature review, Sidani and Fox (2014) reported three specific elements that represented PCC: holistic, collaborative, and responsive care. Even with these varied definitions, "PCC remains one of the most-used and least-understood terms in healthcare" (Weissman, Millenson, & Haring, 2017, p. 1).

D espite the complexity in defining PCC, an obvious similarity among all definitions is the consistent emphasis on patient–clinician relationships. Aspects such as the uniqueness of patient needs, human respect, active participation, and shared decision making are usually used in describing PCC. As Kizer (2002) points out, "This intimate relationship is the medium by which information, feelings, fears, concerns and hope are exchanged between caregiver and patient" (p. 117). Preserving and enhancing the integrity of this relationship is foundational for successful diagnosis, treatment, and satisfying experiences of care (Kizer, 2002).

Although not labeled PCC per se, registered nurses (RNs) have consistently embraced PCC as a primary component of their practice and the essence of their work (Mitchell, 2008). The Quality-Caring Model©'s (QCM) four fundamental relationships and the concept of relationship-centered professional encounters are congruent with contemporary notions of PCC (see Table 5.1).

Elements of the whole person of the patient, the works of the pioneering nurse theorists of the 1950s, 1960s, and the 1970s, and the terms *meeting patient needs, interpersonal relationships between patients and nurses, keeping patients safe*, and *family presence* are common in most nursing curricula, yet we rarely acknowledge their importance in everyday practice. How ironic is it that such long-standing principles of quality nursing care are now part of the national agenda? And sadly, how is it that nursing still isn't driving this work?

Unfortunately, although *patients want and value* PCC, clinicians vary in their practice of it (Stewart, 2001), health systems create barriers to it, and it is not well studied. Some measures, including direct observation of clinical encounters, patient self-reports, and video simulations, have been developed to measure PCC (Epstein et al., 2005), but most have been inadequately validated or have been tested in outpatient settings with physicians. In acute care settings, little effort has been made to evaluate PCC and generate the practice changes needed to improve it. Most agree that the best measures of PCC are those obtained by patients themselves

TABLE 5.1 Congruence of Quality-Caring Model with Experts' Definitions of Patient-Centered Care

Components of Patient-Centered Care as Defined by Various Experts	Related Assumptions, Concepts, Propositional Statements, and the Nursing Role in the Quality-Caring Model
Respect (IOM, 2001; Epstein et al., 2010; IOM, 2001)	Humans are inherently worthy. Humans exist in a relationship with themselves, others, communities or groups, nature (or the environment), and the universe.
Responsiveness to patients' expressed needs, preferences, and values (IOM, 2001; Radwin, 2003; QSEN, 2012)	Initiate, cultivate, and sustain caring relationships with patients and families.
Patient as person, individualization (Mead & Bower, 2000; Radwin, 2003; QSEN, 2012)	Humans are multidimensional beings capable of growth and change. Humans evolve over time and in space.
Therapeutic relationship (healing relationship, therapeutic engagement, caring presence; Epstein et al., 2010; Epstein & Street, 2011; Mead & Bower, 2000; Stewart, Brown, Weston, & Freeman, 2003)	Caring relationships benefit both the caregiver and the one being cared for. When relationships are grounded by caring factors, a human connection occurs that is transpersonal and has the potential to be transformative for all involved. Caring relationships engender "feeling cared for" and arouse persons', groups', and systems' capabilities to change, learn and develop, or self-advance. Caring relationships facilitate growth and change. Relationships characterized as caring contribute to individual, group, and system self-advancement.
Education, information, and support (Epstein et al., 2010; Hobbs, 2009; Shaller, 2007)	Two caring behaviors or processes used during relationship-centered professional encounters, namely, mutual problem solving and encouraging manner, speak to providing information, reframing, helping patients learn, and validating understanding, enthusiasm, support, and empowerment.

(Hudon, Fortin, Haggerty, Lambert, & Poitras, 2011). Recently, an updated systematic review showed an increased reporting of value concordance in measures of PCC. However, large differences existed in the way PCC was defined and calculated, making it difficult to draw conclusions (Winn, Ozanne, & Sepucha, 2015).

EVIDENCE OF THE BENEFITS OF PATIENT-CENTERED CARE

Several studies have demonstrated positive associations between *medically delivered* PCC and improved outcomes (including clinical outcomes, decreased utilization, lower costs, and fewer lawsuits) in outpatient settings (Schall et al., 2009). For example, outcomes such as improved recovery, increased emotional health, fewer diagnostic tests, and referrals at 2 months (Stewart et al., 2000), improved health outcomes and fewer emergency visits (Hack, Degner, Watson, & Sinha, 2006), reduced malpractice claims, greater clinician satisfaction (Beckman, Markakis, Suchman, & Frankel, 1994), decreased postoperative pain, function, and length of stay (Gittell et al., 2000), and improvement of health outcomes in patients with chronic disease have been linked to PCC (Kaplan, Greenfield, & Ware, 1989). In addition, improvements in recall and adherence (Bartlett et al., 1984; Horwitz et al., 1998); blood pressure, blood sugar control, and decreased pain in patients with chronic disease; and improvement in quality of life for those with diabetes have been reported (Wasson, Johnson, Benjamin, Phillips, & MacKenzie, 2006). In a longitudinal study of PCC and hospitalized adults with myocardial infarction (MI), those patients who rated PCC lower had worse health status and more symptoms (chest pain) than other patients during the first year after the MI despite adjusting for severity (Fremont et al., 2001). A follow-up study of 1,858 veterans with MI demonstrated an association between PCC and lower 1-year mortality, even after controlling for patient characteristics and technical quality of care (Meterki, Wright, Lin, Lowy, & Cleary, 2009). Two randomized clinical trials in primary care settings specifically tested a *practice-based PCC intervention*. Greenfield, Kaplan, Ware, Yano, and Frank (1988) developed a 20-minute intervention designed to increase the involvement of patients in medical decision making. Using a randomized clinical trial in two clinic sites, experimental patients reported significantly fewer functional limitations and improved blood sugar control. Cooper et al. (2009) tested a patient-centered, culturally tailored intervention on 279 poor patients with hypertension. They concluded, "There is strong evidence that patient-centered communication behaviors impact patient adherence, patient satisfaction and important health outcomes" (p. 12). Finally and most significantly, Bertakis and Azari (2011) found decreased utilization of healthcare services and lower total annual charges in those patients ($N = 509$) who received higher than average amounts of PCC during outpatient visits over 1 year. The authors demonstrated this finding despite controlling for patient gender, age, education, income, self-reported health status, and health risk behaviors (obesity, alcohol abuse, and smoking). More recently, a combined intervention that included oncologist communication training and coaching for patients with advanced cancer showed statistically significant results in improving communication, but did not affect secondary outcomes (Epstein et al., 2017).

Several *nursing* studies have linked caring patient–nurse relationships (a core component of PCC) to positive health outcomes (such as patient satisfaction, decreased anxiety, increased knowledge, improved functional status, and decreased symptom distress), authentic self-expression, sense of well-being, optimism, and trust in nurses (Burt, 2007; Latham, 1996; Radwin, Cabral, & Wilkes, 2009; Swan, 1998; Wolf, Colahan, & Costello, 1998; Yeakel, Maljanian, Bohannon, & Coulombe, 2003). A nurse-led patient-centered self-management support intervention was also found that showed significantly lowered HbA1c among patients with type 2 diabetes (Jutterström, Hörnsten, Sandström, Stenlund, & Isaksson, 2016). Finally, a Cochrane Review of 17 educational intervention studies targeting PCC demonstrated greater patient satisfaction, well-being, and communication (Lewin, Skea, Entwistle, Zwarenstein, & Dick, 2009).

Despite the emerging and important evidence linking PCC to improved patient and health system outcomes, some existing PCC studies have important limitations. Many were correlational and were conducted in primary care settings with physicians. Only two investigated PCC over time. Few studies focused on RNs, were conducted in acute care settings, or examined teams of health providers delivering PCC. And measures used to operationalize PCC were varied.

The Patient-Centered Outcomes Research Institute (PCORI) was created in 2012 as a result of the Affordable Care Act. PCORI's distinct approach to research involves patients and other stakeholders in all aspects of the research process, from determining which research topics and outcomes should be studied, to helping to develop and conduct the studies, to sharing the results (PCORI, 2017). It now has funded multiple studies designed to improve patient care and outcomes important to patients through patient-centered comparative clinical effectiveness research. In addition, it has established PCORnet, the National Center for Clinical Research Network. This is a large, highly representative, national network of clinical data gathered in a variety of healthcare settings, including hospitals, doctors' offices, and community clinics. The data are stored and shared across the network using strict methods to ensure confidentiality. This patient-centered approach to research is a promising method for systematic, highly applicable findings that matter to patients and families.

Although the meaning and evidence for PCC are emerging, less often stated are the competencies and moral implications (or accountability) for delivering PCC.

In a 2013 article, Bernabeo and Holmboe suggested the following competencies are needed by health professionals to authentically deliver PCC:

- Establish, develop, and adapt a partnership
- Establish or review the patient's preferences for information about his or her health or treatment plan
- Review and establish the patient's preferred role in decision making and any uncertainty about the course of action to take
- Identify choices and evaluate the research evidence in relation to the individual patient
- Present evidence, taking into account the patient's competencies, framing effects, etc.
- Help the patient reflect on and assess the impact of alternative decisions with regard to his or her values and lifestyle; negotiate decisions with the patient, resolve conflict, agree on a care plan, and arrange for follow-up
- Negotiate decisions with the patient, resolve conflict, agree on a care plan, and arrange for follow-up

How many of us have spent time in class or clinical courses perfecting these competencies? How do health systems ensure these capabilities are established and sustained?

Finally, because PCC is based on a deep respect for patients as worthy human beings who live in unique contexts, the professional obligations to care for patients and families in this fashion are readily apparent—they are disciplinary values. Second, a growing body of knowledge suggests an association between PCC, particularly the quality of patient–clinician relationships, and improved patient experiences and other short- and long-term quality indicators across healthcare settings. Respect for and appreciation for the uniqueness of human persons together with the evidence base for PCC provide the foundation for professional obligations and health system actions to measure, improve, and consistently deliver PCC.

Such obligations and actions include consistently offering respect and attention; appreciating and incorporating patients' unique values and preferences; mutually helping patients solve their health problems, including providing information/education; being optimistic and supportive; ensuring that human and affiliation needs are met; and guaranteeing patient safety (also known as caring behaviors). These duties and responsibilities are enmeshed in the Quality-Caring concept, relationship-centered professional encounters.

RELATIONSHIP-CENTERED PROFESSIONAL ENCOUNTERS

In healthcare situations, persons with health needs meet in relationship with health professionals who function independently and collaboratively with them. Independent relationships are those carried out between patients and families and one health professional. Collaborative relationships are those interactions performed among multiple health professionals who work in a complementary nature to cohesively provide coordinated services to patients and families. These three-way encounters (see Chapter 3) are relationship centered when they are grounded in caring processes or behaviors.

> Caring relationships are healing or healthy for both patients and health professionals. Moreover, caring relationships (when cultivated and sustained) generate human connections that transcend the individuals alone and result in an understanding of others that anticipates, guides, provides for, teaches and learns, protects, and advocates. This form of relationship trumps the traditional diagnostic, procedural, disease-based care that usually occurs during illness because it protects the overall health and well-being of whole individuals (not just the treatment of disease) and has the potential to be transforming.

Relationship-centered professional encounters begin between health professionals and potential patients in communities and primary care settings and hopefully follow individuals during episodes of acute care and beyond. Characteristics of relationship-centered professional encounters include the caring processes or behaviors (see Table 5.2) that shift the focus from instrumental or "doing" activities to those that are more in line with "being" or "authentic presence." This is hard to practice for busy healthcare professionals who typically define their identities in terms of helping, assisting, fixing, or resolving problems. Creating a safe

TABLE 5.2 Caring Behaviors, Definitions, Required Knowledge, and Behavioral Skills

Caring Behavior	Definition	Professional Behaviors and Skills	Knowledge Needed by Health Professionals
Mutual problem solving	Professional behaviors that help patients and families understand how to confront, learn, and think about their health and illness; involves a reciprocal, shared approach with resulting decisions acceptable to both	Providing information Reframing Deliver learning opportunities Exploring alternative ways or options for dealing with health Brainstorming together Figuring out questions to ask Validating what patients know Accepting feedback from patients Experimenting with different ways of providing care Adopting patients' ideas Listening skills Fostering the patient's preferred role in decision making Helping patients reflect on and assess the impact of alternative health decisions on lifestyle Ensuring access to understandable information Assessing and using patients' competencies, problem-solving skills, including health literacy	Informed, up to date on the literature Knowledge of searchable databases Comfortable "in relationship" Knowledge of multiple learning approaches How to engage others
Attentive reassurance	Availability of health professionals who display a hopeful outlook, even when the future is not promising (in terms of a cure)	Optimistic; able to convey possibilities Accessible Repeated confirmation of availability Confident Clarifying misperceptions Reassuring	Knowledge of self Self-reliant Positive attitude Assertiveness knowledge Self-aware

Human respect	Honoring the worth of human persons	Unconditional acceptance
		Careful handling of the body
		Recognition of human rights and responsibilities
		Appreciates the integrity of the patient (biopsychosociocultural or "whole person" approach)
		Calls patient by preferred name
		Makes eye and physical contact
		Preserves patient autonomy
		Knows the patient as an individual
			Knowledge of ethical principles
			    Autonomy
			    Beneficence
			    Nonmaleficence
			    Justice
			Knowledge of patients' rights
			Active listening
			Mutual interactions

Encouraging manner	Affective dimension of behavior associated with demeanor/attitude	Supportive verbal demeanor Supportive nonverbal demeanor Enthusiasm Positive feedback Supportive view of the system Empowering, inspiring	Knowledge of effective communication techniques Knowledge of constructive feedback techniques Skillful communication Positive attitudes

(continued)

TABLE 5.2   Caring Behaviors, Definitions, Required Knowledge, and Behavioral Skills *(continued)*

Caring Behavior	Definition	Professional Behaviors and Skills	Knowledge Needed by Health Professionals
Appreciation of unique meanings	Knowing the patient's context and worldview; discerning and then acknowledging the subjective inner value attached to a situation, person, or event; knowing what is important to patients and families, including distinctive sociocultural connections	Active listening Nonjudgmental attitude Tolerance for both positive and negative ideas or expressions Flexibility Elicits patient values and preferences Uses patient values and preferences when designing and delivering care	Knowledge of and appreciation for diversity Personal "knowing" of patient (developed in relationship and over time)
Healing environment	Safe and aesthetically pleasing surroundings	Establishes safe environment Makes frequent checks/surveillance Provides safety information and associated teach-backs Ensures call systems in place Performs accurate, timely, and comprehensive handoffs Maintains privacy and confidentiality Ensures clean and pleasant surroundings	Knowledge of safety standards, benefits, and limitations of selected safety-enhancing technologies Knowledge of the ethical standard, fidelity Knowledge of current evidence related to prevention of adverse outcomes

Basic human needs	Physical, safety, social/relational, self-esteem, and self-actualization needs	Consistent attention to airway, intake, elimination, sleep and rest, mobility, and hygiene needs Attention to emotional, social, and self-esteem needs Regular assessment and maintenance of comfort	Knowledge of basic physiology and pathophysiology Knowledge of human emotions during health and illness Knowledge of human development across the life span Knowledge of pain and suffering, pain interventions, and pain/comfort theories
Affiliation needs	Person's needs for belonging and membership in families or other social contexts	Responsive to families Engages family members in health decisions per patients' wishes Allows family members' presence Involves family Conducts routine family meetings Resources available to families	Knowledge of family theories Knowledge of individual patient's family situation and routines

space for the disclosure of patients' feelings and emotions or mutually deciding the "right" course of action requires that health professionals redefine their practice and self-image from "do-ers" to "be-ers" (listeners and responders with relational knowledge who attend to the quality of the patient–provider relationship as the primary component of care).

The eight caring behaviors or processes are multifaceted, and although comprised of both being and doing, the emphasis is on the genuine caring nature of the relationship that undergirds the activities. The caring behaviors are the basis for relationship-centered professional encounters—both those with patients and families and those among health professionals. In other words, although the relationship with patients and families is primary, relationships with other health professionals should also be based on the caring behaviors. When enacted in this manner, such encounters induce positive feelings and intermediate outcomes in recipients (next chapter) that guide future interactions and ultimately healthy outcomes.

Jamie's Story (narrated here) illustrates the human experience of an RN as she spent time with her ill sister in an ICU:

> *My sister became very ill and was hospitalized for pneumonia. My family, who live out of state, notified me and informed me that her condition was more severe than first thought. With her history of illness and a weakened immune response, I felt a strong urge to go home to check on her—my intuition was speaking to me. By the time I arrived, I was informed that her condition had progressed to acute respiratory distress syndrome (ARDS) and she had been placed on a ventilator. I went to her room and felt overwhelmed at the sight of my sister on a ventilator, fully sedated of course. I was not an ICU nurse, so my limited understanding of ventilators made it even scarier. In fact, at this point, I was not a nurse at all, but a deeply worried sister. What if she didn't pull through? What if I hadn't arrived on time to say goodbye to the little sister I waited so anxiously for my mom to bring home from the hospital when I was just 3 years old? Jamie was 46 now and we shared a remarkable sisterhood, one with such deep and unbreakable bonds that words to describe it elude me.*
>
> *Her hospitalization lasted over a week, most of which was spent unconscious on a ventilator. I stayed in her room most days and my mom and I gave each other breaks. We had been informed that there was no guarantee of a positive outcome for Jamie. We stayed close to her just in case of the unthinkable. We would gently rub her arms and legs and talk to her in a very soft voice, hoping she would somehow feel our presence and love. Nurses came in and out over the course of the week and did their "tasks." Sometimes they would say hello, or smile, but usually it was clear that they were there to do their required "work" and move on. There was no interest or even concern for the family conveyed by the nurses. It seemed to*

be inherently lacking in them. Even when I asked a question, their answers were inadequate, or they would tell me I "need to ask the doctor." I didn't understand the lack of advocacy, and worse yet, their indifference. And if it wasn't bad enough to serve the family so inadequately, it appeared that Jamie was not much more than an object either—no kind words for their unconscious patient, no touch, no notice of her humanness. Furthermore, the nurses failed to notice my desperation and angst, were not in tune to my worry that my sister and I may never communicate again, provided no words of encouragement—just administered meds, and quickly suctioned—in a hurried demeanor. One thing I was certain of—these nurses were either completely lacking in self-awareness or they just did not care.

Days went by with this type of care. It's actually even hard to call it care; it felt so distant and negligible, only tending to the technical aspect of things. About four or five different nurses had been involved in Jamie's care to this point, all gloomy, distant, preoccupied, and removed. Then something wonderful happened . . .

A different nurse arrived in the room the next morning. What a ray of light! She brought hope and even some cheer. She immediately took notice of my state of mind and started asking what I needed, and if I understood what was going on. There was a huge lump in my throat as I was so touched by her genuine concern. Then she said, "I see Jamie has been on the ventilator for a few days. I'm going to decrease the sedation so you can have a few moments together." She stayed for a minute to be sure all was well when Jamie regained some awareness, and then said she'd return in a few minutes to check on us. There were no words to describe my emotions at that moment. I was going to be able to communicate with my sister after all! This nurse was magic to me, an absolute angel, I thought. As Jamie somewhat "came to," we were able to connect and I cried quietly, and when she recognized my voice her tears flowed, too. I wiped both of our eyes with the same tissue and kept it close to me, just in case we shared our last tears. I playfully but gently lifted her eyelids and said, "I know you're in there and I want you to see that we are right here!" Of course she couldn't speak, being intubated, but there was hand holding, well, squeezing, and I was able to hug her and tell her that I loved her, and that I had been there watching over her while she was unaware and that I would stay until she was safely off of the ventilator. I told her to just let this ventilator do the work for her for now so she could rest and heal. Her reactions showed me she heard and understood everything. We had connected! The nurse (or the angel) reappeared with a calm demeanor and a peaceful smile. The meaning of the few moments we had was inde-scribable. I finally had some sense of peace.

The significance of this story is to illustrate that many days passed with a family's needs unmet, creating unnecessary anxiety and fear, an outcome that didn't have to be, an outcome that was positively changed by a nurse *who emphasized caring and relationship over task completion. Although the story shared here is heavy with emotion and rich with meaning, I think it is significant to point out that this profound experience took place over the course of 5 minutes, illuminating the fact that it is not always about "more time."* This nurse did not have any more time in her day than the others with their hurried demeanors and displays of insensitivity. It is what she did with the moments she had that made her different. *I can still see her face like it was yesterday, even though 3 years have passed, and I can describe her hair and the scrubs she was wearing the day she came into that hospital room and reassured us with her genuine care, relieving our angst and totally changing our outlook.*

After this experience, I sometimes wondered, what if Jamie hadn't survived? I can only assume that our chances of having had an opportunity for a last connection may have been unlikely, with the high percentage of task-focused nurses we encountered. Of all of the nurses we encountered, why was only one practicing caring?

(As told to this author by Kim Payne, RN, BSN, Hannibal Regional Hospital, Hannibal, MO)

What caring behaviors were displayed by the "different" nurse? How would you teach the first group of nurses to "see" and attend to the family in this situation?

Contrast the story above with the following exemplar relayed by a nursing unit manager.

A 70-year-old male was admitted for syncopal episodes and frequent falling; this was thought to be related to cardiac arrhythmias and later confirmed so. The patient was alert and oriented throughout his 13-day hospital stay, but complained of ankle pain periodically, with some swelling and bruising beginning on day 3. On the sixth day of his admission, an orthopedic consult was obtained after x-rays revealed a medial malleolus fracture in his left ankle. He was taken to surgery the following day and had an open reduction and internal fixation.

Since admission, the patient had been voiding in a urinal without difficulties and on day 6, the day it was discovered that the patient had a fracture, he attempted to walk across the room to get his urinal to void. He was in too much pain and returned to his bed and called his nurse. No one came. He continued to call the nurse for 30 minutes without success and became incontinent. His nurse placed a diaper on him due to his incontinence and he was told he had to wear them throughout the rest of this stay. Afraid to speak up or cause any problems, he complied.

On the day of discharge, he shared this information with his son-in-law, also a nurse and visiting from another state. Immediately, his son-in-law contacted administration and voiced a complaint. "Administration" (including this nurse manager) visited the patient and heard the heart-breaking story from the voice of the 70-year-old man, who explained that even though he was 70 and wrinkled, "he was still a man and had been humiliated and stripped of his dignity from the moment the diapers were placed on him." It was his perception that his nurse that day was irritated that he messed his bed and assumed he was too lazy to retrieve his urinal. He also shared that when the same nurse would come and change his diaper, she would have him stand, holding onto the bed and yank his diaper to his knees while he was standing—naked, exposed, and humiliated.

Tears poured from this gentleman's eyes as he told the story and from mine as I held his hand and apologized for the lack of human respect shown by his nurse, the lack of mutual problem solving by not exploring alternate ways of assuring his basic human needs were met, the lack of attentive reassurance by not being available to him when he needed to urinate, and reassurance that it was not his fault, the lack of an encouraging manner by not helping him deal with bad feelings that he had become incontinent, the lack of appreciation of unique meanings by not knowing what was important to this man, the lack of a healing environment by not checking on him or ensuring a safe environment (urinal within reach), and the lack of affiliation needs by not encouraging family participation in care.

How did this man's experiences affect his outcomes? What could have been done to avoid this occurrence? How should the nurse be dealt with?

Through the ongoing processes of interaction and mutual relating, patients and health professionals come together, communicate, express their views, and over time, develop a connection based on caring. This connection deepens the relationship and if sustained, leads to knowing who the other is and what matters to them. Sometimes, as the relationship intensifies, one can almost foresee the needs of the other. Knowing another in this way provides the insight needed to detect problems early, to be protective, to provide anticipatory guidance and creative problem solving, and to facilitate healthy future behaviors. Thus, knowing another is dependent on ongoing caring interactions and resultant connections, and this is an important aim for professional practice.

Using the caring relationship to really understand how the ill person feels and then jointly working together to develop individualized processes of care continues the connection. Effective use of the caring behaviors is central to relationship-centered professional encounters (and the delivery of PCC) and requires integration of a health professional's external knowledge and skills with the more internal self-knowledge, beliefs, and attitudes.

> Relationship-centered professional encounters require the ability to remain authentically present and attentive to relationships amid the everyday demands of the clinical environment. Such a stance entails courage on the part of health professionals to advocate for the importance of and expression of caring behaviors as crucial elements of safe and quality care.

PATIENT-CENTERED CARE AND QUALITY CARING

The QCM is aligned with current definitions of PCC, as depicted in Table 5.1. The model concept, relationship-centered professional encounters, is particularly suited for promoting PCC as it specifies explicit processes (caring behaviors) required for caring (or healing) relationships, a core aspect of PCC. As such, it assists health professionals to see, to understand, and then actually interact in a way that matters to patients and families (aka, is patient centered), versus the more current notion of caring relationships as intangible professional ideals. PCC contrasts with health professional or system-centered care that typically revolves around the professional or the organization. In a patient-centered health system, health professionals and patients/families coexist in relationships characterized as caring, where mutuality, shared decision making, and health services are performed with the patient as the authority for care delivered. Thus, the patient's health and the health professional's work satisfaction are dependent on reciprocal caring relationships, in which different perspectives are heard and honored. From this caring foundation, health services are provided that preserve the needs of patients and families while meeting professional standards and guidelines that define health professionals' work.

In spite of the challenges, some visionaries have attempted to incorporate aspects of PCC into some models of care, such as those for older adults (the Chronic Care Model [Wagner, 1998]), NICHE (Mezey et al., 2004), primary care, transitional care (Naylor et al., 1999), and the medical home (National Committee for Quality Assurance, n.d.). Viewed by the general public, healthcare systems, and funding/licensing agencies as an essential component of high-quality healthcare (Berwick, 2015; Patient Protection and Affordable Care Act, 2010; Price et al., 2015), patient-centered care has been touted as a central aim for the nation's health system since 1999. It remains to be seen whether PCC persists as a health system ideal or becomes a real, tangible process that can facilitate individual and health system advancement.

> The Quality-Caring Model, with its emphasis on the caring (or healing) nature of relationships pertinent to health and illness, may offer some hope in the actual implementation of PCC, particularly in acute care settings. Its very nature is patient centered as it is founded on beliefs about the worth of human persons.

The QCM has well-defined assumptions and concepts that can be learned, measured, and improved. It is centered on patients and families, but speaks to health professionals' individual and collective relationships, which are necessary for quality care. The model proposes intermediate and terminal outcomes that might be tested, both in the practice setting and through more rigorous research. Furthermore, it can serve as a unifying approach in health systems in which individual health professionals are forever locked in their own worldview. For those organizations currently and consistently using this professional practice model, it has become an energizing force for sustainable change.

SUMMARY

The history of, characteristics of, and evidence for PCC are described and examined in relation to the current healthcare system. Elements of the QCM, specifically the concept of relationship-centered professional encounters, are compared to PCC and similarities are shown. The eight caring behaviors essential to relationship-centered professional encounters are defined and associated with specific behaviors and required knowledge. The caring relationships among patients and health professionals central to the QCM are linked to the reality of a true patient-centered health system.

> Call to Action
>
> PCC is a professional responsibility and a national directive. **Adopt** relationship-centered professional encounters (caring relationships) as the grounding approach for the delivery of PCC.

REFLECTIVE QUESTIONS/APPLICATIONS

. . . for Students

1. What is patient-centered care? Have you learned about it in your educational program?
2. Analyze the eight caring behaviors with respect to your ability to implement them in real patient settings.
3. Reflect on the evidence for patient-centered care. Can you summarize it?
4. Outline your plans to develop the caring behaviors in yourself. How will you know you have achieved competence?
5. How would you go about evaluating patient-centered care? Provide specific examples.

. . . for Professional Nurses in Clinical Practice

1. Discuss the delivery of authentic patient-centered care in your healthcare institution.
2. Is there an expectation that the caring behaviors are a significant component of an RN's work? If so, how are they evaluated?
3. Reflect on your profession. Is patient-centered care being practiced every day in every patient encounter? If not, what would it take to deliver it?
4. What health outcomes could be enhanced with the delivery of genuine patient-centered care in your institution?
5. What organizing framework or professional practice model ensures the delivery of patient-centered care on your unit? What are its essential components?
6. How do you hold yourself and fellow nurses accountable for the delivery of patient-centered care?

. . . for Professional Nurses in Educational Practice

1. What specific curricular revisions have you developed that address patient-centered care? What evidence did you use to shape them? What teaching/learning strategies will you use to help undergraduate and graduate students learn how to care?
2. Reflect on today's practice environments. How do you think your educational program helps graduates stay focused on relationship-centered professional encounters? In what specific ways does your

program build relational skills among the students? How do you know they are competent in these skills at graduation?

3. What are the necessary thinking patterns that will have to occur in undergraduate and graduate faculty in order to meet the challenges of patient-centered care?

4. How might you suggest using PCORI and its website to educate today's health professional students?

5. Examine Table 5.2. Provide some suggestions for teaching/learning strategies to meet the behavioral skills and knowledge requirements.

. . . for Professional Nurses in Leadership Practice

1. How has patient-centered care improved/worsened over the past 3 years at your institution?

2. How have you specifically articulated and championed patient-centered care at your institution? Is it working?

3. Reflect on the developmental activities in place at your institution. Do they include aspects of relationship building? How do you ensure that professionals are competent in caring relationships?

4. How is patient-centered care monitored and measured to revise practice at your institution? What could you do to enhance this process?

5. How do you help health professionals to stay focused on caring relationships as the central component of professional practice?

6. Does your leadership team embrace patient-centered care? If not, how will you deal with them?

7. Create a plan for dramatically altering RN work such that the patient is truly at the center. Who should be involved? What methodology would be used? How long would it take? What implications for RN practice would occur? How would you ensure that the plan is enacted as developed? How would you evaluate its implementation?

PRACTICE ANALYSIS

A 68-year-old African American woman, who was status post a hyperglycemic episode, went to the outpatient primary care facility for follow-up and medicine management. When she arrived, she was directed to fill out a few forms and wait in the waiting room. The room was decorated in bright colors with paintings on the wall and comfortable chairs. There were health magazines and pamphlets available on a variety of health-related concerns. The patient was told that she would be seen shortly and was offered something to drink while she waited. She was shown the bathroom and provided with an opportunity to verify her records.

After 10 minutes, a nurse practitioner (NP) approached the patient, introduced herself, and asked the patient to follow her to one of the rooms. Once inside, the NP sat down across from the patient, made eye contact, and explained that she would be treating her and wanted to learn a little more about her. The NP asked questions like "I understand you recently became hyperglycemic. Can you tell me how it is living with diabetes?" and "What is your normal day like?" The NP seemed at ease sitting close to the patient while writing her responses in the computer. The patient had a complete view of what the nurse was writing because the computer screen was near. The NP continued her questioning with "What do you want from this visit today?" and seemed genuinely interested in what the patient was saying. She asked a few follow-up questions, but allowed the patient to explain how her diabetes started and what she does to manage her illness. The patient expressed her fears about the long-term consequences of diabetes.

After a physical examination and inspection of recent laboratory values, the NP used her clinical judgment and recent evidence to adjust the patient's medications. Using a collaborative approach, the NP asked the patient, "Do you know what medication you currently take?" and then, "I think it might be best to increase the dosage of this medication to better control your blood sugar and prevent future hyperglycemic episodes." She showed the patient an article about the dosing of the particular medication. But the patient expressed concerns related to some of the side effects of the medication. After discussion, the patient and the NP came to a mutual agreement to increase the dosage a little and monitor the patient's HbA1c in 2 weeks. With that, the patient seemed willing to try this new regime. The NP then reviewed all the patient's medications with her and allowed her to ask questions. The NP shared that at the next visit she wanted to review the patient's diet and exercise plan and asked the patient to keep a log of her eating and exercise habits for the next 2 weeks. The patient agreed and appeared content as she left the clinic for home.

1. Did the NP practice PCC? How do you know?
2. How did the system (or context) of the primary care facility support the practice of PCC? Or did it?
3. What caring behaviors did the NP display? Should she have done something different?

REFERENCES

Audet, A. M., Davies, K., & Schoenbaum, S. C. (2006). Adoption of patient-centered care practices by physicians: Results from a national survey. *Archives of Internal Medicine, 166*(7), 754–759. doi:10.1001/archinte.166.7.754

Balint, E. (1969). The possibilities of patient-centered medicine. *Journal of the Royal College General Practitioners, 17*(82), 269–276.

Bartlett, E. E., Grayson, M., Barker, R., Levine, D. M., Golden, A., & Libber, S. (1984). The effects of physician communications skills on patient satisfaction, recall, and adherence. *Journal of Chronic Diseases, 37*(9–10), 755–764. doi:10.1016/0021-9681(84)90044-4

Beckman, H. B., Markakis, K. M., Suchman, A. L., & Frankel, R. M. (1994). The doctor-patient relationship and malpractice: Lessons from plaintiff depositions. *Archives of Internal Medicine, 154*(12), 1365–1370. doi:10.1001/archinte.1994.00420120093010

Bernabeo, E., & Holmboe, E. S. (2013). Patients, providers, and systems need to acquire a specific set of competencies to achieve truly patient-centered care. *Health Affairs, 32*(2), 250–258. doi:10.1377/hlthaff.2012.1120

Bertakis, K. D., & Azari, R. (2011). Patient-centered care is associated with decreased health care utilization. *Journal of the American Board of Family Medicine, 24*(3), 229–239. doi:10.3122/jabfm.2011.03.100170

Burt, K. (2007). The relationship between nurse caring and selected outcomes of care in hospitalized older adults (Doctoral dissertation). Retrieved from Dissertation Abstracts International (UMI No. 3257620).

Conway, J., Johnson, B., Edgman-Levitan, S., Schlucter, J., Ford, D., Sodomka, P., & Simmon, L. (2006). *Partnering with patients and families to design a patient and family-centered health system: A roadmap for the future, A work in progress.* Bethesda, MD: Institute for Family-Centered Care.

Cooper, L. A., Roter, D. L., Bone, L. R., Larson, S. M., Miller, E. R., Barr, M. S., . . . Levine, D. M. (2009). A randomized controlled trial of interventions to enhance patient-physician partnership, patient adherence and high blood pressure control among ethnic minorities and poor persons: Study protocol NCT00123045. *Implementation Science, 4,* 7. doi:10.1186/1748-5908-4-7

Davies, E., & Cleary, P. D. (2005). Hearing the patient's voice? Factors affecting the use of patient survey data in quality improvement. *BMJ Quality and Safety, 14,* 428–432. doi:10.1136/qshc.2004.012955

Detsky, A. S. (2011). What patients really want from health care. *Journal of the American Medical Association, 306*(22), 2500–2501. doi:10.1001/jama.2011.1819

Dunn, N. (2003). Practical issues around putting the patient at the centre of care. *Journal of the Royal Society of Medicine, 96,* 325–327. Retrieved from https://www.ncbi.nlm.nih.gov/pmc/articles/PMC539534

Entwistle, V. A., & Watt, I. S. (2013). Treating patients as persons: A capabilities approach to support delivery of person-centered care. *The American Journal of Bioethics, 13*(8), 29–39. doi:10.1080/15265161.2013.802060

Epstein, R. M., Duberstein, P. R., Fenton, J. J., Fiscella, K., Hoerger, M., Tancredi, D. J., . . . Kravitz, R. L. (2017). Effect of a patient-centered communication intervention on oncologist-patient communication, quality of life, and health care utilization in advanced cancer: The VOICE randomized clinical trial. *JAMA Oncology, 3*(1), 92–100. doi:10.1001/jamaoncol.2016.4373

Epstein, R. M., Fiscella, K., Lesser, C. S., & Stange, K. C. (2010). Why the nation needs a policy push on patient-centered health care. *Health Affairs, 29*(8), 1489–1495. doi:10.1377/hlthaff.2009.0888

Epstein, R. M., Franks, P., Fiscella, K., Shields, C. G., Meldrum, S. C., Kravitz, R. L., & Duberstein, P. R. (2005). Measuring patient-centered communication in patient-physician consultations: Theoretical and practical issues. *Social Science and Medicine, 61*(7), 1516–1528. doi:10.1016/j.socscimed.2005.02.001

Epstein, R. M., & Street, R. L. (2011). The value and values of patient-centered care. *Annals of Family Medicine, 9*(2), 100–103. doi:10.1370/afm.1239

Fights, S. (2012). Do we really provide patient-centered care? *MedSurg Nursing, 21*(1), 5–6.

Fremont, A. M., Cleary, P. D., Hargrames, J. L., Rowe, R. M., Jacobson, N. B., & Ayanian, J. Z. (2001). Patient centered processes of care and long term outcomes of myocardial infarction. *Journal of General Internal Medicine, 16*(12), 800–808. doi:10.1046/j.1525-1497.2001.10102.x

Gazarian, P. K., Morrison, C. R., Lehmann, L. S., Tamir, O., Bates, D. W., & Rozenblum, R. (2017). Patients' and care partners' perspectives on dignity and respect during acute care hospitalization. *Journal of Patient Safety.* ePub ahead of print. doi:10.1097/PTS.0000000000000353

Gerteis, M. (1993). Coordinating care and integrating services. In M. Gerteis, S. Edgman-Levitan, J. Daley, & T. L. Delbanco (Eds.), *Through the patient's eyes: Understanding and promoting patient-centered care* (pp. 45–71). San Francisco, CA: Jossey-Bass.

Gillespie, R., Florin, D., & Gillam, S. (2004). How is patient-centered care understood by the clinical, managerial and lay stakeholders responsible for promoting this agenda? *Health Expectations, 7*(2), 142–148. doi:10.1111/j.1369-7625.2004.00264.x

Gittell, J. H., Fairfield, K. M., Bierbaum, B., Head, W., Jackson, R., Kelly, M., . . . Zuckerman, J. (2000). Impact of relational coordination on quality of care, postoperative pain and functioning, and length of stay: A nine-hospital study of surgical patients. *Medical Care, 38*(8), 807–819. Retrieved from http://ipls.dk/pdf-filer/gittell_2000.pdf

Greenfield, S., Kaplan, S. H., Ware, J. E., Jr., Yano, E. M., & Frank, H. J. (1988). Patients' participation in medical care: Effects on blood sugar control and quality of life in diabetes. *Journal of General Internal Medicine, 3*(5), 448–457. doi:10.1007/BF02595921

Hack, T. F., Degner, L. F., Watson, P., & Sinha, L. (2006). Do patients benefit from participating in medical decision making? Longitudinal follow-up of women with breast cancer. *Psycho-Oncology, 15*(1), 9–19. doi:10.1002/pon.907

Hobbs, J. L. (2009). A dimensional analysis of patient-centered care. *Nursing Research, 58*, 52–62. doi:10.1097/NNR.0b013e31818c3e79

Horwitz, R. I., Viscoli C. M., Berkman, L., Donaldson, R. M., Horwitz, S. M., Murray, C. J., . . . Sindelar, J. (1990). Treatment adherence and risk of death after a myocardial infarction. *Lancet, 336*, 542–545. doi:10.1016/0140-6736(90)92095-Y

Hudon, C., Fortin, M., Haggerty, J. L., Lambert, M., & Poitras, M. E. (2011). Measuring patients' perceptions of patient-centered care: A systematic review of tools for family medicine. *Annals of Family Medicine, 9*(2), 155–164. doi:10.1370/afm.1226

Institute of Medicine. (2001). *Crossing the quality chasm: A new health system for the 21st century.* Washington, DC: National Academies Press.

Jutterström, L., Hörnsten, Å., Sandström, H., Stenlund, H., & Isaksson, U. (2016). Nurse-led patient-centered self-management support improves HbA1c in patients with type 2 diabetes—A randomized study. *Patient Education and Counseling, 99*(11), 1821–1829. doi:10.1016/j.pec.2016.06.016

Kaba R., & Sooriakumaran, P. (2007). The evolution of the doctor–patient relationship. *International Journal of Surgery, 5*(1), 57–65. doi:10.1016/j.ijsu.2006.01.005

Kaplan, S. H., Greenfield, S., & Ware, J. E. (1989). Assessing the effects of physician-patient interactions on the outcomes of chronic disease. *Medical Care, 27*(7), S110–S127. doi:10.1097/00005650-198903001-00010

Kizer, K. W. (2002). Patient centred care: Essential but probably not sufficient. *Quality and Safety in Health Care, 11*, 117–118. doi:10.1136/qhc.11.2.117

Latham, C. P. (1996). Predictors of patient outcomes following interactions with nurses. *Western Journal of Nursing Research, 18*(5), 548–564. doi:10.1177/019394599601800506

Lewin, S., Skea, Z., Entwistle, V. A., Zwarenstein, M., & Dick, J. (2009). Interventions for providers to promote a patient-centered approach in clinical consultations (Review). *The Cochrane Collaboration, 3.* doi:10.1002/14651858 .CD003267

Lipkin, M., Quill, T. E., & Napodano, R. J. (1984). The medical interview: A core curriculum for residencies in internal medicine. *Annals of Internal Medicine, 100*(2), 277–284. doi:10.7326/0003-4819-100-2-277

Lowes, R. (1998). Patient centeredness for better patient adherence. *Family Practice Management, 51*(5), 46–47. Retrieved from https://www.aafp.org/ fpm/1998/0300/p46.html

Mazor, K. M., Smith, K. M., Fisher, K. A., & Gallagher, T. H. (2016). Speak Up! addressing the paradox plaguing patient-centered care. *Annals of Internal Medicine, 164*(9), 618–619. doi:10.7326/M15-2416

Mead, N., & Bower, P. (2000). The evolution of the doctor-patient relationship. *International Journal of Surgery, 5*(1), 57–65. doi:10.1016/j.ijsu.2006.01.005

Meterki, M., Wright, S., Lin, H., Lowy, E., & Cleary, P. D. (2010). Mortality among patients with acute myocardial infarction: The influences of patient centered care and evidence-based medicine. *Health Services Research, 45*(5), 1188–1204. doi: 10.1111/j.1475-6773.2010.01138.x

Mezey, M., Kobayashi, M., Grossman, S., Firpo, A., Fulmer, T., & Mitty, E. (2004). Nurses improving care to health system elders (NICHE): Implementation of best practice models. *Journal of Nursing Administration, 34*(10), 451–457. doi:10.1097/00005110-200410000-00005

Mitchell, P. (2008). Patient-centered care—A new focus on a time-honored concept. *Nursing Outlook, 56*(5), 197–198. doi:10.1016/j.outlook.2008.08.001

National Committee for Quality Assurance. (n.d.). Patient-centered medical home (PCMH) recognition. Retrieved from http://www.ncqa.org/programs/recognition/practices/patient-centered-medical-home-pcmh

Naylor, M. D., Brooten, D., Campbell, R., Jacobsen, B. S., Nezey, M. D., Pauly, M. V., & Schwartz, J. S. (1999). Comprehensive discharge planning and home follow-up of hospitalized elders: A random clinical trial. *Journal of the American Medical Association, 281*(7), 613–620. doi:10.1001/jama.281.7.613

Patient-Centered Outcomes Research Institute. (2017). PCORnet: The National Patient-Centered Clinical Research Network. Retrieved from http://www.pcori .org/research-results/pcornet-national-patient-centered-clinical-research-network

Patient Protection and Affordable Care Act, Pub. L. No. 111-148, 124 Stat. 119. (2010). Retrieved from http://www.gpo.gov/fdsys/pkg/PLAW-111publ148/pdf/PLAW-111publ148.pdf

Price, R. A., Elliott, M. N., Cleary, P. D., Zaslavsky, A. M., & Hays, R. D. (2015). Should health care providers be accountable for patients' care experiences? *Journal of General Internal Medicine, 30*(2), 253–256. doi:10.1007/s11606-014-3111-7

Quality and Safety Education for Nurses. (2012). Graduate QSEN competencies. Retrieved from http://qsen.org/competencies/graduate-ksas/

Radwin, L. E. (2003). Cancer patients' demographic characteristics and ratings of patient-centered nursing care. *Journal of Nursing Scholarship, 35*(4), 365–370. doi:10.1111/j.1547-5069.2003.00365.x

Radwin, L. E., Cabral, H. J., & Wilkes, G. (2009). Relationships between patient-centered cancer nursing interventions and desired health outcomes in the context of the health care system. *Research in Nursing and Health, 32*, 4–17. doi:10.1002/nur.20302

Schall, M., Sevin, C., & Wasson, J. H. (2009). Making high-quality patient-centered care a reality. *Journal of Ambulatory Care Management, 32*(1), 3–7. doi:10.1097/01. JAC.0000343118.23091.8a

Shaller, D. (2007). Patient-centered care: What does it take? *The Commonwealth Fund.* Retrieved from http://www.commonwealthfund.org/usr_doc/Shaller_patient-centeredcarewhatdoesittake_1067.pdf

Sidani, S., & Fox, M. (2014). Patient-centered care: Clarification of its specific elements to facilitate interprofessional care. *Journal of Interprofessional Care, 28*(2), 134–141. doi:10.3109/13561820.2013.862519

Sokol-Hessner, L., Folcarelli, P. H., & Sands, K. E. (2015). Emotional harm from disrespect: The neglected preventable harm. *BMJ Quality & Safety, 24*, 550–553. doi:10.1136/bmjqs-2015-004034

Stempniak, M. (2015). Don Berwick Offers Health Care 9 Steps to End Era of "Complex Incentives" and "Excessive Measurement." *Hospitals & Health Networks.* Retrieved from http://www.hhnmag.com/articles/6798-don-berwick-offers-health-care-9-steps-to-transform-health-care

Stewart, M., Brown, J. B., Donner, A., McWinney, I., Oates, J., Weston, W. W., & Jordan, J. (2000). The impact of patient-centered care on outcomes. *Journal of*

Family Practice, 49(9), 796–804. Retrieved from https://www.mdedge.com/jfponline/article/60893/impact-patient-centered-care-outcomes

Stewart, M., Brown, J. B., Weston, W. W., & Freeman, T. R. (2003). *Patient-centered medicine: Transforming the clinical method* (2nd ed.). Oxford, UK: Radcliffe Medical Press.

Swan, B. A. (1998). Postoperative nursing care contributions to symptom distress and functional status after ambulatory surgery. *MedSurg Nursing, 7*, 148–158.

Tresolini, C., & The Pew-Fetzer Task Force. (1994). *Health professions education and relationship-centered care*. San Francisco, CA: Pew Health Foundations Communication.

Wagner, E. H. (1998). Chronic disease management: What will it take to improve practice? *Effective Clinical Practice, 1*(1), 2–4. Retrieved from https://ecp.acponline.org/augsep98/cdm.pdf

Wasson, J. (2017). A troubled asset relief program for the patient-centered medical home. *Journal of Ambulatory Care Management, 40*(2), 89–100. doi:10.1097/JAC.0000000000000180

Wasson, J. H., & Baker, N. J. (2009). Balanced measures for patient-centered care. *Journal of Ambulatory Care Management, 32*(1), 44–55. doi:10.1097/01.JAC.0000343123.53585.51

Wasson, J. H., Johnson, D., Benjamin, R., Phillips, J., & MacKenzie, T. A. (2006). Patients report positive impacts of collaborative care. *Journal of Ambulatory Care Management, 29*(3), 199–206. Retrieved from https://journals.lww.com/ambulatorycaremanagement/Abstract/2006/07000/Patients_Report_Positive_Impacts_of_Collaborative.4.aspx

Weissman, J. S., Millenson, M. L., & Haring, R. S. (2017). Patient-centered care: Turning the rhetoric into reality. *The American Journal of Managed Care, 23*(1), e31–e32. Retrieved from http://www.ajmc.com/journals/issue/2017/2017-vol23-n1/patient-centered-care-turning-the-rhetoric-into-reality

Wen, L. S., & Tucker, S. (2015). What do people want from their health care? A qualitative study. *Journal of Participatory Medicine, 7*, e10. Retrieved from https://participatorymedicine.org/journal/evidence/research/2015/06/25/what-do-people-want-from-their-health-care-a-qualitative-study

West, E., Barron, D. N., & Reeves, R. (2005). Overcoming the barriers to patient-centered care: Time, tools, and training. *Issues in Clinical Nursing, 14*, 435–443. doi:10.1111/j.1365-2702.2004.01091.x

Winn, K., Ozanne, E., & Sepucha, K. (2015). Measuring patient-centered care: An updated systematic review of how studies define and report concordance between patients' preferences and medical treatments. *Patient Education and Counseling, 98*(7), 811–821. doi:10.1016/j.pec.2015.03.012

Wolf, Z. R., Colahan, M., & Costello, A. (1998). Relationship between nurse caring and patient satisfaction. *MedSurg Nursing, 7*(2), 99–105.

Yeakel, S., Maljanian, R., Bohannon, R., & Coulombe, K. (2003). Nurse caring behaviors and patient satisfaction: Improvement after a multifaceted staff intervention. *Journal of Nursing Administration, 33*(9), 434–436. doi:10.1097/00005110-200309000-00002

6

Relational Capacity

We all have ability. The difference is how we use it.
—Charlotte Whitten

THE MEANING OF RELATIONAL CAPACITY

Relational capacity in simple terms refers to the ability to relate. More specifically, however, relational capacity includes an individual's, a group of individuals' (a healthcare team), a department's, or the organization's ability to continuously engage people in high-quality connections (see Figure 6.1). It includes various individual and collective factors that together contribute to organizational relational capacity. Relational capacity from whatever stance is increasingly seen as a needed strength in this era of transformational change in healthcare. Relational capacity in complex health systems is especially crucial to attain visions and complete missions, to implement lasting change, and to self-advance.

The development of healthy, creative relationships is a dynamic social process that is by nature self-advancing. People tend to relate to and engage with those who are amiable and who share useful information that is other-focused. Furthermore, relational capacity involves trust and responses that are interesting and appealing versus those that are flat or off-putting. Relationship capacity can be thought of on an individual level, team or department level, and organizational levels (see Figure 6.2).

FIGURE 6.1 Organizational relational capacity.

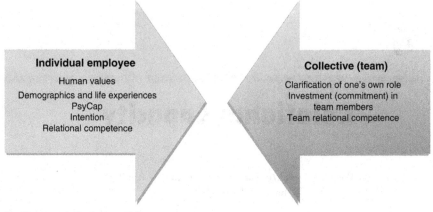

Individual employee
Human values
Demographics and life experiences
PsyCap
Intention
Relational competence

Collective (team)
Clarification of one's own role
Investment (commitment) in
team members
Team relational competence

PsyCap, psychological capital.

FIGURE 6.2 Levels of relational capacity in complex health systems.

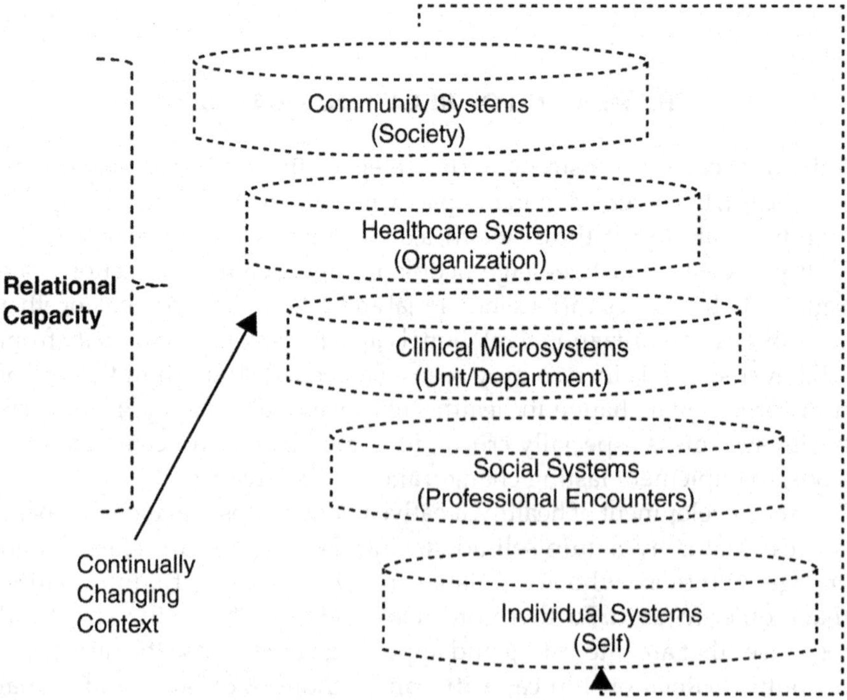

Community Systems
(Society)

Healthcare Systems
(Organization)

**Relational
Capacity**

Clinical Microsystems
(Unit/Department)

Social Systems
(Professional Encounters)

Continually
Changing
Context

Individual Systems
(Self)

INDIVIDUAL RELATIONAL CAPACITY

Obviously, relational capacity varies by individual on a continuum from those who are overwhelmed by or simply cannot connect to others and those who are actively engaged in high-quality relationships. In nursing, modes of being (or caring) with another were well explained by Haldorsdottir (1991) as extending from life-giving or biogenic (caring) on the one hand to life-destroying or biocidic on the other (uncaring). Sandwiched between these two extremes are the categories of life sustaining (bioactive), life neutral (biopassive), and life restraining (biostatic).

At the extreme biocidic end of the spectrum, relationships between patients and nurses were described as depersonalized, distressful, cold, and characterized as robbing joy from patients. At the other biogenic extreme, relationships between patients and nurses were affirming, protective, warm, and growth producing. It is these life-giving relationships that were described as professional, creating the ideal conditions for healing or goal attainment.

To effectively relate, one must consider the individual traits of human values, life experiences and demographics, psychological characteristics (psychological capital [PsyCap]), the intention to relate, and the competence required to relate. Certainly, one's values or belief systems impact the ability to relate. Schwartz's (1994, 2006, 2011, 2012) theory of basic human values suggests that one's dormant or unexpressed values and beliefs guide behavior. More specifically, one's values are abstract and tend to be tied to emotions, not objective facts; thus they are difficult to pinpoint, vary among individuals, and are not necessarily tied to reality. Values provide a motivational aspect as they frequently are attached to individuals' desired goals. As such, values guide our evaluations of people, behaviors, and events, and are ordered in importance. In essence, values serve as guiding principles that direct one's behavior (Schwartz, 2012).

Schwartz has defined 10 motivational values that guide people's behavior and contends that they overlap and compete with each other (see Table 6.1). For example, the power to achieve value (pursuit of self-interests) may conflict with the benevolence value (concern for the welfare and interests of others) at a point in time, impacting behaviors or attitudes tied to high-quality relationships.

Typically, people's demographics and life circumstances or experiences shape the priority attached to their values. For example, a person's age or generation, and his or her education and family structure, will influence to a large extent his or her view of the world and will affect potential behaviors. According to Schwartz and Bardi (1997), changing life experiences influence persons to upgrade the importance attributed to values they can readily attain and downgrade the importance of those whose

TABLE 6.1   Schwartz's Motivational Human Values

Universalism
Benevolence
Conformity
Security
Power
Stimulation
Achievement
Self-direction
Tradition
Hedonism

Source: Adapted from Schwartz, S. H. (1994). Are there universal aspects in the structure and contents of human values? *Journal of Social Issues, 50*, 33. doi:10.1111/j.1540-4560.1994 .tb01196.x

pursuit is blocked. However, this relationship changes when considering the power and security values; when they are easily attained, their importance drops. For example, people who suffer economic hardship and social upheaval attribute more importance to power and security values than those who live in relative comfort and safety (Inglehart, 1997).

In summary, people's age, education, gender, and other characteristics largely determine the life circumstances to which they are exposed. These include their family dynamics, socialization and learning experiences, the social roles they play, the culture they are born into, expectations and sanctions they encounter, and the abilities they develop. Thus, differences in background characteristics represent differences in the life circumstances that ultimately influence the value placed on various priorities (Schwartz, 2011).

The psychological state of individuals, particularly those who exhibit the positive characteristics of hope, resilience, optimism, and self-efficacy, termed *psychological capital*, was first labeled as an important construct by Luthans and Youssef (2004). In their important contributions to human strengths in the workplace, most often identified as *positive psychology*, Luthans defined PsyCap as "a core psychological factor of positivity in general, and . . . the investment/development of 'who you are'" (Luthans, Avolio, Walumbwa, & Li, 2005, p. 253). The four characteristics of PsyCap are considered resources that individually and collectively impact performance (Luthans, 2005; Luthans & Youssef, 2007; Luthans & Youssef-Morgan, 2017).

The characteristic of *optimism* refers to positive acknowledgment of one's immediate and future success. The characteristic of *resiliency* is defined as "when beset by problems and adversity, sustaining and bouncing back and even beyond (resilience) to attain success" (Luthans, Youssef, & Avolio, 2007, p. 3). The concept of *hope* is derived from the work of Snyder (2000), who reported that hope is a multidimensional construct composed of both an individual's determination to set and maintain effort toward goals (described as *willpower* or *agency*) and that individual's ability to discern alternative courses of action to attain those goals (described as *way power* or *pathways thinking*). Finally, as defined by well-known research psychologist Bandura (1997), *self-efficacy* refers to people's convictions about their own capacity for successfully executing a course of action that leads to a desired outcome. Bandura has argued that if adequate levels of ability and motivation exist, self-efficacy will impact an individual's decision to perform a specific task and his or her level of persistence in performing that task despite problems, disconfirming evidence, and even adversity. Weak efficacy beliefs can contribute to behavior avoidance and anxiety, whereas strong efficacy beliefs can promote behavior initiation and persistence.

The concepts of self-efficacy, optimism, hope, and resiliency have been incorporated in an operational definition of the construct PsyCap, and when combined have a synergistic effect. Specifically, researchers have found that PsyCap is a core construct that predicts performance and satisfaction better than any of the individual strengths that make it up (Luthans et al., 2005; Luthans, Avey, Avolio, & Peterson, 2010; Luthans, Norman, Avolio, & Avey, 2008). Using the valid and reliable measure of PsyCap (Psychological Capital Questionnaire [PCQ]; Luthans et al., 2007), a recent meta-analysis including a total of 12,567 employees found the expected significant positive relationships between PsyCap and desirable employee attitudes (job satisfaction, organizational commitment, psychological well-being), desirable employee behaviors (citizenship), and multiple measures of performance (self, supervisor evaluations, and objective measures of performance). There was also a significant negative relationship between PsyCap and undesirable employee attitudes (cynicism, turnover intentions, job stress, and anxiety) and undesirable employee behaviors (deviance). Additionally, no major differences were observed between the types of performance measures used (i.e., between self, subjective, and objective; Avey, Reichard, Luthans, & Mhatre, 2011).

PsyCap can now be measured using a short form (PCQ-12; Avey et al., 2011) that has the advantage of decreased burden and applicability across cultures. As an individual resource, PsyCap can change over time and be developed through training interventions. Importantly, overall PsyCap is correlated with satisfaction and investment in relationships (Luthans & Youssef-Morgan, 2017).

More recently, Heled, Somach, and Waters (2016) studied team PsyCap. Their findings included a positive relationship between the team's PsyCap and the individual employee's job satisfaction and the team's organizational citizenship behavior (OCB). These findings are important for healthcare work environments where implications for team-based care on individual employee job satisfaction may provide leaders with new information that could drive practice changes. Finally, conceptualizing PsyCap at the organizational level is emerging as a potential factor of optimistic organizations, based on cultures of hope (Luthans & Youssef-Morgan, 2017). Thus, based on the emerging evidence, PsyCap is a strong component of relationship capacity that can be leveraged in organizations.

Intention refers to purposeful actions performed to achieve immediate outcomes and future goals. Husserl (1980) identified intention as a phenomenological trait that characterizes a mental state or experience as being "directed toward something." Intention in its simplest form was defined more precisely as a thinking–feeling response that motivates action (Anscombe, 1957/1963). According to Anscombe, the basic building blocks of intention are an identified reason to act, the desire to act, and consideration for the feasibility of acting, all of which converge to form an intention (or choice) to achieve attainable and beneficial goals.

Thus, the intention to relate (or connect) is a combination of individuals' awareness of a reason to act, the resulting desire it influences, the feasibility of an identified set of actions, and finally the choice to act. This combination of factors is a process of thinking and feeling that is subjective in nature and results in a conscious (fully aware) choice to relate.

Perugini and Bagozzi (2004) differentiated intention from desire through two studies. They found that desires are more abstract, less feasible, and less connected to action, whereas intention is related to action and behavior. However, these analyses did point to the fact that desire is an important predictor of intention. In relational terms, one may desire to spend time with others, but the final intention (choice to relate) and perhaps the resultant behavior may vacillate or not occur at all.

Dossey and Keegan (2009) defined intention as "the conscious determination to do a specific thing or to act in a specific manner; the mental state of being committed to, planning to, or trying to perform an action" (p. 21). Intention is behaviorally oriented and is not to be confused with the term *intentionality*. Intentionality refers to a state of being or one's whole frame of reference at a point in time. It signifies a deep or a grounding dimension that sets the stage for *how* one directs his or her thoughts. Acting with intention (relational intention) is enhanced when one is fully aware, purposeful, and centered (see Figure 6.3). Associated

FIGURE 6.3 Caring intention.

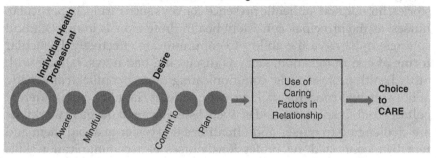

behaviors become more authentic, even reverent. Relational intention is apparent when behavior is positively directed toward the other using the caring factors to initiate, cultivate, and sustain relationships.

Competence refers to one's knowledge, skills, and abilities, but in this case, relational competence is defined as the individual's knowledge, skills, and attitudes for facilitating the acquisition, development, and maintenance of mutually satisfying social relationships (Carpenter, Hansson, Rountree, & Jones, 1983). This ability to move toward another, to develop mutuality, staying open, even enjoying the experience, is a necessary component of relational capacity. According to Carpenter et al. (1983), relational competence consists of five dimensions that predispose individuals to *initiate* relationships and five dimensions that help *enhance* or *maintain* those relationships over time. Initiation skills are assertiveness, dominance (the desire and ability to be in charge of one's own situation and to engage in leadership), and independence and belief in one's ability to relate (Carpenter, 1993). Shyness and social anxiety were seen as factors that were detrimental to initiating relationships. Maintenance factors were intimacy (tendency toward helping and support), ability to trust, interpersonal sensitivity, altruism, and perspective taking (ability to see all sides of an issue). These factors are aligned with the caring behaviors or processes described in Chapter 3 and are often at least superficially dealt with as part of health professional curricula. Proficiency in their use is essential if relational competence is to flourish. Nurses, in particular, are known for the maintenance factors, but assertiveness, dominance, and beliefs about one's abilities to relate are not necessarily discussed, learned, or evaluated.

Communication skills are also considered fundamental dimensions of relational competence. In fact, the majority of activities in health systems involve communication, often among individuals who are not well known to each other. Effective communication begins with caring about the way a message is delivered and caring about the people whom you engage in dialogue (Hertz, 2015). Using simple explanations, personal stories, humor, and authentic presence conveys such caring. In particular, nurses, as the principal, consistent health professionals in most clinical settings, must have the ability to communicate effectively. Particular forms of communication, such as discussing bad news, talking with other health professionals, communicating during conflict, conversing about spiritual concerns, talking with patients/families from different cultures, public speaking, and actively listening amid the busy workflow are challenging to nurses and oftentimes it is easier to avoid them and remain unconnected. Yet, professional nurses learn communication skills such as questioning, reframing, clarifying, using open-ended questions, demonstrating cultural sensitivity, and specialized techniques for communicating with those who cannot actively interact (such as those who are comatose, psychologically impaired, or under the influence of medications). Using these in everyday practice builds trust and teamwork, strengthening relational competence.

COLLECTIVE RELATIONAL CAPACITY (TEAM CARING)

The healthcare needs of today's public demand specialized skills requiring groups of health professionals working together in the best interests of patients and families. For example, patients with diabetes often have problems with chronic overweight and obesity, heart disease, and frequently need assistance with behavioral changes (American Diabetes Association, n.d.). The comprehensive care of patients with diabetes, therefore, is often best met through teams of dietitians, nurses, endocrinologists, cardiologists, primary care physicians, psychology professionals, and others who work together to help the patient meet his or her health goals. Regular interaction among these professionals is not enough; rather, "effective health care teams share common goals, understand each other's roles, demonstrate respect for each other, use clear communication, resolve conflict effectively, and are flexible" (Grumbach & Bodenheimer, 2004, p. 1246). Thus, groups of health professionals who relate in a caring, collaborative manner (team caring) contribute to health organizations and positive patient outcomes (see Chapter 4).

However, situating a discipline such as nursing *within* the interprofessional team with respect to daily processes of care requires clarification of one's own role as a member of the interprofessional team. This way, nurses are able to appreciate their unique contribution as well as those of the other team members. In fact, as interprofessional practice evolves toward the norm in health systems, nurses should be able to demonstrate the significance of their unique perspective and skill sets for different patient populations. Just as relationships with patients and families take time, so do relationships with team members. Investing in team members in terms of committing to ongoing interactions that reach the levels of connection and knowing (Duffy, 2003) is key.

Nurses, however, have documented problems relating to *each other* with known instances of intimidating and disruptive behaviors (Monteau, 2017). Disruptive behaviors include bullying, lateral violence, and verbal abuse. Such factors have been linked to problems in nursing recruitment, turnover, and retention. However, findings from research suggest that the consequences of disruptive behavior go far beyond nurses' job satisfaction and morale, and affect the health of the work environment, including interprofessional collaboration, which may well, in turn, have a negative impact on clinical outcomes, including safety (Houck & Colbert, 2017; The Joint Commission, 2008; Schultz, 2017).

Inadequate professional collaboration among health professionals may cause much distress for patients and their families, who often want consistent information and a sense of certainty about their diagnosis and treatment alternatives. Additionally, relational difficulties among clinicians may impede the recruitment of patients to clinical trials, cause confusion about courses of action, and create a loss of confidence in the team's ability to meet patient needs.

Consider the following:

Kelly is a recent baccalaureate graduate who is working her first job on an orthopedic floor of a general community hospital. One of her patients, Mrs. Powers, a 58-year-old White female, is experiencing newly developed shortness of breath postop day 2 after a total knee replacement. Kelly becomes concerned and calls the orthopedic surgeon to report Mrs. Powers' status change. She becomes nervous on the phone and cannot deliver a clear, concise report. The physician becomes irritated, and asks for detailed information (lab results, lung sounds) that Kelly cannot produce. He finally tells her to call him back "when she can do her job thoroughly and has her information straight."

Kelly, visibly shaken by this encounter, approaches an experienced nurse, Joan, to ask for help. Kelly is inexperienced in assessments and the possible complications of knee surgery and feels dispirited after the phone conversation with the physician. Joan, who is busy with her own patients, does not appreciate the meaning of this experience for Kelly and dismisses her concerns saying, "You will have to wait—I am up to my eyeballs with this patient." Under her breath, she says, "I don't get these new baccalaureate grads—you'd think that after 4 years, they could listen to a few lung sounds, check lab results, and call a physician. I am so sick of doing their job for them."

Kelly walks away and does her own assessment, this time listening for lung sounds and checking the chart for lab results. Nothing seems amiss. Mrs. Powers' shortness of breath is abating and Kelly attributes the whole episode to her own lack of experience. She calls the physician back and reports that everything seems okay now.

Two hours later, Mrs. Powers' shortness of breath returned but it was worse and she needed to sit straight up in bed to catch her breath. She looked sweaty and a little off color as well. Kelly called another senior nurse (Mary) who came into the room took down the patient's bedclothes and examined both legs. The one unaffected by the surgery was swollen and slightly reddened. Mary assessed Mrs. Powers' lungs and applied oxygen all the while explaining to Kelly what she was doing. Simultaneously, she reassured Mrs. Powers, who was getting more and more upset. Convinced that the patient was stable for the immediate future, Mary took Kelly out- side the room and explained what was going on, why she did what she did, and then she coached Kelly on what to say and how to convey her concerns (organize her thoughts) during the subsequent phone call to the physician. She allowed Kelly to "teach back" her report and then stayed with her during the phone call. This conversation went a little smoother and the physician ordered some blood work and a CT scan and assured Kelly she would be there soon. After the call, Mary reviewed the entire experience with Kelly, offering further advice on complete assessments and complications after orthopedic surgery.

This case is typical, particularly during summer months, when new nurses take their first positions after graduation. Can you characterize the type of behaviors used by Joan, the experienced nurse, and by the physician in the beginning of the case? How do you think they con- tributed to Kelly's sense of efficacy as a nurse or her desire to remain employed on that unit? How did they contribute to the patient's sense of safety or confidence in her recovery? The second nurse, Mary, was also busy, but understood the importance of this "teaching moment" and used her caring knowledge, skills, and attitudes to relate profes- sionally to Kelly, the patient, and the physician, all the while keeping her focus on "what's best for the patient." She role-modeled certain behaviors, relayed information, reassured the patient, and allowed Kelly to ask questions and practice her reporting skills—Mary under- stood her unique role as an experienced nurse on this team. She also invested in Kelly by supporting her during the conversation and mak- ing time for her.

Or reflect on this account in which a senior nurse was "floated" to help on another unit, a typical anxiety-provoking situation in nursing:

> *It is customary in this health system for nurses working on the inpatient hospice unit to provide support and expertise with subcutaneous access ports in patients who are housed on other units. On the day shift in such an organization, the hospice unit was called to provide a routine flush for an access port in a patient on a medical–surgical unit. An experienced hospice nurse went to the unit in another building. Upon arrival, she introduced herself to the unit secretary, told her why she was there and asked her to find the charge nurse, so she could find out who the patient was and where supplies and equipment were kept. The charge nurse responded that she was busy with another patient and the hospice nurse would have to wait about 10 minutes. Fifteen minutes later, the charge nurse still was not available, leaving the hospice nurse unaware of the patient, or where to find the sup-plies for the procedure. Finally, when the charge nurse became available, she said it was the patient in bed 79B, leaving the hospice nurse to fetch the supplies—an uncomfortable situation since she did not know the unit. She went about collecting the necessary equipment rather haphazardly and performed the flush as requested, documented it, and told the secretary she had finished. The whole episode took far longer than an hour.*
>
> *Two weeks later she was asked to do the same procedure, and when she arrived on the unit, a licensed practical nurse (LPN) greeted her, took her to see the patient, and helped collect the needed supplies; then she stayed and assisted. It was an easy and efficient experience that lasted 20 minutes.*

For an expert nurse providing services in an unknown unit, the first incident was unpleasant and inefficient; in the second incident, the LPN collaborated with the hospice nurse, contributing to an efficient and pleas-ant work experience. The LPN used her relationship skills to affirm the hospice nurse, facilitating a calm experience, and an efficient procedure. It is no wonder that many nurses don't like to "float"!

In addition to understanding one's role and working hard to generate quality relationships on an interprofessional team, a third aspect of col-lective relational competence is the teams' shared relational competence. Earlier in this chapter, relational competence was described in terms of initiation and maintenance of relationships. The senior nurse, Mary, in the previous example, exuded relational competence. She was assertive yet caring, dominant (understood and exercised her leadership role in this situation), and confident (viewed herself as able). Mary also understood the work or had a strong knowledge base in the care of postop orthopedic patients and communicated well, imparting information, supporting the new nurse, and soliciting feedback. Thus, effective relational capacity in health teams consists of clarification of one's individual role as a contributing member of a team, investment in each team member, and collective relational competence (see Figure 6.1).

> Relational competence is the glue that holds a health team together and ensures its success in meeting patient and team member needs. It helps ease friction during conflict, calm difficult personalities, persuade, soften the sadness of disappointing moments, and, most important, guarantees that the team's work is focused on the patient and family.

Interprofessional teams can function for a short while without relational capacity, but eventually they will break down and unknowingly distress team members and potentially place patients in jeopardy. Individual health professionals depend on their larger and multidisciplined work group for support in handling the hard relational work that is central to healthcare. In such teams, members trust each other, hold productive mini-meetings (called *rounds* in healthcare), have fun together, feel safe and acknowledged—overall they use collective relational capacity to get the work done. The more an interprofessional work group is conscious of itself as a collective that serves important functions in supporting the individual work of its members, the more successful that group will be in its overall role of meeting the health needs of patients and families, and, by default, health systems.

ORGANIZATIONAL RELATIONAL CAPACITY

In health systems, relational capacity is a meaningful asset that is based on developing, cultivating, and sustaining high-quality individual and collective relationships. It can be further described to include external organizations or work groups that influence or impact the business of healthcare, including customers, suppliers, employees, accrediting organizations, governments (including international), partners, other stakeholders, and, sometimes, even competitors. Health systems with relational capacity often have wide networks of relationships with others who impact healthcare and healthy ties with all of its key stakeholders. This relational strength, if nurtured and allowed to emerge, is naturally self-advancing, directly impacting performance.

In health systems, it is relationships that drive the work. Relationships people have with their peers, their bosses, their patients, families, and even the organization, all impact the quality and costs of services provided. Relationships are commonplace in health services and oftentimes they are so implicit that they go unnoticed. For example, despite the fact that health professionals spend the majority of their time "relating," this is not routinely acknowledged, studied, or attended to. At the core of organizations, however, are the specific ways individuals are tied to and interact with one another and the organization itself. In fact, Gittell (2009) states that "shared goals and mutual respect form the basis for collected coordinated action" (p. 14). Such relationships uniquely characterize and provide a framework for organizational work.

The essence of organizational relating is more than just getting along with people and attaining goals; it is about realizing that we are not alone in this work and that, together, people create, grow and develop, and are productive workers. This relationship factor is almost a hidden asset for it is not readily seen, but it sure goes a long way toward healthy performance. For example, employees' level of engagement, willingness to go above and beyond, and relational competence with patients and families are not easy to observe but directly impact patients' experiences (a reimbursable outcome), other employees' satisfaction with work, and the bottom line.

Building organizational relational capacity is a major responsibility of health systems leaders. Typically, health systems leaders are judged based on quality, safety, and system (financial) outcomes, the assumption being that this is good for patients and good for the system. Yet, the quality of relationships in an organization may be a key driver of these organizational metrics. As leaders, then, it is vital to notice the quality of relationships and how you are contributing and benefiting from them. Leaders who spend time with their staff, share common interests, ask them how they are doing, what they are working on, and use a sense of humor have a good chance of gaining a level of respect that will form the basis for future relationships. Valuing relationships with coworkers is also important as a source of ongoing learning. Although we are all busy, allocating time to nurture relationships is an essential aspect of leadership.

To assess the relational capacity with a health system, the leader could start by asking questions (the root of learning). For example, leaders might ask:

- Does the system invest time and effort in selecting employees with the right relational competences?

- Do the socialization practices in the system reflect the relational values and culture of the organization? Are these practices well thought out? Or are they considered a waste of time?
- What type of orientation and mentoring is available to new employees?
- Do leaders focus on relationships as their primary work activity?
- Are leaders of meetings in this organization capable of engaging members and do the members interdependently rely on each other to get the work done?
- Are there systems in place to help employees (all employees) deal with work–family dynamics?
- Does the system honor individuals' and teams' needs for reflection and conscious awareness?
- What meaningful rewards are in place to recognize high-quality relationships?

After all, leadership development is a dynamic *process* encompassing self-awareness, practicing one's values and beliefs, applying meaningful motivations, developing and using a supportive team, and living an integrated life. In essence, leadership is a way of being versus just doing a job. Thus, for those who teach leadership in health systems, helping students learn how to evolve leadership capacity is paramount.

Likewise, health educators have a responsibility to teach and help students learn the importance of relationships to healthcare practice. Particularly in online courses, maintaining and nurturing high-quality faculty–student relationships is key. Educating in this way requires faculty members who are comfortable and relationally competent themselves and who understand the benefits of such learning. Frankel, Eddin-Folinsbee, and Inui (2011) proposed three areas necessary for faculty development. Although directed toward medical education, these ideas are important for all health professionals, especially in light of the high dependency and teamwork required in modern-day health services. The three areas for faculty development are mindful practice, formation (ethical development), and communication skills. Future recommendations for faculty development include (a) making patient- and relationship-centered care a central competency in all healthcare interactions, (b) developing a national curriculum framework with input from patients, (c) requiring performance metrics for professional development, (d) partnering with national healthcare organizations to disseminate the curriculum framework, and (e) preserving face-to-face educational methods for delivering key elements of the curriculum.

Although it may be painful for health educators to acknowledge that time-honored approaches to learning and curricula need major revision, articulating the relational outcomes we most desire and asking which methods will best help us to achieve them are important first steps in reconstructing educational programs that will produce graduates with individual and collective relational capacity.

As organizational relational capacity also includes relationships with external partners, it is significant that health systems in recent years have placed an increased focus on academic–service partnerships. For example, many schools of nursing are now formally partnering with clinical sites for teaching and research, improving care, and instilling principles of lifelong learning (Beal, 2012). Conceptually, such partnerships entail sharing power and resources, and some empirical evidence is available related to their success. For example, Duffy et al. (2015) and Duffy, Culp, Sand-Jecklin, Stroupe, and Lucke-Wold (2016) used a formal caring-based partnership model to evaluate research knowledge and research productivity, showing some positive results. Barriers and facilitators to the partnership were also identified. Likewise, Highfield et al. (2016) used an academic–service partnership to promote evidence-based practice over several areas of practice. And Howard and Williams (2016) used a partnership approach to facilitate the preparation of Doctor of Nursing Practice graduates for advanced practice to meet the health needs of their community. Others have evaluated academic–practice partnerships to build alliances, fulfill health needs of communities, and advance the professional nursing workforce. The strength of the relationships among the partners has been key to their success.

Building organization relational capacity is enabled by the individual and collective relational capacity of employees. Nurses, in particular, have a unique opportunity to make a profound difference in patient and system outcomes based on the highly relational characteristics of their discipline. However, continued reliance on mechanistic or disease-based models of care detracts from this opportunity. It is high time to use our collective relational capacity to enhance the health of patients, health systems, and ourselves.

SUMMARY

Relational capacity, a resource necessary for quality caring at the individual, collective, and organizational levels, is explored. Human values, life experiences, intentions, PsyCap, and relational competence are described as important elements of individual relational capacity. Team or collective relational capacity, including the disruptive behavior reported in nursing, is exposed as a detractor to authentic collective relational capacity. Case studies illuminate the importance of relational capacity on patient and employee outcomes. Finally, organizational relational capacity is highlighted as an often unseen asset that positively impacts performance. Examples for leadership and education are used.

Call to Action

Relational capacity is an individual and collective trait, and an organizational strength that impacts self-advancement. Relational capacity is everyone's responsibility. **Assess** your own relational capacity—include your underlying values, PsyCap, caring intention, and relational competence. Shared relational capacity among health teams contributes to organizational relational capacity. **Build** relationships, particularly those with yourself, with patients and families, with other health professionals, and with the health system.

REFLECTIVE QUESTIONS/APPLICATIONS

. . . for Students

1. What is relational capacity? How have you developed it in your educational program?
2. Analyze the components of individual relational capacity. How do you fare?
3. Reflect on the case studies presented in this chapter. As a student, did these raise your awareness of an issue that you might face as a new nurse? What would you have done differently? Can you develop some actions that would help you relate to the first experienced nurse?

4. Outline your plans to develop interprofessional relational capacity. How will you know you have achieved it?
5. How do you go about building relationships? Or do you? Provide specific examples.

... for Professional Nurses in Clinical Practice

1. Discuss the interprofessional practice among nurses on your unit. Is it of high quality? Why or why not?
2. Is there an expectation that relational capacity is necessary for registered nurse (RN) work at your institution? If so, how is it evaluated?
3. Reflect on your own individual relational capacity using the components presented in this chapter. Where do you stand? What do you need to do to improve it?
4. What patient outcomes do you think might be enhanced with more relational capacity?
5. Which experienced nurse would you have been in the case study? Joan or Mary? Why?
6. Take a minute and think back to a team that you absolutely loved being a part of. Did that have anything to do with the relational capacity of the team? How did you contribute to that team's relational capacity?

... for Professional Nurses in Educational Practice

1. What specific curricular revisions have you developed that address individual, collective (team), and organizational relational capacity? How do you evaluate it? What teaching/learning strategies do you use to help undergraduate and graduate students learn how to relate?
2. Reflect on the need for relational capacity among teams of health professionals. How does your educational program facilitate graduates' capacity to work effectively in teams?
3. What can you do to select, develop, and mentor students to enhance their individual relational capacity? Specifically, how can they best learn how to listen, be optimistic, communicate, understand their unique contribution to healthcare, and *do* the ongoing work necessary to build relational capacity?

4. How might you suggest incorporating relational capacity building into your online courses?
5. Provide some suggestions for exposing students' values and belief systems that would provide them some insight into their behavior.

. . . for Professional Nurses in Leadership Practice

1. What is the state of relational capacity at your organization? How do you know?
2. How do you specifically hold yourself accountable to build relational capacity at work?
3. Reflect on the hiring process in place at your institution. Does it include assessment of individuals' relational capacity? What would it take to revise this?
4. How is collective (team) relational capacity monitored and measured at your institution? What could you do to enhance this process?
5. How do you facilitate the individual relational capacity of health professionals under your supervision? What specific activities (orientation, mentoring, career development, etc.) support this?
6. Does your leadership team understand the importance of relational capacity at all levels as it relates to the bottom line? If not, how will you facilitate their development?
7. Create a plan for dramatically altering the selection, orientation, socialization process, and ongoing career development of employees to enhance organization relational capacity. Who should be involved? What methodology would be used? How long will it take? What implications for RN practice would occur? How would you ensure that the plan is enacted as developed? How would you evaluate its implementation?

PRACTICE ANALYSIS

Bill, a 60-year-old male with pancreatic cancer, has been hospitalized for almost 2 weeks and in the intensive care unit for the past 5 days. His physical deterioration and suffering had created anguish in his wife and in the healthcare team. The attending physician discussed with the wife the likelihood of her husband having a cardiac and/or respiratory arrest, described the actions the team would take for a full resuscitation as well as the varying levels of resuscitation approved by the treatment setting, which included a do-not-resuscitate option, and asked her to express her preferences regarding resuscitation. The wife initially chose the do-not-resuscitate status for her husband and completed all of the official paperwork to implement that decision. During the next 12 hours, the wife actively solicited from nursing and medical staff their definitions of do-not-resuscitate. She then contacted the attending physician to rescind her decision, choosing instead to have a full resuscitation order in place. She explained her decision change as, "When I saw that the nurses and doctors did not all define resuscitation in the same way, I decided that I would not leave that in their hands. I am my husband's wife and will be to the end." This new decision was enacted and over the next 4 days, the patient showed clear signs of dying. His wife stayed with him in the intensive care unit and witnessed the changes in her husband's physical appearance. She began commenting on those changes and on her husband's obvious suffering. Within 2 hours of his death, the wife told the nurse that she did not want her husband to be resuscitated. This information was immediately conveyed to the physician who once again, changed the order in the electronic health record.

1. What individual and collective (team) relational capacity was exhibited in this case?
2. What was the state of organizational relational capacity in this unit? How might the nurse leader in this unit evaluate and improve organizational relationship capacity?
3. What could have been done differently by the health professionals in this situation?

REFERENCES

American Diabestes Association. (n.d.). Living with Diabetes. Retreived from http://www.diabetes.org/living-with-diabetes

Anscombe, G. E. M. (1957/1963). *Intention*. Cambridge, MA: Harvard University Press.

Avey, J., Reichard, R. J., Luthans, F., & Mhatre, K. H. (2011). Meta-analysis of the impact of positive psychological capital on employee attitudes, behaviors, and performance. *Human Resource Development Quarterly*, 22(2), 127–152. doi:10.1002/hrdq.20070

Bandura, A. (1997). *Self-efficacy: The exercise of control*. New York, NY: Freeman.

Beal, J. (2012). Academic-service partnership in nursing: An integrative review. *Nursing Research and Practice*, 2012, 501564. doi:10.1155/2012/501564

Carpenter, B. N. (1993). Relational competence. In D. Perlman & W. H. Jones (Eds.), *Advances in personal relationships, a research manual* (Vol. 4, pp. 1–28). London, UK: Jessica Kingsley.

Carpenter, B. N., Hansson, R. O., Rountree, R., & Jones, W. H. (1983). Relational competence and adjustment in diabetic patients. *Journal of Social and Clinical Psychology, 1*(4), 359–369. doi:10.1521/jscp.1983.1.4.359

Dossey, B., & Keegan, L. (2009). *Holistic nursing: A handbook for practice* (p. 21). Sudbury, MA: Jones & Bartlett.

Duffy, J. (2003). Caring relationships and evidence-based practice: Can they co-exist? *International Journal for Human Caring, 7*(3), 45–50.

Duffy, J. R., Culp, S., Sand-Jecklin, K., Stroupe, L., & Lucke-Wold, N. (2016). Nurses' research capacity, use of evidence, and research productivity in acute care: Year 1 findings from a partnership study. *Journal of Nursing Administration, 46*(1), 12–17. doi:10.1097/NNA.0000000000000287

Duffy, J. R., Culp, S., Yarberry, C., Stroupe, L., Sand-Jecklin, K., & Coburn, A. S. (2015). Nurses' research capacity and use of evidence in acute care: Baseline findings from a partnership study. *Journal of Nursing Administration, 45*(3), 158–164. doi:10.1097/NNA.0000000000000176

Frankel, R. M., Eddin-Folensbee, F., & Inui, T. S. (2011). Crossing the patient-centered divide: Transforming health care quality through enhanced faculty development. *Academic Medicine, 86*(4), 445–452. doi:10.1097/ACM.0b013e31820e7e6e

Gittell, J. H. (2009). *High performance healthcare: Using the power of relationships to achieve quality, efficiency and resilience.* New York, NY: McGraw-Hill.

Grumbach, K., & Bodenheimer, T. (2004). Can health care teams improve primary care practice? *Journal of the American Medical Association, 291,* 1246–1251. doi:10.1001/jama.291.10.1246

Haldorsdottir, S. (1991). Five basic modes of being with another. In D. Gaut & M. Leininger (Eds.), *Caring: The compassionate healer* (pp. 37–49). New York, NY: The National League for Nursing.

Heled, E., Somech, A., & Waters, L. (2016). Psychological capital as a team phenomenon: Mediating the relationship between learning climate and outcomes at the individual and team levels. *The Journal of Positive Psychology, 11*(3), 303–314. doi:10.1080/17439760.2015.1058971

Hertz, H. (2015). Effective communication requires caring, explaining, listening, and living the role. Retrieved from https://www.nist.gov/baldrige/effective-communication-requires-caring-explaining-listening-and-living-role

Highfield, M. E., Collier, A., Collins, M., & Crowley, M. (2016). Partnering to promote evidence-based practice in a community hospital: Implications for nursing professional development specialists. *Journal for Nurses in Professional Development, 32*(3), 130–136. doi:10.1097/NND.0000000000000227

Houck, N. M., & Colbert, A. M. (2017). Patient safety and workplace bullying: An integrative review. *Journal of Nursing Care Quality, 32*(2), 164–171. doi:10.1097/NCQ.0000000000000209

Howard, P. B., & Williams, T. E. (2016). An academic–practice partnership to advance DNP education and practice. *Journal of Professional Nursing, 33*(2), 86–94. doi:10.1016/j.profnurs.2016.08.010

Husserl, E. (1980). *Ideas pertaining to a pure phenomenology and to a phenomenological philosophy: Second book: Studies in the phenomenology of constitution.* Dordrecht, The Netherlands: Kluwer Academic.

Inglehart, R. (1997). *Modernization and postmodernization: Cultural, economic, and political change in 43 societies.* Princeton, NJ: Princeton University Press.

The Joint Commission. (2008). Behaviors that undermine a culture of safety. Retrieved from http://www.jointcommission.org/assets/1/18/SEA_40.PDF

Luthans, F. (2005). *Organizational behaviour* (10th ed.). New York, NY: McGraw-Hill International Edition.

Luthans, F., Avey, J. B., Avolio, B. J., & Peterson, S. J. (2010). The development and resulting performance impact of positive psychological capital. *Human Resource Development Quarterly, 21,* 41–67. doi:10.1002/hrdq.20034

Luthans, F., Avolio, B., Walumbwa, F., & Li, W. (2005). The psychological capital of Chinese workers: Exploring the relationship with performance. *Management and Organization Review, 1,* 247–269. doi:10.1111/j.1740-8784.2005.00011.x

Luthans, F., Norman, S. M., Avolio, B. J., & Avey, J. B. (2008). The mediating role of psychological capital in the supportive organizational climate–employee performance relationship. *Journal of Organizational Behavior, 29,* 219–238. doi:10.1002/job.507

Luthans, F., & Youssef, C. M. (2004). Human, social, and now positive psychological capital management. *Organizational Dynamics, 33,* 143–160. doi:10.1016/j.orgdyn.2004.01.003

Luthans, F., & Youssef, C. M. (2007). Emerging positive organizational behavior. *Journal of Management, 33*(3), 321–349. doi:10.1177/0149206307300814

Luthans, F., Youssef, C. M., & Avolio, B. J. (2007). *Psychological capital.* New York, NY: Oxford University Press.

Luthans, F., & Youssef-Morgan, C. M. (2017). Psychological capital: An evidence-based positive approach. *Annual Review of Organizational Psychology and Organizational Behavior, 4,* 339–366. doi:10.1146/annurev-orgpsych-032516-113324

Monteau, M. (2017). Eliminating intimidating and disruptive behavior. *The American Journal of Nursing, 117*(4), 13. doi:10.1097/01.NAJ.0000515212.62097.57

Perugini, M., & Bagozzi, R. P. (2004). The distinction between desires and intentions. *European Journal of Psychology, 34,* 69–84. doi:10.1002/ejsp.186

Schultz, C. K. (2017, March 17–20). Nurses experiences with behaviors that compromise a healthy work environment within the hospital setting. In *Creating Healthy Work Environments.* Indianapolis, IN: STTI.

Schwartz, S. H. (1994). Are there universal aspects in the structure and contents of human values? *Journal of Social Issues, 50,* 19–45. doi:10.1111/j.1540-4560.1994.tb01196.x

Schwartz, S. H. (2006). Basic human values: An overview. Retrieved from http://segr-did2.fmag.unict.it/Allegati/convegno%207-8-10-05/Schwartzpaper.pdf

Schwartz, S. H. (2011). Studying values: Personal adventure, future directions. *Journal of Cross-Cultural Psychology, 42*(2), 307–319. doi:10.1177/0022022110396925

Schwartz, S. H. (2012). An overview of the Schwartz Theory of Basic Values. *Online Readings in Psychology and Culture, 2*(1). doi:10.9707/2307-0919.1116

Schwartz, S. H., & Bardi, A. (1997). Influences of adaptation to communist rule on value priorities in Eastern Europe. *Political Psychology, 18*, 385–410. doi:10.1111/0162-895X.00062

Snyder, C. R. (2000). *Handbook of hope: Theory, measures, and applications.* New York, NY: Academic Press.

7

Feeling "Cared For"

They may forget your name but they will never forget how you made them feel.

—Maya Angelou

THE POSITIVE EMOTION OF "FEELING CARED FOR"

Feeling "cared for" is a positive emotion that develops over time through connected, caring relationships. In 1962, the philosopher Heidegger described "feeling cared for" as a universal phenomenon involving meaningful closeness with others. In a later phenomenological nursing study, Bunkers (2004) found the meaning of "feeling cared for" among 10 poor women to be "contentment with intimate affiliations arising with salutary endeavors, while honoring uniqueness amid adversity" (p. 63). An important finding in Bunker's research was that "feeling cared for" emerged as a separate phenomenon from the caring process itself. It included acknowledgment of the unique individual who has the freedom to choose connection as well as separation. This is consistent with the Quality-Caring Model© (QCM), which views "feeling cared for" as a consequence of (separate from) the caring process.

Repeated connections between patients and health professionals that are of a caring nature foster this affirmative feeling of being "cared for." Nurses, through their intimate attention to basic human needs, as an example, interact with patients and families and, with repetition, create connections that ultimately result in knowing the other. This transformative process facilitates "feeling cared for," enabling patients and families to relax, feel safe, learn, rest, participate, and cope with illness.

"Feeling cared for" during illness is especially important today as families are often scattered over many miles and may be further separated by technology and generational or age-related differences. Most patients and families desire this emotion, yet hospitalization often places people at risk for noncaring relationships, resulting in anxiety, isolation, prolonged recovery, and sometimes pain or discomfort unrelated to disease. In fact, these negative emotions have been tied to increased heart rate and blood pressure, increased cortisol levels, and may alter the immune system (Adler, 2002). In a systematic review of healthcare neglect in three countries, Reader and Gillespie found feelings of not being cared for in hospitalized patients, and in particular, caring neglect was described as "being rude, not responding to patient complaints of pain, purposefully delaying help for patients, intentionally ignoring patients, avoiding contact with patients, preferring to socialise with colleagues rather than treat patients, and prioritising some patients over other others due to liking them more" (2013, p. 8). Furthermore, there were wide discrepancies in patient perceptions of not feeling cared for compared to nurses' perceptions, with physical and emotional harms resulting. Such harms are incongruent with current ethical and quality standards!

Feeling cared for is a positive reaction that has been associated with improved social connectedness and some physiological alterations. In fact, recent studies have shown that positive emotions were significantly connected to health and, in some cases, actually protected against and slowed the progression of cardiovascular disease (Boehm & Kubzansky, 2012; Falk et al., 2015; Kok et al., 2013; Park et al., 2016; Thong, Tan, & Jensen, 2017; Weng et al., 2013). Other studies have shown positive relationships between positive emotions and psychological health and team performance (Kiken, Lundberg, & Fredrickson, 2017; Meneghel, Salanova, & Martínez, 2016; Wingo et al., 2017). Finally, in a recent qualitative nursing study, participants reported outcomes associated with feeling cared for during stroke hospitalization. These included a safe transfer home, optimal recovery, speedy discharge, and loyalty to the institution (Baggett et al., 2016).

Feeling "cared for" by health professionals provides patients with the energy or drive to continue treatment or make behavioral changes, interact, learn, and maybe even follow through; in other words, it may be tied to one's ability to engage, progress, or advance. It seems to buffer stress, promote resilience, relieve the burden of expectations, lessen some uncertainty, and increase confidence and comfort. This reaction is a necessary antecedent to future interactions and more terminal outcomes. Thus, it is imperative that nurses appreciate their role in motivating this important intermediate outcome.

Because of the continuous and highly emotional involvement with patients and other health professionals, demanding patient situations, required competencies, fluctuating workflow, and stressful system-related issues, "feeling cared for" from the perspective of the health professional is significant to healthy work environments. In fact, when employees feel cared for, the meaning of their work may deepen, they may feel a heightened sense of belonging, experience psychological safety, feel affirmed, and become more emotionally available, providing the energy that allows for greater engagement and teamwork (Kahn & Heaphy, 2014). Yet, allowing oneself to "feel cared for" is often difficult for some health professionals. As experts in caring, nurses know how to care for others but find it strange to receive such regard. At one organization, the notion of team caring was formalized in a 45-minute group meeting that regularly convened once a week to process the week's work. A few rules were established, such as only positive or affirming words could be used, everyone was to be heard, and members were to actively listen. This group time allowed members to recognize the collective work of the group, solve emergent problems, celebrate successes, work on affirming projects, receive caring from each other, and share resources to face the challenges of the upcoming week. Unknowingly, the consequences of this group process resulted in "feeling cared for," strengthening individual members and allowing them to better see their possibilities. Another interesting result was the gradual reevaluation of individual members about their unique strengths and contribution to the work.

There is a reciprocal nature to caring. When one truly cares for others, others tend to care in return (and when caring is withheld, the converse occurs). Thus, "feeling cared for" is enhanced when caring is extended to others. As a professional charged with the safety of vulnerable individuals, it is the nurse's role to extend caring first.

THE UNIQUE ROLE OF THE NURSE

Feeling cared for is a significant and differentiating nursing-sensitive intermediate outcome that can be observed and measured. Thus, it could be considered a "marker" of quality nursing care. As a result of caring relationship–centered professional encounters, patients develop this positive emotion that connotes "I matter; I am viewed as capable; I belong." The importance that patients attribute to feeling recognized as worthy and capable individuals with the potential for decision making is significant to "feeling cared for" and influences future interactions, intermediate health outcomes, and ultimately self-advancement (see Figure 7.1).

Typically, in healthcare situations, authority gradients (or hierarchies of power) exist that place patients and families in dependent relationships (with respect to clinicians) with well-meaning health professionals assuming the power during healthcare interactions (see Figure 7.2). Authority gradients have been frequently described in healthcare safety situations where various workers, with differences in status, perceive power or authority pressures that result in failure to relay important information or failure to act (Cosby & Croskerry, 2004). Consider the following case:

> *A new graduate nurse is working on a busy pulmonary acute care unit. She notices that one of her patients with asthma is more dyspneic and a little tachycardic. The new graduate nurse knows she should communicate this to the physician, but he has a reputation for getting agitated when interrupted. So she decides to communicate it to the charge nurse, but when approached, the charge nurse, who is very busy, appears annoyed. Because of her lack of confidence and the perceived lack of caring by those in power, the new graduate decides to wait. Unfortunately, the patient worsens and has a near-respiratory arrest, requiring intubation, mechanical ventilation, and a visit to the ICU.*

What could have been done differently in this situation? Who could have attended to this new graduate's need for feeling cared for?

Authority gradients often create unintended barriers that, in high-risk environments, may lead to errors and even sentinel events. Thus, preventing or neutralizing them as soon as recognized is essential.

Likewise, when well-meaning health professionals exert authority over or are perceived by patients to be the ones with power, the result may be situations in which patients are afraid to speak up, impeding communication and the transfer of important information (and in some cases, the occurrence of error). This lopsided and somewhat conditional patient–health professional relationship does not honor the shared partnership that should exist between patients and health professionals, but

FIGURE 7.1   Consequences of feeling "cared for."

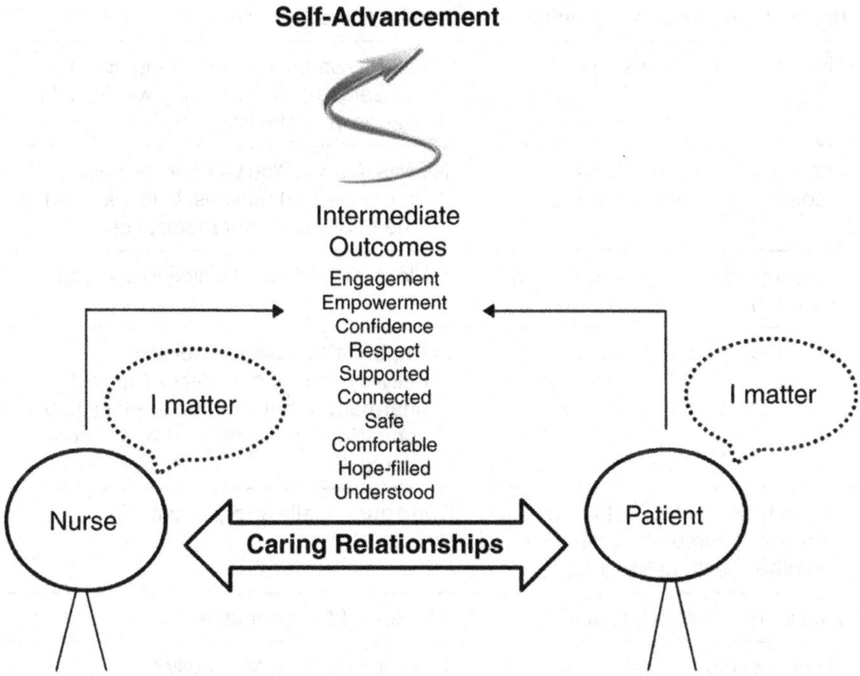

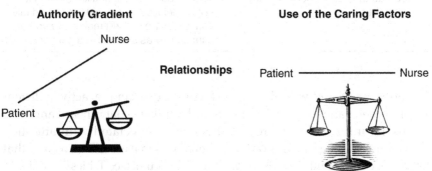

Self-Advancement

Intermediate
Outcomes
Engagement
Empowerment
Confidence
Respect
Supported
Connected
Safe
Comfortable
Hope-filled
Understood

I matter

I matter

Nurse

Patient

Caring Relationships

FIGURE 7.2   Nature of relationships between patients and nurses.

Authority Gradient   **Use of the Caring Factors**

Nurse

Relationships   Patient ———————— Nurse

Patient

rather creates an imbalance of power that many times is experienced as degradation, sometimes damaging to present and future interactions.

Nurses who are experts in the caring behaviors routinely use them to convey mutuality and reciprocity in relationships (see Figure 7.1), thereby equalizing authority between patients and health professionals (see Figure 7.2). Such actions are conveyed verbally and nonverbally through words, use and timing of language, facial expressions, human physical contact, tone of voice, distance, head nodding, eye contact—basically behaviors and

TABLE 7.1   Differences in Verbal Messages Based on Authority

Health Professional Is the Authority	Patient Is the Authority
Time to do your dressing.	Hello, Mr. Smith. I am checking up on you as I said I would. Is it okay with you if I change your dressing now?
I have so many patients today, I couldn't get here any sooner.	Hi, Mrs. Mallon. You've been on my mind for the past 30 minutes. Is this a good time to discuss your medication?
Hi honey—you seem to be doing fine today.	Hello, Mrs. Lanoue. It's nice to see you today.
Your meds have not come up yet.	Jane, there has been a delay in the delivery of your medications from the pharmacy. What can I do to make you comfortable while we wait a few more minutes?
I know how you feel but I have been busy with three other patients and another nurse called in sick.	You sound really angry about this.
That won't work on this unit.	Mr. Horn, I like your idea!
I know how to do this!	How do you do it, Mrs. Kelly?
Calm down—they will take you as soon as they can. They are busy down there.	Mr. Gannon, your test was scheduled for 10 a.m. but they just notified me that it will be delayed. They said they could take you about 1 p.m. I will make sure you get a lunch tray as soon as you get back.

attitudes associated with the caring factors. For example, actively listening and then validating with patients and families what is heard and then clarifying information represents behaviors associated with attentive reassurance. Using caring words and behaviors that are affirming and that acknowledge the authority of the patient is important (see Tables 7.1 and 7.2). Engaging families in actual care or care decisions attends to the caring behaviors, appreciation of unique meanings and affiliation needs, and conveys the family's significance in helping family members to get well.

Once the authority gradient is counterbalanced through caring behaviors, skills, and attitudes, nurses further facilitate "feeling cared for" by:

- Inspiring patients to activate their own resources
- Advocating for patients and families
- Staying genuine (honest, forthright)

- Being responsive (tuned in to the patient versus the health professional or system)
- Extending oneself (going the extra mile when necessary)
- Being present
- Displaying technical competence
- Remaining self-aware
- Embracing the support of a caring team

Professional nurses manifest caring and the resultant positive emotion of "feeling cared for" as they assist healthcare consumers and other health professionals in preventing or healing health problems. Giving and receiving another's attention, respect, support, and protection while assisting in human and affiliation needs builds relationships versus tearing them down. Listening to one's personal and professional wisdom and learning how to grow despite negative emotions and events enables others to accept and *"feel* cared for." By doing so, nurses benefit as well, feeling as if they matter; are more secure in their role; more caring to self, coworkers, and families; calmer and more centered; connected to the values inherent in professional nursing; and part of a larger whole (see Figure 7.1).

TABLE 7.2 Nonverbal Messages That Convey Caring

Maintain eye contact

Smile

Sit comfortably and not too far away

Face the patient, always

Pay attention—while someone is dialoguing with you, don't do any other activity

Do not allow interruptions—phone calls, people—unless it is an emergency

Excuse and explain yourself, *if* it is an emergency and you have to leave

Be enthusiastic and energetic

Allow patients to talk without interruption

Listen for cues to underlying feelings

Dress professionally

Use soft, gentle touch

Use relaxed body posture, even leaning in

Acknowledge patients' words—nod head, say "yes"

MEASURING "FEELING CARED FOR"

Evaluation and demonstration of the influence of caring processes (or behaviors) on specific health outcomes reveals the value of caring relationships not only to the nursing profession but to patients, their families, health systems, and policy makers. Both qualitative and quantitative data can assist in assessing "feeling cared for." For example, patient interviews and focus groups are often used to gather data from patients. Using such techniques, interview guides that ask specific questions about feeling cared for could provide useful data for decision making or to improve practice. Quantitative data are useful to assess and improve practice as well as to provide evidence for decision making. They are also used in research to generate connections among variables, test caring interventions, and validate and refine theory. Because the phenomenon of "feeling cared for" has been conceptualized and defined, it *is* measurable, albeit with recommendations.

Measurement, a fundamental aspect of quantitative analysis, is generally understood as a process by which attributes or dimensions of a phenomenon are assigned a value (to eliminate guessing or uncertainty). "Feeling cared for" can be measured in terms of its degree, its observed current state, improvements over time, what it is associated with, how it compares among groups, and patients' opinions of it. Using a systematic method of collecting data (to ensure accurate and consistent application) and employing focused instruments is implicit in measurement. Measuring phenomena is commonly associated with some error—either in the instrument itself, how the data were collected, or in the characteristics of the sample. Reducing this error is a major goal of high-quality instruments. Understanding how an instrument was developed is important because it has implications for its accuracy, application in practice, and interpretation of results.

Although many have attempted to measure caring (Watson, 2002, 2008a, 2008b), the emotion of "feeling cared for" as a consequence of caring actions assumes that the patient is the authority for care received and the resultant unit of analysis. Although many tools are available to measure caring, there are few that measure this phenomenon from the patient's point of view, explicitly reveal the conceptual definition of caring that guided item development, are valid and reliable, are low in burden, and were tested in diverse populations with large sample sizes.

Thus, there is much confusion about what and how to measure "feeling cared for." For further information on measurement and methods of assessment, see Grove, Burns, and Gray (2017). This text provides a good overview of quantifying variables, including reducing measurement error and ensuring accurate, reliable, and sensitive assessment. In the context of this brief background regarding measurement and assessment of "feeling cared for," the importance of choosing appropriate instruments with the most credibility is stressed.

First, recognizing the definition or conceptual framework from which the items in an instrument were generated is paramount. The emotion of "feeling cared for" in a patient is a consequence of health professionals' caring actions and suggests a preconceived notion of what caring means and an assessment of its outcomes from the patient's point of view. In the QCM, the meaning of caring is derived from the caring behaviors, which were developed from multiple theories (see Chapter 2), and the measurement of "feeling cared for" is recommended to be generated from the patient's point of view. It is likewise important to understand the context in which an instrument was developed to better assess its usefulness in a particular setting. For example, the patient population, setting, age group of respondents, emotional states of respondents, and severity of illness all have a bearing on the results. If an instrument was developed in acute care, administering the same instrument in a community setting would not necessarily yield the same results, unless it was later tested in that population.

Next, clarity of items, including the degree of readability, is important. If an item was meant to measure mutual problem solving, for example (a caring behavior), but the way it was worded connoted trust, the answers would not be valid. Additionally, if items on a caring instrument were worded in language that was difficult to understand, respondents may not accurately be able to answer it. How an instrument is administered impacts its results—for example, potential biases of the data collector, burden to the patient (e.g., how long it took), consistency of administration, and interrater reliability (multiple data collectors using the same approach) all affect how an instrument performs. Burden to the patient and the evaluation team is also important as they may affect accuracy of responses and availability of results. Obviously, validity (accuracy) and reliability (consistency) of instruments are a major concern, and these properties should be explicitly made known to potential users. (See Table 7.3 for a list of criteria from which to judge caring instruments.)

Of the multiple instruments that measure aspects of caring in Watson (2008a, 2008b), several measure the importance of caring, others measure caring from the nurses' point of view, others measure caring in specific

TABLE 7.3   Criteria for Choosing Caring Instruments

Criteria	Questions for Consideration
Conceptual framework	On whose theory of conceptual base were the items developed?
Purpose	What was the original purpose of the instrument?
Context	In what patient population or setting has the instrument been tested and used?
Perspective	From whose viewpoint is the tool seeking information—patients, families, students, or nurses?
Clarity	Are the items understandable? Are the directions easy?
Administration	How is the questionnaire administered—paper and pencil, electronically, over the Internet? What is the time required for completion? How is scoring accomplished?
Psychometrics	Is the tool valid and reliable? How was this established? Was it established in a similar population? Are the forms of validity and reliability consistent with your purpose?
Burden	How easy is it for patients to complete?

patient populations, and some conceptual definitions from which items were developed are missing. Furthermore, methods for testing reliability and validity were not always explicit and methods, including sampling procedures, were oftentimes not available. Information on subject burden and use in different settings were also problematic. Thus, although many have contributed to assessing and measuring caring, accurately evaluating "feeling cared for" remains challenging.

The Caring Assessment Tool (CAT) is a 27-item instrument designed to capture patients' perceptions of feeling cared for by nurses (Duffy, Brewer, & Weaver, 2014; Duffy, Hoskins, & Seifert, 2007). A confirmatory factor analysis with 1,111 randomly selected patients from 12 U.S. hospitals found a single-factor solution, explaining 73% of the variance in the construct. The instrument contains 27 easy to understand items with high internal consistency (alpha = 0.97) and acceptable fit indices (comparative fit index = 0.989; Tucker-Lewis index = 0.988; Duffy et al., 2014). It has been used extensively in studies of patient–nurse interactions and as an indicator of patient-centered care.

The electronic version of the CAT (e-CAT) was piloted in a group of hospitalized older adults with positive feasibility results (Duffy, Kooken, Wolverton, & Weaver, 2012). The e-CAT was displayed on a mobile device with functionality to gather (through the touch screen) data and score the

FIGURE 7.3 Sample e-CAT.

Since I have been a patient here, the nurses					
Are responsive to my family	NEVER 1	RARELY 2	OCCASIONALLY 3	FREQUENTLY 4	ALWAYS 5
Pay attention to me when I am talking	NEVER 1	RARELY 2	OCCASIONALLY 3	FREQUENTLY 4	ALWAYS 5
Support me with my beliefs	NEVER 1	RARELY 2	OCCASIONALLY 3	FREQUENTLY 4	ALWAYS 5
Respect me	NEVER 1	RARELY 2	OCCASIONALLY 3	FREQUENTLY 4	ALWAYS 5
Help me feel less worried	NEVER 1	RARELY 2	OCCASIONALLY 3	FREQUENTLY 4	ALWAYS 5

results (see Figure 7.3). The majority of participants (88%) agreed or strongly agreed that the display was easy to use, and 81% of participants agreed or strongly agreed that they were satisfied with this way of completing the CAT. Seventy percent said they would complete the questionnaire again using this format. Completion time averaged 31 minutes and 74% of the participants said they would do it again. The CAT and the e-CAT are available in English, Spanish, and Japanese and offer a means of measuring nurse caring behaviors from patients' point of view. The instrument is theory derived, has been evaluated in multiple studies, and is accurate, reliable, easy to administer, low in burden, and easily interpreted.

Although a growing knowledge base regarding the measurement of caring is emerging, there continue to be issues related to the conceptual base of the instruments, adequate psychometrics, and the perspective of the evaluator. With regard to the latter factor, the recipient of caring (most often the patient) is the most direct source of "feeling cared for" in clinical situations. This perspective is always the most advantageous because patients' and nurses' perceptions of caring have been known to differ (Duffy, 2009; Swanson, 1999). Likewise, when measuring caring among nursing students, families or caregivers, or nurses themselves, it is important to collect the data from those being "cared for."

Since caring patient–nurse relationships flourish in environments where leaders create and sustain caring cultures, the measurement and continual improvement of nurse manager caring behaviors is also essential to advancing excellence. The Caring Assessment Tool-administrative version (CAT-adm©; Duffy, 2008; Wolverton, 2016) is available to provide internal evidence for practice improvement. This recently revised tool was adapted from the CAT (and thus uses the same theoretical foundation), assesses nurse manager caring behaviors from the perspective of staff nurses, contains 25 items, and has minimum burden. Examples of its use for ongoing quality assessment and research are listed below:

- For many years now, the CAT-adm has been applied annually at MD Anderson Cancer Center to assess nurse manager caring behaviors and used to structure ongoing leadership development.
- The CAT-adm is currently being used at a New Jersey hospital to evaluate improvement in nurse manager caring behaviors in a pre–post study of a caring-based educational intervention targeted to department-level leaders.
- At a hospital on the west coast, the CAT-adm is being used as a performance indicator during 360 nurse leader evaluations.

No doubt, as more and more institutions begin to see the enabling value of caring cultures, the CAT-adm will be further employed.

IMPROVING "FEELING CARED FOR"

Measuring "feeling cared for" refers to quantifying the concept and is most often linked to research. Improving "feeling cared for" refers to using evidence to make judgments about a phenomenon and then revising practice accordingly. Evidence about the quality of "feeling cared for" can be derived internally and externally. Internally, health professionals' clinical experience (awareness gained from reflection on practice), narratives from patients and families, and specific performance improvement evaluations generate data from which to make revisions in practice. Externally, regional and national benchmarks, research, and dissemination of results through presentations and publications provide evidence needed for actionable practice changes. For example, in a 12-hospital quality collaborative, the participating hospitals measured "feeling cared for" quarterly using the CAT and then benchmarked their data against the remaining hospitals (Duffy et al., 2010). Staff nurses were involved in data collection, results were analyzed centrally, and then disseminated via reports to individual hospitals. The evidence generated was interpreted, compared, and used to make improvements in caring knowledge and behaviors. Using knowledge in this manner (best evidence) to make shared decisions about how caring relationships are perceived is an important activity that often gets left undone. In fact, patient–RN relationships are often not assessed at all or are conducted by proxy through questionnaires conducted *after* hospitalization. Yet, regularly evaluating and using evidence to improve "feeling cared for" is a first step in its improvement.

Internal to health systems, health professionals engage patients and families in caring relationships but patients themselves are considered the best authority for evaluating the relationship; thus, efforts to measure and improve "feeling cared for" should include their voice (Hudon, Fortin, Haggerty, Lambert, & Poitras, 2011). Generally, improvement requires a process designed to help reach conclusions about clinicians' practice or health systems' attainment of certain objectives or behaviors. Measurement is inherent in quality improvement because criteria are identified, quantified, and assessed according to some scale to make decisions. Improvement processes provide the basis for performance reviews, continuation or revisions of programs, and improvements in services. Data are collected, both ongoing (formative) or at the conclusion (summative), of an initiative and are used to make informed decisions.

Because "feeling cared for" is theorized to result from caring professional practice, the caring factors provide practical guidance on "how to care" (see Chapter 3 for some examples). In the context of a caring relationship, the health professional uses instrumental and relational values, knowledge, and skills to meet specific health outcomes. The knowledge, skills, and behaviors tied to caring relationships vary among health professionals and settings and fluctuate further by system characteristics. Thus, to ensure that patients and families as well as health professionals themselves "feel cared for," an ongoing process of evaluation, analysis of data, reflection on data, and practice revisions are needed. Unfortunately, well-designed caring improvement programs are overlooked or not conducted because of the perceived complexity of the process, including the collection of data while simultaneously caring for patients. Healthcare professionals, in particular, seem to rely on patients' comments or their own passion and feelings to conclude that their practice is meeting patients' needs. However, without proper evaluation and improvement, the value or usefulness of caring relationships cannot be known.

An evaluation model provides a framework to guide the process. In the context of a caring professional practice, the QCM provides an overarching framework from which to guide quality improvement efforts. Using this model, structural components of professional practice include characteristics of the participants. In this case, patients, providers, or organizational demographic data provide important information that may impact the processes or outcomes of practice and need to be captured. For example, patients who are more severely ill or have multiple comorbidities may influence how professional nurses use the caring factors and what outcomes can be realistically attained. Likewise, nurses with certain credentials (i.e., education, certifications) may provide care that varies from their peers—this may impact the results. And organizations that use specific staffing models or that provide more educational opportunities for professional nurses may inadvertently impact the processes and outcomes of care. Taking these factors into consideration during improvement processes allows one to modify the resulting data, lending credibility to the outcomes.

Evaluating the process of caring (use of the caring behaviors) by assessing "feeling cared for" provides evidence related to *how* professional practice is working. This assessment is useful when staff and patients' opinions about care vary, to engage in evidence-based discussions about recommendations for improvement, or to make adjustments or decisions about continuation of certain practices. In the acute care environment, it is especially important to capture these perceptions as close to real time as possible to be able to knowledgably change practice so individual patients and families will benefit. Regularly assessing caring processes allows clinicians and administrators to monitor improvements in nursing practice, to link caring processes with nursing-sensitive outcome measures, to study ways that structural indicators such as staffing patterns or nurse credentials affect caring processes, and to examine trends over time.

RESEARCHING "FEELING CARED FOR"

To extend the understanding and strengthen the evidence of caring relationships as a significant variable in the healthcare process, much more research must be conducted and disseminated. Continuing to build on the rich foundation of caring science using multiple methods will enrich the knowledge base. Refining existing measures of "feeling cared for" using appropriate conceptual definitions and adequate psychometric properties, with a particular emphasis on the patient's view, will allow for correlational studies and multisite comparisons. Qualitative studies permitting in-depth assessment of "feeling cared for" and its immediate consequences, cultural influences and "feeling cared for," the complexities of caring relationships, how caring capacity develops, and requirements for caring relationships are necessary. Using approaches such as observation, interviews, focus groups, narratives, and other interpretive methods will enrich the science.

Quantitative methods linking "feeling cared for" to specific patient, nurse, and system outcomes will strengthen the evidence regarding the value of caring in clinical practice. Likewise, linking "feeling cared for" to student learning outcomes and administrative caring to healthy work environments for professional nurses will provide the basis for innovation in these settings. Most importantly, developing caring-based interventions for testing in quantitative studies is necessary to provide high levels of evidence for caring-based nursing practice and to validate caring theory.

Caring-based interventions designed to elicit "feeling cared for" in recipients are complicated to design and the practical implications for testing can be challenging. Nevertheless, caring-based interventions must be tested to better understand how they contribute to overall healthcare outcomes. Choosing a caring-based conceptual framework to support the intervention followed by an application based on prior research and organized to meet the needs of the population under study is paramount. Developing a protocol describing the content, strength, and frequency of the intervention allows for replication. Using probability sampling and longitudinal studies, questions such as "What is the effect of the intervention on specific outcomes of care?" can be answered. Integrating cost-effectiveness components will add to the understanding of the intervention's worth.

The Patient-Centered Outcomes Research Institute (PCORI, 2014) has designated five priority areas for research. They are:

1. Assessment of Prevention, Diagnosis, and Treatment Options: Comparing the effectiveness and safety of alternative prevention, diagnosis, and treatment options to see which ones work best for different people with a particular health problem.
2. Improving Healthcare Systems: Comparing health system–level approaches to improving access, supporting patient self-care, innovative use of health information technology, coordinating care for complex conditions, and deploying workforce effectively.
3. Communication and Dissemination Research: Comparing approaches to providing comparative effectiveness research information, empowering people to ask for and use the information, and supporting shared decision making between patients and their providers.
4. Addressing Disparities: Identifying potential differences in prevention, diagnosis, or treatment effectiveness, or preferred clinical outcomes across patient populations and the healthcare required to achieve best outcomes in each population.
5. Accelerating Patient-Centered Outcomes Research and Methodological Research: Improving the nation's capacity to conduct patient-centered outcomes research by building data infrastructure, improving analytic methods, and training researchers, patients, and other stakeholders to participate in this research (PCORI, 2014).

Since 2012, PCORI has funded more than $1.4 billion in research projects, many of which pertain to the patient's inclusion and decision making about his or her care. "Feeling cared for" as a positive consequence of caring professional relationships may fit into one of these priorities and provide an approach for ongoing studies.

Likewise, the National Institute of Nursing Research (NINR) has designated several areas of clinical research emphasis that may provide pathways for future research. Identified priority areas include:

- Symptom Science
- Wellness
- Self-Management
- End-of-Life and Palliative Care
- Technology and Training

Caring-based interventions could be designed for specific populations in many of these priority areas. For example, in school-age children, promoting wellness might be improved through targeted interventions provided in the context of caring relationships with school nurses or counselors. Or, increasing regular exercise among elderly women living in assisted-living facilities might be tested using a walking group with consistently assigned nurses. The management of symptoms might be augmented by caring studies that use holistic approaches toward symptom management. Nonpharmacologic interventions, such as optimizing sleep patterns, frequent reorientation, decreasing environmental triggers, massage, family engagement, healing aesthetics, and individualized comfort measures provided in the context of caring relationships are examples of holistic approaches. Identifying barriers to symptom management, correlating "feeling cared for" with reduction of specific symptoms, testing patient-defined comfort, and using qualitative methods to elicit lived experiences or culturally congruent ideas related to symptom management will meet this mandate.

Self-caring, a form of self-management, builds on a person's strengths and uses positive thoughts or intentions to accept encouragement and assistance from others (when necessary) to adopt healthy behaviors and maintain independence. Caring-based interventions that seek to increase self-caring or studies that identify factors associated with self-caring practices are warranted. How self-caring impacts quality of life or maintenance of independence, especially in those with chronic illnesses, is important. Supporting caregivers, especially those caring for patients with chronic disease, with long-term caring-based interventions and demonstration projects that honor the importance of caregivers to the health of loved ones are issues of deep concern for nursing. Research questions such as "Do caring relationships with health professionals improve self-caring and quality of life?" or "How well does a caregiver–care recipient caring relationship sustain time?" are important to answer.

Studying caring end-of-life interventions based on patient preferences would provide evidence of nursing's value in this vulnerable population. In addition, understanding how enhancing communication among health professionals (collective relational capacity) might improve decision making or decrease physical and psychological burden to patients and families would greatly enhance our knowledge base. Creative technological innovations that incorporate "feeling cared for" among patients, caregivers, and the healthcare team may enhance nursing's value by first evaluating the concept and second, by applying analyses in ways that enhance clinical outcomes. For example, evaluation of "feeling cared for" in real time (using technological solutions) may help investigators develop interventions that enhance nurses' delivery of patient-centered care and subsequently improve patient outcomes. Finally, ongoing and accelerating preparation of nursing scientists who are especially passionate about the value of "feeling cared for" as it relates to these priority areas is important.

In education, the National League for Nursing (NLN) has prioritized building the science of nursing education through discovery and translation of innovative evidence-based strategies linking student learning to sentinel health indicators to promote health, prevent disease, and manage the symptomatology of illness and in the academic context related to health transitions in their 2016–2019 research priorities (NLN, 2016). Understanding the impact of caring-based pedagogies on student learning, how caring relationships are best learned in simulated teaching environments, evaluation of caring competence, the student–teacher relationship, building meaningful connections between learning and patient outcomes, identification of teaching strategies for learning and practicing interprofessionalism, mechanisms for lifelong learning, better understanding of how caring relationships influence grief and loss, extensions of caring relationships during healthcare transitions, and preparation of nurse faculty for teaching caring relationships as the basis for professional practice are all research questions that would enhance the educational environment and possibly student learning.

Important to the discussion of educational research is the preparation of the next generation of scientists. Without role models conducting research in health professions schools, graduate students will not get the chance to participate in advancing the notion of "feeling cared for" and its link to important health outcomes. Researchers involved in such research must involve students at all levels, explain their methods and results during class discussions, invite participation in specific projects, demonstrate the consistency between conceptual frameworks and specific research variables, and model the process of conducting research. Examples of this include undergraduate student honors programs, research practicums, joint publications, and faculty–service partnerships in which research is a component.

At the systems level, it is important to know how best to adopt and improve relationship-centered professional encounters such that "feeling cared for" in recipients can be tied to important and reimbursable outcomes (e.g., patient engagement, 30-day readmission rates, adverse outcomes). The benefits of carefully evaluating clinician–patient relationships in real time and using results to make actionable practice changes; evaluating the impact of caring cultures on health professionals' work satisfaction, retention, and turnover; identifying ways to improve relationship-centered interprofessional teams; understanding how use of information technology might assist patients and families to provide feedback about their care; identifying ways to reprioritize relationships in the professional workflow; comparing departments in an organization in terms of how leadership impacts caring relationships; and evaluating the benefits of academic–service partnerships for improving "feeling cared for" among recipients are examples of important research questions that must be answered. The American Organization for Nurse Executives' (AONE, 2017) Institute for Patient Care Research & Education provides seed money to fund small studies about leadership, excellence in patient care, and health policy. And the U.S. Health Resources and Services Administration (HRSA) offers funding under the mechanism Nurse Education, Practice, Quality, and Retention Program (NEPQR) that administrators and their educational partners can tap into to examine such questions.

Using strategies such as interprofessional research teams (team science); applying methods in which data are pooled from multiple sites; and integrating biological, behavioral, and cost-effectiveness strategies will eventually enable us to make predictions about how health professionals with certain characteristics perform the caring processes, the proper "dose" required for "feeling cared for" in particular patient populations, the most effective ways to learn caring, and the relative worth of caring practices. Dissemination of findings through publications and presentations and their use in the revision of policy will help translate credible results to the bedside and hopefully transform the work environment such that health professionals find added meaning in the work they do. Understanding how "feeling cared for" improves health outcomes and contributes to evolving theory will provide a rationale for new patient care delivery systems that honor caring relationships as a valuable asset.

SUMMARY

Feeling cared for is a positive emotion that occurs as a separate consequence of caring relationships and is theorized to influence important intermediate and terminal health outcomes. The importance of "feeling cared for" to health outcomes is reviewed, as are the benefits to health professionals themselves. The unique role of the nurse in facilitating "feeling cared for" is reviewed in terms of specific attitudes and behaviors. Measuring "feeling cared for" using well-designed and effectively applied instruments is crucial to evaluating and improving caring practice. The criteria for judging instruments are presented along with a discussion of those important characteristics. The CAT is presented and examples are provided of its use in clinical settings with emphasis on the patient's voice. Research on "feeling cared for" is considered and emphasis is placed on advancing the science through multiple methods and approaches. National research priorities are reviewed. Building on the existing research, and developing caring-based interventions combined with advanced investigational strategies, will eventually enable predictions and validate evolving theory. Dissemination of results and quickly translating credible findings to practice environments provides encouragement for the future.

Call to Action

Positive emotions are connected to health. "Feeling cared for" is a positive emotion that positively influences patients' well-being. **Generate** "feeling cared for" in your patients. Evaluating "feeling cared for" and using those results to improve professional practice, linking it to important outcomes, explaining differences among groups and individuals, and accelerating health systems' adoption of relationship-centered professional encounters is the responsibility of health professionals and leaders. **Compare** and then **choose** ways to best measure "feeling cared for" in your setting. Regularly **evaluate** and use results to improve "feeling cared for." **Brainstorm** potential research questions that could be conducted, including how you would **participate.**

REFLECTIVE QUESTIONS/APPLICATIONS

. . . for Students

1. Describe "feeling cared for." Why is it important to patients and families? What about you?

2. Analyze the nurse's role in facilitating "feeling cared for." How do you measure up?
3. Choose two instruments that measure "feeling cared for" and evaluate them based on the criteria presented in this chapter. Which one would you choose to evaluate this phenomenon in an acute care setting, in a school, and in a nursing home?
4. Outline your plans to use research on "feeling cared for" to advance your practice.
5. Explore the PCORI website. What is your reaction? Should we spend our federal dollars on this research? Why or why not?
6. Contrast qualitative and quantitative approaches to research. How would each of them contribute to understanding "feeling cared for"?

. . . for Professional Nurses in Clinical Practice

1. Discuss your views on whether patients in your organization "feel cared for." Why do you think you have answered this way?
2. Is there an expectation that facilitating "feeling cared for" is a necessary component of RN work at your institution? If so, how is it evaluated?
3. Reflect on your own individual ability to receive "feeling cared for" by members of the health team. Where do you stand? How could you better accept this positive emotion from others?
4. What patient outcomes do you attribute to "feeling cared for?" Why?
5. What have you learned about measurement as a result of reading this chapter?
6. Appraise one qualitative and one quantitative research study on caring relationships. What are the variables? How are they measured? Are the results credible? Would you adopt the findings in practice? Why or why not?
7. How do you participate in research? Take a minute and create a PICO (Patient problem or population, Intervention, Comparison, and Outcome[s]) question that might advance your understanding of "feeling cared for." What will you do with this question?

. . . for Professional Nurses in Educational Practice

1. What specific curricular activities have you developed to enhance the unique role of the nurse in facilitating "feeling cared for" among patients and families and among the health team? How do you evaluate them?

2. Reflect on the need for acceptance of "feeling cared for" among the interprofessional team. How does your educational program facilitate graduates' capacity to accept positive emotions from team members?
3. What can you do to advance the understanding of measurement among undergraduate students and among graduate students?
4. How might you suggest facilitating team caring during educational programs?
5. Provide some suggestions for exposing students to national research priorities and publication/presentation opportunities.
6. Identify two or three research priorities from those discussed in this chapter. How can the study of "feeling cared for" contribute to these priorities? Be specific.
7. Develop a caring-based intervention to facilitate "feeling cared for" among a population of your choice.
8. Design a study to examine the impact of nursing intervention on "feeling cared for" among junior high students with asthma.

. . . for Professional Nurses in Leadership Practice

1. What is the state of "feeling cared for" among patients at your organization? How do you know?
2. How do you specifically hold yourself and your staff accountable for "feeling cared for" among patients and families? Should they be?
3. Reflect on the quality improvement process in place at your institution. Does it include assessment of "feeling cared for"? Why or why not? What would it take to revise this?
4. How do you facilitate research at your organization? What specific research questions are you investigating?
5. Does your leadership team understand the importance of "feeling cared for" as it relates to the bottom line? If not, how will you facilitate their development?
6. Discuss how you would go about partnering with a health professions school to provide research/quality improvement consultation to your staff, design studies that measure "feeling cared for," and submit proposals to potential funders.
7. Create a plan to dramatically alter the quality improvement process to include the routine evaluation of "feeling cared for" from the patient's point of view. What methodology would be used? How long will it take? What implications for RN practice would occur? How would you ensure that the plan is enacted as developed? How would you evaluate its implementation?

PRACTICE ANALYSIS

Alicia is a 37-year-old female who was admitted to an outpatient surgery center for a breast biopsy. She is observed sitting with her husband in the waiting area rapidly moving her crossed right leg and staring straight ahead by a nurse. The perioperative nurse approaches her, introduces herself, and brings her into the operating suite in preparation for surgery. The nurse sits down with Alicia, asks her how she would like to be addressed, and begins explaining the procedure. The nurse then stops talking and allows Alicia and her husband to ask questions. Alicia begins by responding that she is scared and asks if her husband can accompany her. She reassures Alicia and affirms that her husband can accompany her. Then she explains how she had the same procedure and relayed to her how it went. She stayed with Alicia through the procedure and when she was in the recovery area, she talked to her husband about Alicia's progress. When Alicia was ready, she explained the discharge instructions and follow-up care. The couple remained anxious about the impending pathology results. The nurse provided them with her phone number should they have any further questions.

1. Do you think Alicia and her husband felt "cared for?" How could you be sure? Would you have felt this way in this scenario?
2. What specifically does the nurse do to help Alicia feel "cared for?" What did she miss?
3. Did the nurse use any of the caring behaviors in her interactions with this couple? If so, what were they?

REFERENCES

Adler, H. M. (2002). The sociophysiology of caring in the doctor-patient relationships. *Journal of General Internal Medicine, 17*(11), 883–890. doi:10.1046/j.1525-1497.2002.10640.x

American Organization of Nurse Executives. (2017). Seed grants. Retrieved from http://www.aone.org/aone-foundation/research/smallgrant.shtml

Baggett, M., Giambattista, L., Lobbestael, L., Pfeiffer, J., Madani, C., Modir, R., . . . Davidson, J. E. (2016). Exploring the human emotion of feeling cared for in the workplace. *Journal of Nursing Management, 24*(6), 816–824. doi:10.1111/jonm.12388

Boehm, J. K., & Kubzansky, L. D. (2012). The heart's content: The association between positive psychological well-being and cardiovascular health. *Psychological Bulletin, 138*(4), 655–691. doi:10.1037/a0027448

Bunkers, S. S. (2004). The lived experience of feeling cared for: A human becoming perspective. *Nursing Science Quarterly, 17*(1), 63–71. doi:10.1177/0894318403260472

Cosby, K., & Croskerry, P. (2004). Profiles in patient safety: Authority gradients in medical error. *Academy of Emergency Medicine, 12,* 1341–1345. doi:10.1197/j.aem.2004.07.005

Duffy, J. (2008). The caring assessment tools—Administrative version. In J. Watson (Ed.), *Assessing and measuring caring in nursing* (2nd ed.). New York, NY: Springer Publishing.

Duffy, J. (2009). *Quality caring in nursing and health systems: Applying theory to clinical practice, education, and leadership.* New York, NY: Springer Publishing.

Duffy, J., Brewer, B., & Weaver, M. (2014). Revision and psychometric properties of the Caring Assessment Tool. *Clinical Nursing Research, 23*(1), 80–93. doi:10.1177/1054773810369827

Duffy, J., Hoskins, L. M., & Seifert, R. F. (2007). Dimensions of caring: Psychometric properties of the Caring Assessment Tool. *Advances in Nursing Science, 30*(3), 235–245. doi:10.1097/01.ANS.0000286622.84763.a9

Duffy, J., Kooken, W., Wolverton, C., & Weaver, M. (2012). Evaluating patient-centered care: Feasibility of electronic data collection in hospitalized older adults. *Journal of Nursing Care Quality, 27*(4), 307–315. doi:10.1097/NCQ.0b013e31825ba9d4

Falk, E. B., O'Donnell, M. B., Cascio, C. N., Tinney, F., Kang, Y., Lieberman, M. D., . . . Strecher, V. J. (2015). Self-affirmation alters the brain's response to health messages and subsequent behavior change. *Proceedings of the National Academy of Sciences of the United States of America, 112*(7), 1977–1982. doi:10.1073/pnas.1500247112

Grove, S. K., Burns, S., & Gray, J. (2017). *The practice of nursing research* (8th ed.). New York, NY: Saunders.

Hudon, C., Fortin, M., Haggerty, J. L., Lambert, M., & Poitras, M. E. (2011). Measuring patients' perceptions of patient-centered care: A systematic review of tools for family medicine. *Annals of Family Medicine, 9*(2), 155–164. doi:10.1370/afm.1226

Kahn, W. A., & Heaphy, E. D. (2014). Relational contexts of personal engagement at work. In C. Truss, K. Alfes, R. Delbridge, A. Shantz, & E. Soane (Ed.), *Employee engagement in theory and practice* (pp. 82–96). London, UK: Routledge.

Kiken, L. G., Lundberg, K. B., & Fredrickson, B. L. (2017). Being present and enjoying it: Dispositional mindfulness and savoring the moment are distinct, interactive predictors of positive emotions and psychological health. *Mindfulness, 8*(5), 1280–1290. doi:10.1007/s12671-017-0704-3

Kok, B. E., Coffey, K. A., Cohn, M. A., Catalino, L. I., Vacharkulksemsuk, T., Algoe, S. B., . . . Fredrickson, B. L. (2013). How positive emotions build physical health: Perceived positive social connections account for the upward spiral between positive emotions and vagal tone. *Psychological Science, 24*(7), 1123–1132. doi:10.1177/0956797612470827

Meneghel, I., Salanova, M., & Martínez, I. M. (2016). Feeling good makes us stronger: How team resilience mediates the effect of positive emotions on team performance. *Journal of Happiness Studies, 17*(1), 239–255. doi:10.1007/s10902-014-9592-6

National League for Nursing. (2016). NLN Research priorities in nursing education 2016–2019. Retrieved from http://www.nln.org/docs/default-source/professional-development-programs/nln-research-priorities-in-nursing-education-single-pages.pdf?sfvrsn=2

Park, N., Peterson, C., Szvarca, D., Vander Molen, R. J., Kim, E. S., & Collon, K. (2016). Positive psychology and physical health research and applications. *American Journal of Lifestyle Medicine, 10*(3), 200–206. doi:10.1177/1559827614550277

Patient-Centered Outcomes Research Institute. (2014). National priorities and research agenda. Retrieved from http://www.pcori.org/research-results/research-we-support/national-priorities-and-research-agenda

Reader, T. W., & Gillespie, A. (2013). Patient neglect in healthcare institutions: A systematic review and conceptual model. *BMC Health Services Research, 13*, 156. doi:10.1186/1472-6963-13-156

Swanson, K. M. (1999). What is known about caring in nursing science. In A. S. Hinshaw, S. Feetham, & J. Shaver (Eds.), *Handbook of clinical nursing research* (pp. 31–60). Thousand Oaks, CA: Sage.

Thong, I. S., Tan, G., & Jensen, M. P. (2017). The buffering role of positive affect on the association between pain intensity and pain related outcomes. *Scandinavian Journal of Pain, 14*, 91–97. doi:10.1016/j.sjpain.2016.09.008

Watson, J. (2002). *Instruments for assessing and measuring caring in nursing and health sciences.* New York, NY: Springer Publishing.

Watson, J. (2008a). *Instruments for assessing and measuring caring in nursing and health sciences* (2nd ed.). New York, NY: Springer Publishing.

Watson, J. (2008b). *The philosophy and science of caring* (Rev. ed.). Boulder: University of Colorado Press.

Weng, H. Y., Fox, A. S., Shackman, A. J., Stodola, D. E., Caldwell, J. Z., Olson, M. C., . . . Davidson, R. J. (2013). Compassion training alters altruism and neural responses to suffering. *Psychological Science, 24*(7), 1171–1180. doi:10.1177/0956797612469537

Wingo, A. P., Briscione, M., Norrholm, S. D., Jovanovic, T., McCullough, S. A., Skelton, K., & Bradley, B. (2017). Psychological resilience is associated with more intact social functioning in veterans with post-traumatic stress disorder and depression. *Psychiatry Research, 249*, 206–211. doi:10.1016/j.psychres.2017.01.022

Wolverton, C. L. (2016). *Staff nurse perceptions' of nurse manager caring behaviors: Psychometric testing of the Caring Assessment Tool–Administration* (CAT-adm©; Doctoral dissertation, Faculty of the University Graduate School in partial fulfillment of the requirements for the degree Doctor of Philosophy in the School of Nursing, Indiana University).

8

Practice Improvement

Heavy lifting is out; brains are in.
—Tom Peters

THE NATURE OF PROFESSIONAL PRACTICE

Most work roles defined as practices highlight the importance of activity, performance, and creative processes. In fact, a practice has been defined as "a routinized type of behavior which consists of several elements, interconnected to one another: forms of bodily activities, forms of mental activities, 'things' and their use, a background knowledge in the form of understanding, know-how, states of emotion and motivational knowledge" (Reckwitz, 2002, p. 249).

Effective professional practice comprises actual clinical practice, supported by education and leadership practices, all unified by knowledge generated from research, theory, and practical experiences (see Figure 8.1). Using internal and external evidence, health professionals continuously learn about and use knowledge to improve their individual practices, lifting the overall profession's accomplishments. Health professionals take in and use data daily (e.g., patient assessments, performance evaluations, administrative and financial documents) and acquire and apply information through procedures, protocols, and policies. They converse, share documents, and record data and information. However, they often do not take the time to reflect on these data (or information) either alone or in groups, limiting the knowledge available that could be used in a

FIGURE 8.1   Professional practice.

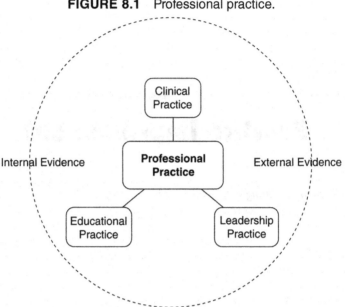

meaningful way to improve practice. For example, in a Magnet®-designated hospital, a patient falls performance improvement (PI) committee meets monthly to review the past month's falls and recommend practice changes. Yet the prevalence of falls continues to rise. Members of the committee are tasked with unit-level monthly audits; however, the audit data are available by unit only in paper and pencil form. The nurse researcher recently suggested that the audit data, when properly aggregated and trended in an ongoing database, might yield important information about practice that might prevent falls. Unfortunately, the committee members, including the master-prepared chairperson, did not see the necessity for such information and elected to continue in the same old pattern. Yet by examining trends and evaluating available information, practice revisions can be designed that integrate this new knowledge into the work and ultimately the underlying beliefs about the work. Additionally, preliminary data reveal that employees who participate in such practices find renewed meaning from the work (Johnson & Jiang, 2017). Health professionals' connections to patients, families, and each other are powerful opportunities to reflect on acquired data and information; yet few take advantage of these interdependencies to improve practice.

At the systems level, the practice of healthcare is complicated, unpredictable, sometimes unfriendly, and often mysterious to patients, families, health professionals, and even top executives. In this complex system (see Chapter 3), new information and knowledge are available each day (some would say each minute). Yet, often, health professionals are not up to date on new knowledge or may be confused by multiple alternatives. But translating empirical evidence into clinical practice is a professional obligation that fulfills our commitment to society, while creating value for health systems. And continuously improving practice is associated with the last concept of the Quality-Caring Model: self-advancing health systems.

In a recent survey, implementation of evidence-based practice (EBP) by nurses was reported to be relatively low (Melnyk et al., 2016). And even though almost one-third of the hospitals were above national core measures benchmarks, such as falls and pressure ulcers, more than one-third of the hospitals were not meeting National Database of Nursing Quality Indicators (NDNQI) performance metrics. Even more alarming, chief nurse executives reported that EBP was ranked lower in terms of budgetary priorities! As a result, evidence-based nursing innovations may not be available for patients when needed, and varying practice patterns among health providers and systems may lead to poorer health outcomes, increased costs, and disparities in care (Soni, Giboney, & Yee, 2016). For example, nursing practice regarding vascular access devices varies tremendously and may lead to creative interventions that are not necessarily evidence based, increasing the risk for central line-associated bloodstream infections (CLABSIs; Conley, Buckley, Magarace, Hsieh, & Pedulla, 2017). In the instance of preventing falls, individual nurses use a variety of practices to ensure patients don't fall. Departments in the same organization may use different policies for urinary catheter care or the management of pain, both within the domain of nursing. Such variations in practice not only influence safety and quality but are costly as well.

Over the last 20 years, the health system has focused on designing elaborate quality improvement and decision-support departments; employed numerous consultants; bought sophisticated software programs; engaged in benchmarking; sent employees to expensive training programs; and constructed policies, reports, and data collection mechanisms to foster internal practice improvement. Each of these mechanisms, although inherently beneficial, has been implemented peripherally to clinical practice, as separate or discrete activities whose goal is to improve the system's performance overall. Furthermore, patients and families are frequently not included in healthcare evaluations of the care received, limiting this important contribution to practice improvement. In some organizations, tensions exist between organizational PI initiatives and departments and the practical application of care. This is a critical challenge for busy health professionals who are doing their best to provide safe, quality patient care. To meet the Institute of Medicine's (IOM) 2020 goal for 90% of clinical decisions supported by accurate, timely, and up-to-date clinical information, including best available evidence, it is crucial that we find ways to empower health professionals and patients to rapidly improve the care they offer and receive (IOM, 2009).

Clinical practice evolves over time and is influenced by supportive practices and the context of the working environment. For example, interactions among employees; imitating high-performing clinicians; reflecting together during rounds; sharing tools, care plans, flow-charts and articles; and ongoing experimentation with new strategies and technology occur every day but are rarely thought of as practice improvement.

Consider the following:

It is lunchtime at Memorial Hospital. A nurse from the heart failure clinic and a medical resident are discussing Mr. T, a patient with Class IV heart failure (HF) who has recently become blind as a result of diabetes and is new to the clinic. The nurse is concerned about his ability to remember to take his medications. Soon they are joined by an occupational therapist and an aide from rehab. "I guess I don't understand what is so worrisome," says the resident. "Just talk to his daughter; she lives with him and she can make sure he takes it."

"But she may not always be available when his meds are due," explains the occupational therapist, "and besides, that means making someone else responsible for his care. The point is to keep patients as self-reliant as possible for as long as possible."

"Mr. T is very independent," says the nurse. "It's almost hard for him to accept help, even in areas where he needs it." "We had a woman coming in for treatments who kept forgetting to take her pills," an aide from rehab recalls. "The nurses asked her to go through the exact story of how she took her meds, every detail—from opening the bottle, taking the cap off, and so on—so that she could imagine it in her mind, and 'see' herself taking the pills as part of it." "That's interesting," said the nurse. "We used a similar technique with someone else in the clinic, and it worked really well."

By now they had been joined by another nurse, this one from the intensive care unit, who had been listening quietly to the conversation. "I used to work as a home health nurse," she says, "and we sometimes used audio recordings for blind patients. Maybe you could produce a tape for this man, and he could use it to remind himself of his meds and other things as well." "Yes," responds the clinic nurse. "Maybe he could even make the tape himself. And that kind of tape could be useful for other patients as well." The conversation becomes animated. "Why not ask Mr. T what he'd like to do?" "Why not ask other HF patients, too?"

"Maybe we could do a survey of HF patients in the clinic, collect their medication stories and their techniques for remembering to take

their pills, and then share those on the tape," says the clinic nurse. "Hey, that is beginning to sound like a nice research project. I think I'll call Jackie (the nurse researcher) and discuss this with her. Who wants to be involved?"

This kind of interaction among many health professionals occurs every day in healthcare settings, yet it is not considered practice improvement. Why not? This group was concerned about a situation with a patient and came up with a possible solution (one that is innovative and included the patient in the process). Through their group dialogue about similar situations and the collective knowledge about blind patients taking medications, they designed a practice improvement project that may help others in the institution as well. Their relational process of sharing a clinical experience resulted in collective learning. In fact, high-quality relationships among health workers actually enable learning through mutual relating, sharing of current evidence, solving problems, appreciation of complementary roles, and the shared purpose of "what's best for the patient."

In health systems, caring relationships among employees and health professionals (relational capacity), together with continuous active engagement in learning (practice improvement), directly influence the quality and rate of self-advancement (see Figure 8.2).

FIGURE 8.2 Practice improvement in self-advancing health systems.

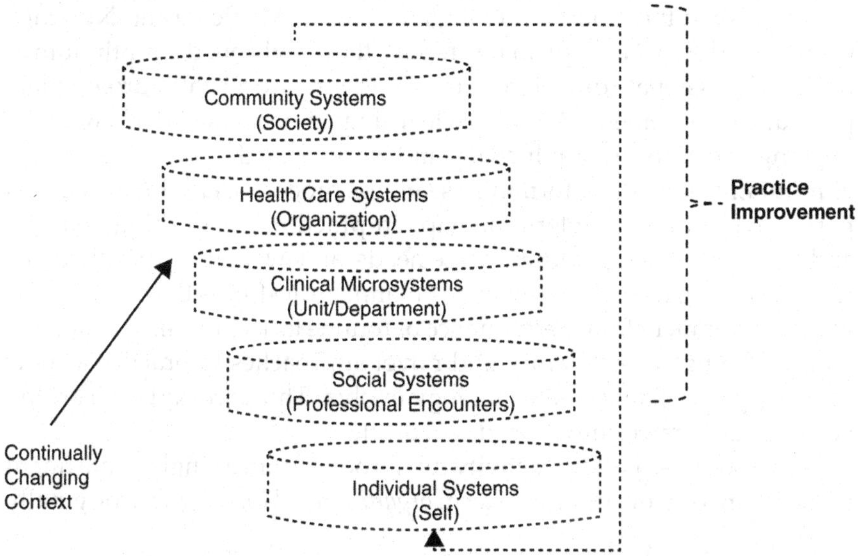

LEARNING IN PRACTICE

Learning typically refers to acquiring new knowledge or skills and sometimes developing new worldviews (values and beliefs). In the individual, new knowledge is equated with new behaviors; at the group level, it is equated with improved communication and interactions; and at the organizational level, it is equated with changes in vision, structure, policies, and new products or services/programs. Usually, learning is characterized as an isolated event—such as going back to school, taking a course, obtaining a certification, completing annual competency testing. As such, it often occurs *before* one does the work and is fragmented from it, sometimes not connected at all. Such learning, although important, does not honor the important relationship between the new knowledge gained and its translation into clinical practice. However, the term *continuous learning* is associated with a deeper and more purposeful learning that is aimed at ongoing development, change, or improvement (most notably at the department or organizational level). Because of the nature of health systems, lifelong learning (also known as continuous learning at the individual level) is a learning outcome of most health professional programs. Thus, individual lifelong learning approaches together with organizational continuous learning processes may facilitate *learning from the work*, a method desperately needed at this time in history.

The American Association of Colleges of Nursing (AACN) Board of Directors and the Association of American Medical Colleges (AAMC) Council of Deans Advisory Board convened a consensus panel in 2009 and published the report "Lifelong Learning in Medicine and Nursing" (AAMC and AACN, 2010). In this report, they envisioned a continuum of health professional education from admission into a health professional program to retirement. Workplace learning, in particular, deals with the ongoing efforts to "unite education and work . . . in the clinical setting . . . as mutually dependent, forming a seamless process of employing clinical performance data to determine gaps in practice, establishing learning and other strategies to address these needs, and evaluating the outcome" (p. 6). Learning from the work in this manner transforms the nature of the work environment from performance of routine tasks to adding, changing, and designing contemporary and novel approaches to practice as new knowledge or changes in technology evolve. Thus, workplace learning becomes integrated into everyday workflow.

On a larger scale, such activity mushrooms from a single department to the entire organization. The term *organizational learning* was originally coined by Senge (1990) in the *Fifth Discipline* and later became focused as a professional discipline through the Organizational Learning Center (OLC) at Massachusetts Institute of Technology. Later, the organization formed the Society for Organizational Learning (SOL). More recently, the continued gap between data and action provided the impetus for the developing subfield of *emergent learning*, which refers to learning about, from, and within the work itself to improve future practice and articulate thinking (Jonas-Simpson, Mitchell, & Cross, 2015). Emergent learning is a relational form of learning that gradually emerges from collective dialogue and work-related activities. As such, it is often unique and unpredictable; however, it enables employees and organizations to adapt their strategies and action plans, in the course of doing work, to achieve the results they want. Taking this approach often produces new and powerful learning while simultaneously making headway on key performance goals. Emergent learning facilitates the complex and fast-moving climates of healthcare organizations, providing employees and leaders with time and space to focus full attention on learning. Further, by weaving learning into real-time work challenges of a business unit or team, an emergent learning approach bypasses the need to stop what we're doing in order to learn. In fact, a team may develop extraordinary emergent learning practices without ever thinking of it as "learning" by self-organizing to focus on improving their performance, rather than stepping into a classroom setting. In this way of learning, performance occurs in context and over time.

Most sociologists would argue that learning is a collective, social, and situated activity.

Emergent learning is considered a social process that challenges the assumptions of traditional performance improvement methods to a learning approach that is dynamic, embedded in daily work, and uses data and analyses in real time. It assumes that health professionals pay attention to what happens in practice, share their experiences, reflect on practice both alone and in groups, develop practice changes, and informally evaluate them for future practice.

Such an environment is characterized by curious employees who feel safe enough to "wonder out loud" and who can see the big picture. Individually, health professionals view themselves as "works in progress" and can use problems, disruptions, and confusion at work in a positive way to fashion new strategies. Such individuals pay attention—and allow themselves to sense, feel, and notice the context. They are also able to respond to data; in so doing, learning is initiated and embedded in the work.

Furthermore, teams of professionals who trust each other, share a mental model of "what's best for the patient," work transparently, and who are cohesive are best able to learn from practice. Leaders in such systems foster learning as a priority and encourage dialogue and the testing of new ideas. Furthermore, leaders who value emergent learning principles are finding ways to make the approach more concrete, infusing it in the work. For example, rather than waiting for patient experience reports (that are often produced 6 months after the fact), some health systems are gathering data on patient–nurse relationships during hospitalization and using real-time results to change practice (Duffy, Kooken, Wolverton, & Weaver, 2012). Others perform real-time debriefing (Nadir et al., 2017), use the electronic health record (EHR), and apply various tracker tools and alert systems to gather real-time data for practice improvement. Such approaches accelerate the learning cycle and makes data available to the clinicians who are actually providing the care. It also focuses more on processes of care *while they are being delivered* versus the more common practice of examining outcomes data after care is delivered.

Focusing more on the here and now is a fundamental change in a system that has been emphasizing, collecting, and disseminating outcomes data for nearly two decades. The adoption of a *learning* health system that incorporates health professionals' lifelong learning, real-time information, including patients' perspectives and measures of patient-centeredness, performance transparency, and leaders who build supportive infrastructures for learning are recommendations from the report "Best Care at Lower Costs: The Path to Continuously Learning Health Care in America" (IOM, 2012). Today, According to Maddox et al. (2017):

> . . . learning health systems (LHS) use health information technology and health data infrastructure to apply scientific evidence at the point of clinical care, while simultaneously collecting insights from that care to promote innovation in optimal health care delivery and to fuel new scientific discovery. Thus, LHS enables rapid, iterative learning in which evidence informs practice and practice informs evidence. (p. e826)

Refocusing on care processes as they are being delivered and revising them in real time demands integrating data access and collection into everyday workflow, using technology for rapid analysis, and reflecting on the results. Reflection involves dialogue and deep thinking about practice and is a way for health professionals to judge the implications of the data, to generate ideas for change, and to take action on those ideas. Labeled *sensemaking* by Kitzmiller, Anderson, and McDaniel (2010), "sensemaking is a social process of searching for answers and meaning that drives the actions people take" (p. 96).

M aking and valuing the time to regularly reflect on care processes (this is not an ad hoc process) and using the time to not only take action but to deeply think about and question former behaviors and their relationships to the underlying professional practice model helps employees make wiser choices in the future. A facilitator can help a group stay connected to clinical practice and find ways to practically apply new knowledge (Harvey & Lynch, 2017). This approach builds learning into the workflow, helps systems learn from mistakes, ensures internal knowledge complements external knowledge, and can generate real impact.

Emergent learning is pragmatic and emerges from the work itself; furthermore, it shifts thinking from reactive to proactive. Emergent learning is intentional, ongoing, and uses approaches that help individuals and small groups learn "through" experience, ultimately improving their performance. Taking this approach requires high-quality relationships and team member interactivity as key interventions to enable health professionals to make the best use of opportunities to improve practice (Parboosingh, Reed, Palmer, & Bernstein, 2011). For example, storytelling aligns current practice with new information, which can trigger group learning and resulting behavioral changes. Working on a project together that is pertinent to the local practice generates new information that might justify practice changes. This approach to practice improvement requires a trusting environment and lifelong learning skills that encourage practitioners to hear each other's perspectives and create ideas for improvement at the microsystem level (examples of how leadership and educational practices support clinical practice). Emergent learning frames organizational learning from the bottom up versus top down and in so doing facilitates individual health professional lifelong learning. Table 8.1 highlights differences in traditional versus contemporary practice improvement.

TABLE 8.1   Differences Between Traditional and Contemporary Practice Improvement

	Traditional Practice Improvement	Contemporary Practice Improvement
Label(s)	Quality improvement (QI)/performance improvement	Practice improvement/emergent learning/continuous learning
Drivers	Corporate needs assessments	Local patient/clinical needs
Emphasis	Discipline specific; focused on externally derived outcomes	Context specific, practice based (department); focused on daily processes
Knowledge acquisition	Centralized, structured approach with predictable outcomes	Decentralized, small work groups learning through relating in everyday practice
Involved individuals	QI professionals, leadership/management	All employees, health professionals, leaders
Role of leadership	Problem identification, policy development, and implementation	Focused on purpose (improvement is the fabric of the work); attention to process; fosters safety culture
Role of patients/ families	Minimal participation	Direct and active patient involvement
Training	QI personnel; leadership	Selective hiring of staff; multiple avenues for training
Value added	Improvement occurs in batches	Practice improvement is embedded in the work; improvement is continuous

MICROSYSTEMS AND COMMUNITIES OF PRACTICE

Since the Dartmouth-based work of Nelson, Batalden, and Godfrey (2007), the concept of microsystems has emerged as a way to envision small work units where various health professionals work together on a regular basis providing care to discrete populations of patients. In the acute care environment, for example, microsystems are organized around similar patient populations or types of procedures (e.g., interventional radiology) or even patient demographics (e.g., pediatrics). Microsystems coexist with others in the system as well as the larger community and when supported may enable self-advancement at a more rapid pace than traditional PI (see Figure 8.2).

This approach capitalizes on the *context* and shared relational purpose aspects of healthcare to foster knowledge and practice improvement/innovation. Furthermore, it uses situation-specific language and understanding of the unique patient population to advance practice. The Dartmouth team developed the popular Joint Commission Journal on Quality Improvement, *Microsystems in Healthcare*, originally a nine-part series (2002–2003). In Part I, Nelson et al. (2002) developed a list of nine clinical microsystem success characteristics, which they published in the journal. They are:

- Leadership
- Culture
- Organizational support
- Patient focus
- Staff focus
- Interdependence of care team
- Information and information technology
- Process improvement
- Performance patterns

Today, the Dartmouth Institute for Health Policy and Clinical Practice has advanced the team's original work on clinical microsystems to offer leadership and coaching development workshops, certificates in value-based care, and online courses to help health professionals in practice improvement approaches (see www.tdiprofessionaleducation.org). Using the clinical microsystems framework enables healthcare clinicians to take collective responsibility for managing the knowledge they need to improve practice. After all, aren't they in the best position to do this?

Similar to clinical microsystems, "communities of practice (CoP) are (voluntary) groups of people who share a concern or a passion for something they do and learn how to do it better as they interact regularly" (Wenger, McDermott, & Snyder, 2002, p. 4). Features of a CoP include a *community* that enables interaction (such as discussions, collaborative activities, and relationship building); a *shared domain of interest* (such as injury prevention); and a *shared practice of experiences*, stories, tools, and ways of addressing recurring problems (Centers for Disease Control and Prevention, 2015). CoPs have been used to support professional practice change in healthcare, including knowledge translation, to support collaboration in diverse groups, and to advance health policy (Bertone et al., 2013; Gagnon, 2013; Yousefi-Nooraie, Dobbins, Brouwers, & Wakefield, 2012). This approach enables health professionals to grow and mature in their disciplines while focusing on efforts to share knowledge and solve problems. Over time, individual members become a community (holding shared meanings) by interacting regularly in relation to each other and their domain. According to Wenger, members don't necessarily work together on a day-to-day basis, but their interactions must have continuity. CoPs are self-governing and group members determine the process.

For example, in a health system, a group of nurses who initially met on the practice council might decide to meet outside the council to discuss the merits of three unique interventions for decreasing delirium in older adults. Perusing the three interventions further, the group of nurses analyzes the advantages and difficulties of each, challenging each other on their effectiveness and efficiencies, and testing their assumptions regarding nurse acceptance and patient outcomes. In the end, they make a case for their point of view. The meetings lasted over several months and were at times challenging and highly emotional. Despite their differences, however, the meetings were engaging and energizing to the members and eventually led to a consensus of a newly adopted delirium intervention. This example characterizes a community of practice.

> Although communities of practice are voluntary, whereas the clinical microsystem approach uses naturally occurring settings, they share a common passion—improving practice—and rely on regular interaction among members to accomplish their goals.

THE VALUE OF PRACTICE IMPROVEMENT

Practice improvement involves health professionals using best evidence (both PI and research) to design actionable practice changes that improve the work. It includes the capacity to give and receive scientific information on behalf of good patient care, to integrate information and technology into the workflow, to balance inquiry and action wisely in daily caregiving, to work interdependently with team members through caring relationships, to engage patients and families, and to use measurement and data to revise patient care (see Table 8.2). Although traditional research, EBP, and various quality improvement strategies have been shown to improve safety and quality, health professionals, their relationships, and the challenges of their work are readily visible and provide rich ground for learning, *if only they would notice their practice and turn it into opportunities for learning.* Embedding learning in the work by fostering caring relationships among team members and tuning in to work-related observations, sensations, and objective data may provide added value to health systems by connecting the dots between everyday clinical practice

TABLE 8.2 Components of Practice Improvement

Give and receive scientific information

Integrate information and technology into the workflow

Balance inquiry and action wisely

Work interdependently "in relationship"

Engage patients and families

Use measurement and data to revise patient care

---

and practice improvement. For example, using the expertise of team members to meet the complete needs of patients (and involving them in the process), solving clinical problems *before* they become catastrophes (receiving immediate answers from expert team members), and increasing individual health professionals' knowledge and performance through sharing collective knowledge, all add meaning to the work, honor patient preferences, and may improve patient outcomes (or at least reduce adverse outcomes). The importance of including patients in the process of practice improvement cannot be overstated. Patients' unique perspectives (which may be surprisingly different from health professionals) provide a reasonable stance from which to evaluate the care received in terms of whether their needs and preferences were met or not. In one Canadian study, where patients were recognized for their experiential knowledge and treated as full members of a PI committee, they identified themselves as real partners in the care process and were grateful for the opportunity to improve care (Pomey et al., 2015). Incidentally, they also become better acquainted with the complexity of the health system and reported a positive change in their relationship with their health professionals as a direct result of their participation.

Practice improvement is important to patients and families not only because they expect safe, quality care but also because it may increase their sense of autonomy and participation in health decisions. As patients view mutual problem solving as caring (a positive emotion), it provides the energy for future interactions with health professionals. Furthermore, the caring behaviors may also translate to healthy behaviors and meet the conditions for self-advancement—learning, growing, changing, taking risks, progressing, coping, and integrating (self-caring).

From the health professional's perspective, learning from the work enhances (uplifts) clinical practice from routine, mundane, repetitive activities to meaningful, knowledge-based work. Knowledge-based practice or EBP is essential to safe, high-quality patient outcomes. Such practice eliminates confusion and ambiguity regarding interventions and may also act to diffuse conflicting situations. Learning from the work may enhance health professionals' self-confidence and feelings of accomplishment necessary for self-advancement—learning, growing, changing, taking risks, progressing, coping, and integrating (self-caring).

Although these are significant examples of the value of contemporary practice improvement, greater potential value lies in members' *use* of new knowledge to try out an approach (innovation value) or change their ways of doing business (change practice) as a result. Additionally, value may be realized when a measurable positive effect occurs within the work team or the organization as a result of a changed practice—for example, practice variation and resultant costs are decreased or patient experiences improved. Value is further added when routine practice improvement is aligned with the academic pursuits of team members, enhancing efficiency and rewarding individual team members (e.g., using group learning in course-related assignments, disseminating group learning through external publications and presentations). When the interactions of the learning team have influenced the participants (and the organization) to reexamine the definition of success, value is added. Finally, when learning from the work becomes integrated into the workflow and practice is continuously improved from the inside out, work becomes meaningful and organizational value is sustained.

SUMMARY

The dynamic nature of professional practice generates new information and knowledge that are almost impossible to efficiently acquire otherwise. Yet clinical, educational, and leadership practice require the use of internal and external evidence to drive practice improvement, resulting in safe, quality care. Learning in practice takes advantage of the relational nature of healthcare, its context, and includes patients in the process. Emergent learning refers to acquiring knowledge and skills in the present moment and using it to take action relative to practice improvement. Such learning assists health professionals to make sense of their actions, to question their ways of doing business, and to use each other's expertise to continually improve. Clinical microsystems and CoP are two approaches that enable emergent learning by exploiting the interdependencies of the health team. The value added by emergent learning meets the conditions for patients and families, health professionals themselves, and health system self-advancement.

Call to Action

Improving professional practice is a complex and relational process. Facilitating emergent learning and resultant practice changes depends on caring-based teams of health professionals who actively learn from their work, generating energy and meaning in the process. **Learn** from your professional colleagues by paying attention to practice, sharing your own expertise, and **use** the knowledge gained to improve.

REFLECTIVE QUESTIONS/APPLICATIONS

. . . for Students

1. When you think of yourself as a continuous or lifelong learner, how does that make you feel? Are you excited about this prospect or are you anxious? Why is it important?
2. Analyze your role in emergent learning. How do you measure up?
3. Contrast the clinical microsystems approach and communities of practice. Choose one and describe how you would use its principles to improve your practice.
4. Design a case study that includes "learning from the work."
5. Explore the Society of Learning and/or the Dartmouth Institute for Health Policy and Clinical Practice website(s). What is your reaction? What did you learn?

. . . for Professional Nurses in Clinical Practice

1. Describe how practice is improved in your organization. Why do you think you have answered this way? Are patients included? What is the role of the staff nurse?
2. Is there an expectation that practice improvement is a necessary component of RN work at your institution? If so, how is it done? How is it evaluated?
3. Reflect on your own individual ability to learn from practice. How do you do it? What do you do with the knowledge and skills you acquire? How could you better integrate this into the workflow?

4. What positive outcomes in health professionals do you attribute to the process of "emergent learning"? Why? What positive outcomes in patients do you attribute to the process of emergent learning? Why?
5. What have you learned about practice improvement as a result of reading this chapter?
6. Evaluate the quality improvement process at your institution. What is specified in the overall plan? What is the role of individual health professionals?
7. Do communities of practice exist at your institution? How do you know? What do they do? How could you participate?

. . . for Professional Nurses in Educational Practice

1. How does emergent learning occur in your university? How does this differ in undergraduate and graduate programs?
2. Reflect on the need for lifelong learning as an outcome of your program. How does your educational program facilitate this outcome? How do you evaluate it?
3. What can you do to advance the understanding of practice improvement among undergraduate students and among graduate students?
4. How might you suggest facilitating emergent learning during your educational programs?
5. Provide some suggestions for exposing students to clinical microsystems and communities of practice.
6. As a health professions educator, discuss how you use an emergent learning stance. Suggest three possible educational research questions involving emergent learning principles. Be specific.
7. Develop an intervention aimed at practice improvement among your professional discipline. How could you make it interprofessional?

. . . for Professional Nurses in Leadership Practice

1. What is the state of practice improvement at your organization? How do you know?
2. How do you specifically hold yourself and your peers accountable for providing the infrastructure necessary for emergent learning among the staff?
3. Reflect on the quality improvement process in place at your institution. Does it take advantage of team relationships and principles

of clinical microsystems? Why or why not? What would it take to revise this?

4. How do you facilitate practice improvement at your organization? What specific methods are used?

5. Does your leadership team understand the value of emergent learning? If not, how will you facilitate their development?

6. What communities of practice are apparent in your organization? What domain are they organized around? Who are the members? How is their work incorporated into the overall performance improvement structure at the organization?

PRACTICE ANALYSIS

The executive team of a large regional health system expressed its frustration at once again needing to consolidate clinical units because of escalating costs. In years past, members had completed the painful work of identifying possible staffing and program cuts. After painstaking processes, they had at least felt a sense of accomplishment at having taken hard but necessary steps to solve the problem.

But, after the third downsizing in 7 years, the team decided to limit the vicious cycle of downsizing and upsizing by taking steps to shift their focus from short-term crisis resolution to a more long-term solution using emergent learning principles. Facing obvious and painful failures in trying to solve recurring financial problems, members recognized how little they really understood about their costs and decided to focus on better understanding it. They made a commitment to develop a deeper and shared understanding of what drives costs, how they were calculated and reimbursed, and to proactively and consistently manage them. They dialogued about the key variables or criteria that would indicate their success.

The team then identified that their weekly staff meetings and reporting documents might offer opportunities for reflections on costs. Because the staff meetings were already on their schedules, they provided a relatively quick and easy way for team members to dialogue about what was driving costs, provide the basis for suggestions and innovations, and gradually evolve into some tangible learning on the issue. This subtle shift to using an already established meeting to "learn" from their joint practice was enlightening.

To start with, team members shared their beliefs and understanding about what contributed to the system's cost structure. Then they very deliberately turned these statements into hypotheses to test with each member considering what he or she was involved in or what data he or she had that would serve as the basis for learning. For example, the director of the cardiovascular program was curious about whether his assumptions about the direct relationship between volume of procedures and overtime costs would hold up. The director of facilities had questions about whether previous cuts in staffing might have actually resulted in increased maintenance costs.

Initially, they simply added brief reviews of cost trends (such as compensation and supplies) to their weekly meetings and included cost patterns to the monthly and quarterly executive reports. Over time, through several iterations, they began to see new relationships and investigate such dynamics as the relationship between patient acuity, compensation, and legal costs. In staff meetings, they reflected on these findings and how they adjusted costs and described different approaches that they had tried to reduce associated costs. (At one meeting, the cardiovascular director reported about asking his team what they would do if high-risk ablation procedures were abolished for a year. The creative responses that he received inspired some of his peers to try the same experiment.)

At each iteration, the group saw that the combined results of their different approaches to learning about costs became the topic on which they reflected. With the benefit of their peer-to-peer relationships, team members teased out unspoken assumptions, lessons learned, and so on. They began to question the actions they had chosen in the past and realized that they needed more powerful and timely cost indicators. They acknowledged how delays in feedback—in the form of unanticipated cost increases—affected their ability to proactively manage expenses. These sessions inevitably led to new questions and novel ideas.

1. What specific approaches did the team use to "learn" about costs? How are they different from or the same as traditional performance improvement approaches?
2. What about the team's interaction did you notice that was new or novel?
3. How might this work lead to even more practice improvement?

REFERENCES

Association of American Medical Colleges and American Association of Colleges of Nursing. (2010). Lifelong learning in medicine and nursing. Retrieved from http://www.aacn.nche.edu/education-resources/MacyReport.pdf

Bertone, M. P., Meessen, B., Clarysse, G., Hercot, D., Kelley, A., Kafando, Y., . . . Sophie Witter, S. (2013). Assessing communities of practice in health policy:

A conceptual framework as a first step towards empirical research. *Health Research, Policy, and Systems, 11*, 39. doi:10.1186/1478-4505-11-39

Centers for Disease Control and Prevention. (2015). Communities of Practices (CoPs). Retrieved from https://www.cdc.gov/phcommunities

Conley, S. B., Buckley, P., Magarace, L., Hsieh, C., & Pedulla, L. V. (2017). Standardizing best nursing practice for implanted ports: Applying evidence-based professional guidelines to prevent central line-associated bloodstream infections. *Journal of Infusion Nursing, 40*(3), 165–174. doi:10.1097/NAN.0000000000000217

Duffy, J., Kooken, W., Wolverton, C., & Weaver, M. (2012). Evaluating patient-centered care: Feasibility of electronic data collection in hospitalized older adults. *Journal of Nursing Care Quality, 27*(4), 307–315. doi:10.1097/NCQ.0b013e31825ba9d4

Gagnon, M. (2013). Moving knowledge to action through dissemination and exchange. *Journal of Clinical Epidemiology, 64*, 25–31. doi:10.1016/j.jclinepi.2009.08.013

Harvey, G., & Lynch, E. (2017). Enabling continuous quality improvement in practice: The role and contribution of facilitation. *Frontiers in Public Health, 5*, 27. doi:10.3389/fpubh.2017.00027

Institute of Medicine. (2009). *Roundtable on evidence-based medicine*. Washington, DC: National Academies Press.

Institute of Medicine. (2012). Best care at lower cost: The path to continuously learning health care in America. Retrieved from http://www.nationalacademies.org/hmd/Reports/2012/Best-Care-at-Lower-Cost-The-Path-to-Continuously-Learning-Health-Care-in-America.aspx

Johnson, M. J., & Jiang, L. (2017). Reaping the benefits of meaningful work: The mediating versus moderating role of work engagement. *Stress and Health, 33*(3), 288–297. doi:10.1002/smi.2710

Jonas-Simpson, C., Mitchell, G., & Cross, N. (2015). Emergence: Complexity pedagogy in action. *Nursing Research and Practice, 2015*, Article ID 235075, 6 pages. doi:10.1155/2015/235075

Kitzmiller, R. A., Anderson, R. A., & McDaniel, R. R. (2010). Making sense of health information technology implementation: A qualitative study protocol. *Implementation Science, 5*, 95. doi:10.1186/1748-5908-5-95

Maddox, T. M., Albert, N. M., Borden, W. B., Curtis, L. H., Ferguson, T. B., Kao, D. P., . . . Shah, N. D. (2017). The learning healthcare system and cardiovascular care: A scientific statement from the American Heart Association. *Circulation, 135*(14), e826–e857. doi:10.1161/CIR.0000000000000480

Melnyk, B. M, Gallagher-Ford, L., Thomas, B. K., Troseth, M., Wyngarden, K., & Szalacha, L. (2016). A study of chief nurse executives indicates low prioritization of evidence-based practice and shortcomings in hospital performance metrics across the United States. *Worldviews on Evidence-Based Nursing, 13*(1), 6–14. doi:10.1111/wvn.12133

Nadir, N. A., Bentley, S., Papanagnou, D., Bajaj, K., Rinnert, S., & Sinert, R. (2017). Characteristics of real-time, non-critical incident debriefing practices in the

Emergency Department. *Western Journal of Emergency Medicine, 18*(1), 146–151. doi:10.5811/westjem.2016.10.31467

Nelson, E. C., Batalden, P. B., & Godfrey, M. M. (2007). *Quality by design: A clinical microsystems approach.* San Francisco, CA: Jossey-Bass.

Nelson, E. C., Batalden, P. B., Huber, T. P., Mohr, J. J., Godfrey, M. M., Headrick, L. A., & Wasson, J. H. (2002). Microsystems in health care: Part 1. Learning from high-performing front-line clinical units. *The Joint Commission Journal on Quality Improvement, 28*(9), 472–493. doi:10.1016/S1070-3241(02)28051-7

Parboosingh, I. J., Reed, V. A., Palmer, J. C., & Bernstein, H. H. (2011). Enhancing practice improvement by facilitating practitioner interactivity: New roles for providers. *Journal of Continuing Education in the Health Professions, 31*(2), 122–127. doi:10.1002/chp.20116

Pomey, M., Hihat, H., Khalifa, M., Lebel, P., Néron, A., & Dumez, V. (2015). Patient partnership in quality improvement of healthcare services: Patients' inputs and challenges faced. *Patient Experience Journal, 2*(1). Retrieved from http://pxjournal.org/journal/vol2/iss1/6

Reckwitz, A. (2002). Toward a theory of social practices. A development in culturalist theorizing, *European Journal of Social Theory, 5*, 243–263. doi:10.1177/13684310222225432

Senge, P. (1990). *The fifth discipline.* New York, NY: Doubleday.

Soni, S. M., Giboney, P., & Yee, H. F. (2016). Development and implementation of expected practices to reduce inappropriate variations in clinical practice. *JAMA, 315*(20), 2163–2164. doi:10.1001/jama.2016.4255

Wenger, E., McDermott, R., & Snyder, W. M. (2002). Cultivating communities of practice: A quick start-up guide. Retrieved from https://icohn.org/uploads/ckeditor/attachments/4/Wenger._Cultivating_CoP_Book.pdf

Yousefi-Nooraie, R., Dobbins, M., Brouwers, M., & Wakefield, P. (2012). Information seeking for making evidence-informed decisions: A social network analysis on the staff of a public health department in Canada. *BMC Health Services Research, 12*, 118. doi:10.1186/1472-6963-12-118

9

Self-Advancing Systems

Natural processes should be judged different from mechanical ones because they are self-organizing.
—Immanuel Kant

THE MEANING OF SELF-ADVANCING SYSTEMS

Self-advancing systems is the last concept in the Quality-Caring Model© (QCM), and the words were specifically chosen. In complexity science, the language of evolution and self-organization is frequently used to signify the combined effects of multiple interacting parts that over time emerge in new creative ways. The direction of the new behaviors or practices is not specified; rather the context and feedback received are theorized to advance certain outcomes. The number of interactions in complex systems emphasizes their dynamic nature, with continuing interactions at the lowest levels forming patterns that provide structure to the system. The environment or context provides the conditions of the interactions but the feedback received sensitizes agents to the conditions. For example, positive feedback may result in greater sensitivity to conditions, perhaps intensifying random variabilities, resulting in unique, unanticipated outcomes. Contrarily, negative feedback may result in less sensitivity to conditions, with typical or standard outcomes as a result.

The word *advancement* signifies forward movement, progress, elevation, growth, change, development, and expansion. Self-advancing systems are quality systems in that they reflect dynamic, positive progress that enhances the system's performance. Caring relationships (with self, patients, and families, among health professionals, and in communities) are forms of positive, energizing feedback that support individuals', groups', and systems' capacities to change, learn, or respond to their fluctuating conditions. Put another way, living systems (including persons, groups, and the organizations in which they work) are alive, interact locally, are capable of discovering new possibilities, co-create patterns that inform behaviors and repeatedly self-organize (promote order), without conscious planning or control. The multiple connections among the individuals (agents) in a complex system are critical and their relationships provide important feedback that informs collective new order. There is no hierarchy of command and control in these living systems, but the context and feedback received from the many relationships among the agents fuel reorganization. This phenomenon of self-organization is pervasive, but subtle, and often goes unnoticed. If the context and feedback are nourishing, the potential for reorganization is great; if not, that same potential may be limited.

In clinical environments, humans and their social interactions are distinctively self-determining and full of promise (assumptions of the QCM). Thus it is reasonable to expect that through ongoing interactions and feedback over time and within a caring—a.k.a. *nourishing*—context, new patterns (habits, conduct, behaviors, methods, approaches, practices) that emerge are optimistically oriented and arise without the need for outside control. And since organizations, as living systems like individuals, have a natural tendency to organize, if ongoing interactions are nurtured (cared for), new patterns or novel forms (e.g., changes in function or behaviors) emerge *on their own* as forward movement; thus they are self-advancing. Acknowledging and even exploiting this complexity, instead of reducing it, is key to advancement.

> Advancement, therefore, is a natural human phenomenon that begins as a local process and is a *product of that process*, not external manipulation. Thus the use of the word *self* in the term self-advancing systems is fitting.

Self-advancing systems are not linear but have highs and lows and emerge gradually over time and are influenced by context. Through multiple interactions between and among individuals and the environment, interdependencies develop, creating small differences or changes that can grow exponentially, *if* nurtured. These small, but positive, differences may enhance the lives of patients and families, health professionals and systems at the local level, and ultimately lead to larger scale advancement. Furthermore, new forms of behavior and resulting changes cannot be predicted, as they occur over time as a result of uncontrollable and numerous connections—drastically changing how we think about progress (or results, outcomes).

For example, our continued focus on quality outcomes several weeks (or months) after care has been delivered is too far removed from the ongoing interactions of those delivering the care and is not able to keep up with the unpredictable complexity in the system and its context. Because of this phenomenon, improvement is often sluggish or weak and frequently does not endure. Rather, if the focus is shifted quickly and locally (at the clinical microsystem level) to the *process* of care before a problem/situation has a chance to spread, it can be very effective. That is, the process can become effective provided the multiple agents (individuals) in the system have a repertoire of ideas or actions to draw from, are free to dialog about them, and then are able to trial and enact them in a context that is supportive and encouraging. Moreover, if a robust frame of reference (e.g., a professional practice model) grounds the practice, individuals can extract concepts from that foundation to modify their ideas and actions, better aligning them with the overall purpose of the discipline or health system.

In health systems, professionals are autonomous individuals with unique knowledge and sets of skills that complement each other. Through ongoing interactions and feedback, their individual expertise becomes integrated in the overall care of patients and families. Successful self-advancing systems use knowledge and anticipation of events to modify their behavior (or functions) and prepare for changes. Those that are grounded in strongly held principles are better able to withstand periods of instability or disruptions in the work.

> Thus well-balanced groups of health professionals who are grounded in a shared purpose and who continually interact and learn from each other (in caring relationships) can self-advance (themselves, their patients, and health systems) without compromising their individual functionality.

Self-advancement, however, doesn't happen quickly—rather, it is incremental and best accomplished through simple processes involving interactions operating locally. For example, simple changes in how a handoff is performed, or ways in which patient mobility is enhanced, or postoperative patients are received onto surgical units can lead to large-scale improvements. An example of this is a hospital associated with a larger health system in a diverse area of New York City. Knowing that pressure ulcers were a problem on a unit, the nurses on their own developed a skin care cart (with supplies and equipment) and set up a protocol of accountability for use by all nurses in the unit. A written communication system was established for use by all RNs on the unit and within a few weeks, skin breakdown was reduced by 50% and staff members' engagement improved. Although the unit intended to improve incidences of skin breakdown, they did not anticipate the improved staff engagement and pride experienced by the nursing staff. Shortly thereafter, other units started imitating the idea.

Without knowledge of their ultimate effects, however, changing practices in nursing (or other health professions) are often left obscure, without tangible evidence of their outcomes. Good ideas can also be impractical, too expensive, or not acceptable (too difficult to implement) to patients or staff. So, pilot studies or demonstration projects are reasonable ways of determining the feasibility of suggested improvements. This approach is performed at the local level (unit) and its evaluation should assess local *and* system variables; thus it represents a shared method that preserves the original idea(s) generated at the local level (and credits them accordingly). The objective is to generate systems capable of adaptation, change, and even novelty by focusing on relevant smaller processes that take place primarily in their natural environment, enabling the system to adapt to real-world tasks, despite the differences in individuals, the environment, and their interactions over time.

Consider the following:

> *A nursing administrator is concerned about the failing Hospital Consumer Assessment of Healthcare Providers and Systems (HCAHPS®; Goldstein, Farquhar, Crofton, Darby, & Garfinkel, 2005) survey scores on several of his units. After attending a conference in which he heard a presenter talk about how they were able to raise their scores through the use of a popular healthcare consultant's approach, he hires the consultant to do the same work at his institution. Over several months (and several thousand dollars), the HCAHPS scores are only a little improved and not improved at all on some units.*

Was the use of a single approach too rigid for the particular context or limiting to the staff? Could the nursing administrator have used a more innovative approach? What if the nursing staff were presented with the problem and expected to find solutions themselves? Even better, what if the nursing staff already knew about the scores (rapid feedback) and used group reflection to design a practice improvement by themselves? Better yet, what if they included patients in the process? The first approach is predictable, orderly, and keeps the administrator in control. The second is flexible, messy, and uncontrolled. Will it work? The only way to know is to implement the staff's recommendation and find out. After all, in the near future, when patients are truly in control of their care, health professional–designed approaches may be obsolete anyway!

Interestingly, despite the interest in advancement and innovation in health systems, diffusion of alternative approaches has been slow. Just like clinical work, it tends to be task oriented (discrete little parts), driven by cost containment, with little discussion about the many interdependent relationships that characterize its complexity. The dominant paradigm is still the sum-of-the-parts mentality in which a health system is viewed as a combination of multiple parts. The problem with such an approach is that health professionals have a tendency to think that if central line infections or falls have been reduced, the job has been done and the larger concept of safety has been reached. Rather, quality or excellence is an *umbrella* term that is really about forward movement. It consists of multiple dimensions—safety, reliability, accuracy, costs, the overall experience, and so on. In complex health systems, superior system outcomes (advancement) are not final solutions but part of a systematic, continuous learning process that leads to alternative decisions about practice by the clinicians and patients themselves. This is a much different approach from the mechanistic quality improvement paradigm of specialized personnel measuring and analyzing specified outcomes and reporting them back to department heads.

The notion of groups of interdependent, creative health professionals interacting and finding ways to improve practice *on their own* runs counter to traditional organizational thinking that emphasizes the ability of systems to be engineered toward predefined goals within a framework of incentives and punishments.

Self-advancing systems naturally evolve as everyone (including patients and families) shares in the *process* of small practice change (improvement)—as part of the work. The challenge for leadership in this time of rapid change is to encourage and expect multiple interactions among health professionals through ongoing collaboration, dialoguing, networking, reflecting, and collective learning about patient care such that it becomes enculturated, enabling rich solutions—and then to trust and get out of their way!

PROCESS, PROCESS, PROCESS

It's relatively easy to advance (deliver safe, high-quality care) when resources are plentiful or there is little competition. But today's environment is atypical, demanding alternative strategies for progression. In the companies with sustained high reliability (self-advancing systems), Weick and Sutcliffe (2015) examined sense making, interacting, and language, digging deep into the human side of organizations for clues about their performance. Sense making is the process through which individuals work to understand novel, unexpected, or even confusing events (Weick, 1995), and it has been defined as a social process that occurs between people, as meaning is negotiated, challenged, and mutually co-created. Organizational members and their customers actively use their underlying interactions with each other to interpret their work, find meaning, and collectively shape the world around them. In this way, employees and customers are involved with the *real work* of organizations. It is clear that self-advancing in today's environment requires optimal sense making, ongoing and thoughtful interaction, and accurate and timely communication—the *processes*—of high-quality healthcare. These processes are best found on local clinical units (or departments) and involve patients, families, and health professionals.

In our current task-focused environment, the emphasis is centered on the health professional or the health system—what needs to be done, who needs to do it, and how and when will it get done? This continued focus on tasks and assignments (and their payment) as well as how they individually contribute to reimbursable outcomes ("if I do this, X will occur") is a linear way of thinking. On the other hand, attention to the relational aspects of healthcare is big-picture, patient centered, comprehensive, and interdependent, more typical of the dynamic nature of complex organizations. In nursing, that means holistic, interpersonal, connected, and complete nursing care that is evidence based and provided collaboratively with other health professionals (well-coordinated).

Such care is always patient centered, with caring relationships as the foundation, and encompasses assessment, ongoing monitoring and surveillance, attention to hygiene (one's own and the patient's), mobility, breathing and circulation, nutritional intake and elimination (including the measurement of intake and output), sleep and rest, planning for transitions, attending to the emotional aspects of illness, education, simple interventions that yield high impact—such as repositioning, anticipating and relieving discomfort, teaching, ambulating or range-of-motion activities, routine spot checking, and regular handwashing.

These simple but fundamental nursing acts are essential for optimal comfort, skin integrity, reasonable functional status, positive patient experiences, reductions in hospital or emergency department readmissions, and longer term independence in the community—all high-impact and *reimbursable* outcomes!

Integrated with basic or fundamental healthcare processes, evidence-based clinical practice guidelines provide health professionals with recommendations for practice that positively influence outcomes. However, how guidelines (which are formulated for the average patient) are implemented for individual patients requires team consideration and patient input. To be useful, guidelines should be well referenced, evaluated regularly, and revised often based on research and sharing of lessons learned. Most importantly, dialog and collaborative decision making among health professionals and patients regarding the use of guidelines in particular situations and the impact of their use have an effect on important outcomes.

After years of focusing on the pessimistic terms, adverse outcomes, and medical errors, most health systems and health professionals still believe that monitoring them intently will help them improve. Our perpetual attention to measuring adverse outcomes has unintentionally taken us away from the fundamental *processes* of good patient care (such a simple idea, but counterintuitive to modern-day thinking). The big difference between a process-focused health system (or health professional) and an outcome-focused one is that during patient care, the outcome-focused health professional's attention is devoted to concerns about what outcomes will result. With this in mind, the health professional may question whether she or he is doing the intervention right, or worry that she or he is taking too long, or what other health professionals might think, or how the boss will evaluate her or him. Each of these outcome-focused thoughts interferes with the care ultimately provided! Concerns about the outcome distract one from being present and aware of the uniqueness of the patient and his or her health situation; they may also cause one to doubt one's capability and take away from the capacity to perform optimally. Many health professionals employed in health systems who take this outcomes stance create outcomes-focused organizations. Over time, outcomes-focused organizations lose focus on the *processes* of good patient care. It is time to consider simply letting go of the outcomes for a while and concentrate closely and attentively on the processes of healthcare.

The *processes* of care are really all we can control in the constantly changing internal and external environment. Focusing on the process—the fundamental practice of good patient care—and trusting that we can perform it well increases the chances of advancement.

Clinical practice that is caring, comprehensive, and accurately and reliably delivered will naturally generate positive outcomes and benefit patients and families, health professionals, and health systems.

THE MEANING OF SELF-ADVANCEMENT FOR PATIENTS AND FAMILIES

Each individual patient has a unique experience with various health professionals and health systems along the healthcare continuum ranging from primary care to episodic acute care, restorative care to long-term or even palliative or hospice care. But services provided in fragmented chunks are usually geographically placed and linked to specific disease states. Each of these disease states has associated outcomes indicators (e.g., survival, HbA1c levels, O_2 levels, intervention success rates) and care is usually delivered in the clinician's office requiring multiple visits. The clinician addresses his or her area of expertise without much thought to the overall events the patient undergoes or the multiple interactions occurring within the larger health system. This leads to unpredictable, changing, conflicting, and sometimes dissatisfying healthcare experiences.

Consider this scenario from Dr. Berwick's (2016) presentation:

> On the day before I get ill, I am an autonomous, capable citizen. I can fill out my tax returns. I can ply my craft. I can make terrific Italian meatballs. I can counsel my adult daughter on how to handle her son's new fears at school. I can finish the Saturday New York Times crossword puzzle. I can binge on three episodes of Game of Thrones while answering 50 emails at the same time.
>
> And then I show up at health care's dinner party and health care strips me. It silences me; it dresses me in a sheet; it takes away my work; it takes away my pleasures, my family; it tells me exactly what to do. "Take a breath, hold your breath." What if, instead, health care asked me what I can do, and thanked me for doing it? What if, instead, health care asked me if I would like to sit or stand . . . if I would like to speak or remain quiet? What if health care asked me for instructions, not doctor's orders, but people's orders?

Experiences of care refer to patients' perspectives on the responsiveness of health providers to their specific needs and include the manner in which care is provided (Institute for Healthcare Improvement [IHI], 2009). Patients' perspectives of their healthcare experiences are essential to providing clinicians with information on how care processes affect responses to illness, and are considered a unique and independent dimension of quality. When validly and reliably measured, experiences of care have been linked to specific quality and business outcomes such as adherence to guideline-based care for myocardial infarction, pneumonia, heart failure, and surgical complications; decreased malpractice claims; better coordinated care; and better preventive care screenings and disease management for chronic conditions (Jha, Orav, Zhen, & Epstein, 2008; Press Ganey Associates Inc., 2008; Sequist et al., 2008; Wennberg, Bronner, Skinner, Fisher, & Goodman, 2009). Moreover, in a systematic review that examined evidence from 55 studies, a consistent positive association was reported between patient experience, patient safety, and clinical effectiveness for a wide range of disease areas, settings, outcome measures, and study designs (Doyle, Lennox, & Bell, 2013).

Using the national HCAHPS Survey (Goldstein et al., 2005), standardized, publicly reported data about patients' experiences of care are collected that allow for meaningful comparison of hospitals and serve as a basis for reimbursement. However, in a study examining patient experience from 2008 to 2014, patient experience improved only modestly at U.S. hospitals—with the majority of improvement concentrated in the period before the reimbursement program was implemented. The authors concluded that no evidence of a beneficial effect was found! As policy makers continue to promote value-based payment, it is critical that health professionals attend to patients' unique needs, responding with compassion and allowance for mutual decision making.

Take the case of a newly diagnosed patient with diabetes who is disadvantaged. Often this is a person who relies on a relative or caregiver, has few resources, and may be unable to understand the meaning of his or her diabetes (health illiteracy). The individual suffers from glucose highs and lows, may not be able to engage in social activities (due to lifestyle changes), may be depressed, must take multiple medications that have untoward side effects, is on dietary restrictions, may suffer from sleep interruptions, may have associated diseases, and must adhere to daily symptom monitoring. Episodically, the individual may be hospitalized and returns home each time often with new medications and the same old routine, with visits to the physician's office periodically. There is no ongoing, convenient, reimbursable mechanism for learning about new medications, dealing with the emotional aspects of the illness, receiving encouragement and positive reinforcement to modify behaviors (e.g., ambulate, eat well), receive suggestions on improving sleep, or dealing with the side effects of multiple medications, or even how to get dressed in the morning! Yet, this is the daily experience of living with chronic diabetes.

In an ideal world, this patient could consistently receive such services in the convenience of his or her own home (the actual delivery mechanism may include telephone, electronic devices, in-person encounters, and the Internet). It is highly likely that such processes of care would better provide patients with the caring relationship he or she needs to learn about the illness, become an expert in symptom control, adhere to diet and ambulation recommendations, sleep better, and detect early warning signs of exacerbation *before* there is a need for hospitalization. Such caring processes influence intermediate and longer term outcomes, such as quality of life and hospital readmissions. In essence, the patient eventually becomes self-caring (able to listen, take responsibility for, repair, and affirm oneself). Isn't this the essence of self-advancement?

THE MEANING OF SELF-ADVANCEMENT FOR HEALTH PROFESSIONALS

Health professionals work in various environments and disciplines; endure demanding jobs with little opportunity for continuing education; work with personnel who may lack commitment or just don't follow through; deal with multiple sources of conflict; sometimes practice in environments that don't recognize or value employee's contributions; or experience periodic burnout, boredom, and even disillusionment. Recently, the American Nurses Association (ANA, n.d.) has endorsed the Healthy Nurse, Healthy Nation™ grand challenge. Since research shows that, in general, nurses are less healthy than average Americans (more likely to be overweight, have higher levels of stress, and get less sleep), the ANA is advocating that facilitating nurses' health is critical to the health of the nation.

Likewise, reports of burnout, symptoms of depression, and substance abuse disorders plague physicians as well (Oreskovich et al., 2014; West et al., 2014). Interestingly, these reports sound like they were written by nurses and most likely by some other health professionals as well (inattention to personal health, demanding work schedules). Yet most health professionals report that they like their work!

In spite of the disciplinary differences and sometimes discouraging work conditions, there are several positive universal principles that present health professionals with opportunities for growth, energy, creativity, an enhanced worldview, improved clinical skills, and even personal and professional fun. For example, in addition to a decent income, many health professional careers are flexible in terms of scheduling and provide opportunities for different types of employment in multiple settings, as well as promotional prospects.

Working in the health professions allows one to meet and learn from talented coworkers who encourage and support growth. It also provides an identity that is valued in society, opening doors that might otherwise be closed. Most importantly, working in the health professions offers many opportunities to make a difference in the lives of others and in so doing learn about one's own life, *provided we stay awake and apply what we learn from our work on ourselves.*

On a daily basis, health professionals encounter situations that cause them great fear—pain, a new cancer diagnosis, chronic disease, loss of function, death. Over time, such situations can lead to feelings of numbness or even paralysis, as health professionals try to protect themselves from the suffering they see every day. Cassel (1982) described suffering as "the state of severe distress associated with events that threaten the intactness or wholeness of the person" (p. 639). Cassel further adds that "suffering is a consequence of personhood—bodies do not suffer, persons do" (1992, p. 3). Thus, suffering is a human experience that affects all beings and health professionals; with their special knowledge and skills, health professionals have unique opportunities to consider and learn from the suffering experiences of their patients and families.

Health professionals also encounter situations that cause them great joy—the birth of a healthy baby, the ability of a formerly bedridden individual to walk, a pain-ridden patient who is now comfortable, or a surgical patient who is able to rejoin the workforce. The process of caring with and for others offers us a unique opportunity to see reality, direct our attention toward the human experience of illness (and its associated joys and suffering), and move toward possibilities that have been in front of us all along—learning how to cope in the face of human suffering, enjoyment, personal development, and self-wisdom. Caring relationships with oneself, patients and families, other health professionals, and communities provide the medium for feeling cared for, and for health professionals this becomes apparent through work engagement, organizational citizenship, belonging, feeling confident, and so forth (see Figure 9.1).

FIGURE 9.1   Intermediate outcomes subsequent to "feeling cared for" among health professionals.

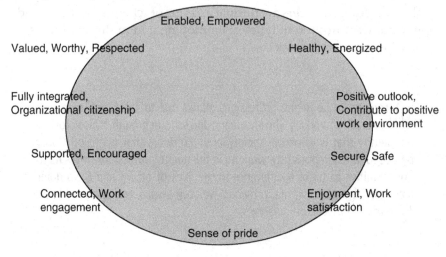

> eing open to the many meanings of clinical practice, rather that rushing past them, shifts our worldview toward the more optimistic aspects of the work. In turn, health professionals find that their work has meaning that transcends income, status, flexible scheduling, and an identity that provides clarity and affirmation.

A perfect example occurred to this author many years ago as a young nurse who hadn't yet fully confronted death.

After being "pulled" off the critical care unit and "floated" to an oncology floor, I was assigned a 58-year-old woman with breast cancer. She had metastasis to the bone and was in severe pain every time she moved or changed her position; she was alert and oriented, receiving intravenous chemo, and had terrible sores in her mouth. In all, she was suffering tremendously and close to death. She had two grown daughters about my age who were quite fearful of their mother's prognosis and in their anxiety could not stay long in the room—they could often be found pacing in the hall. Witnessing this scenario was hard for me as I had never dealt with death in this manner (my critically ill patients were usually unconscious and I hadn't yet experienced death in my personal life). I was anxious and didn't know how to interact well with the patient or the family. Somehow the patient sensed this (could it be that she had children about my age?) and called me over to her bed and asked me to sit down on it. Uncomfortably, I did as I was asked and the woman took my hand, looked right at me, and began to tell me how she had led a wonderful life (she recounted several stories), that she knew she was dying, and that she was okay with it! She did not seem to be in pain as she told me her story and after she was finished, I was in tears. She was smiling. This beautiful lady taught me the powerful lesson that the process of patient care is rich with life lessons that are to be honored and that even those patients and families who are the most distressed (or suffering) can offer us healing.

According to Steger (2017), meaningful work "speaks to people's subjective experience that their jobs, work, or careers are purposeful and significant, that their work is harmoniously and energetically synergistic with the meaning and purpose in their broader lives, and that they are enabled and empowered to benefit the greater good through their work" (p. 60). Thus, if meaningful, the processes and relationships encountered during clinical practice create an overall sense of purpose and significance, consistent with the larger meaning of their lives. In Pavlisch and Hunt's (2012) qualitative study of 13 acute care nurses, narratives were collected to describe meaningful work. Nurses readily participated and 10 of their narratives were categorized as stories of connection, 8 were stories of contribution, and 6 described moments of appreciation. Interestingly, all participants identified relationships with patients and family members as particularly meaningful. Participants also described the importance of seeing patients improve—seeing patients walking out the door, improved physical comfort, or anxiety reduction. Some participants described meaningfulness as being recognized for their expertise, accomplishments, or humane care. Interestingly, all participants described stories that involved the relational aspect of work in which they were heavily involved in *processes* such as being a caring presence, advocating for patients and families, and gently guiding them through the healthcare process.

Most health professionals like their work (personal conversations), but often get caught up in the negative culture of some health systems where employees who do not readily see the importance of their work or who can't/don't slow down enough to really feel the benefits of the care process express displeasure and unhappiness at work. Furthermore, many health professionals work endless shifts (often back to back) or work two or more jobs, sometimes increasing their own stress. Identifying the stresses of the work is good, but dwelling on them without accepting some responsibility for that stress is unwise.

Recently, this author spent some time with a 35-plus years RN who has had her own health problems and works 12-hour shifts in a hospice inpatient department. She complained fiercely about her work, including upper leadership, assistive staff, other nursing and physician staff, and the long hours. Then she proceeded to share how she had just signed up for 14 hours of overtime, went to bed with a bag of potato chips and a Creamsicle® (instead of eating dinner), and proceeded to stay up until 3 a.m. because she was "hyped up" from the work.

Although there is no magic formula for *using what we learn from our work on ourselves,* slowing down a little to listen, to feel, and to appreciate how those meaningful moments encountered in clinical practice enrich our lives is crucial. After all, we are also human. Finding meaning by authentically relating to patients and families and other health professionals through the process of clinical practice facilitates feeling cared for in ourselves and can lead to some highly significant consequences: increased work commitment and engagement, personal health, self-efficacy, and empowerment. The nature of clinical practice is complex and often tiring, but it seems as if the more health professionals "roll up their sleeves," linger a little, stay embedded in the important work they do, and pay attention to the *process* of clinical work, the more meaning that work provides. In turn, the impact of that work on the health professional results in feelings of accomplishment, enjoyment, disciplinary knowledge, belonging, and skill development, personal life and work satisfaction, even a sense of pride—that is, self-advancement.

THE MEANING OF SELF-ADVANCEMENT FOR HEALTH SYSTEMS

As discussed earlier in this chapter, many health systems today are preoccupied with measuring outcomes or their failure to achieve high-level outcomes, still have bureaucratic structures and rigid rules, ignore the contextual factors that impact patient care, and most importantly, are reluctant to really examine, simplify, and fix the *processes* of care. Yet processes of care are theoretically and empirically linked to important health outcomes (Brooks-Carthon, Lasater, Rearden, Holland, & Sloane, 2016; Donabedian, 1966; Linetzky, Jiang, Funnell, Curtis, & Polonsky, 2017; Song et al., 2016). Most health systems characterized this way, however, offer various reasons for their inattention to the obvious—for example, complexity of the work, poor reimbursement (and not enough resources), the younger workforce—and do not see the potential near-misses, accidents waiting to happen, or poor processes that impact their outcomes. Curry et al. (2011) suggest that the daily experience of patients reflects the well-being of a health system and those experiences depend on the organization's culture more than its policies and procedures and may be more reliable than evidence-based protocols. The patient experience below illustrates this point:

> As the husband of a university professor who recently "encountered" the health system, I was horrified by the lack of attention to the basic human needs for information, compassion, and problem solving. Here is our story. I am a software analyst, father of one little girl with a learning disability and another teen-aged son, and am married to a wonderful woman named Laura who is 48. She was a music professor at a prestigious university in Pennsylvania. She started having lower abdominal pain and intermittent nausea in May 2010, and then it progressed to her back. She went to her physician multiple times and was told it was stress or muscle tension. The physician prescribed pain meds and muscle relaxants. Then, finally, in August, she was hospitalized for continued pain and multiple tests. While in the hospital, she called me and said, "They told me I have tumors in my ovaries and abdomen and are sending in an oncologist." By the time I got there, the oncologist had visited and gone, not fully explaining to my wife what her diagnosis, treatment plan, or prognosis was. She was anxious, confused, and needed answers. I asked the nurses what was going on and they said to wait for the oncologist to return.
>
> For 2 days we waited for the oncologist to come in and explain what he found in my wife. When he did appear, he very systematically suggested that they would treat the pain effectively with medication and my wife could go home soon. He still didn't explain the diagnosis. I was so exasperated that I asked the nurses for the medical record. They sent me to the Medical Records Department and I was told it would be a 72-hour wait and I would be charged for a copy of the chart. Although my wife continued to be medicated for pain when she asked for it and the technicians periodically took her blood pressure, no health professional routinely checked in on her or helped us solve our lack-of-information problem.
>
> I continued to ask for information and as our primary physician did not have privileges at this hospital, I asked if the oncologist could at least call him and discuss the case. I also asked for a second opinion and a transfer because I did not like the care my wife was receiving—it was matter of fact and procedure based. When we were transferred, my wife's medical record and transfer summary was incomplete, which meant the new facility could not provide care for several hours as they tried to recreate it using a phone and a fax—the Health Insurance Portability and Accountability Act (HIPAA; United States Department of Health and Human Services, 1996) prevents sending health information over the Internet. They couldn't provide pain

relief or even food during this time. I had to go down to the cafeteria and get her a little something so she could eat.

Finally, they came up with the completed medical record, read it, and then let me read it. It was full of information that would have helped my wife and I receive her poor prognosis better. I sat there astounded that it took 4 days to learn that my beautiful wife had inoperable ovarian cancer with metastasis throughout the abdomen and that no one apparently cared that our lives were almost instantaneously turned upside down. No business would operate this way. Why does the healthcare system get away with such poor service? How can health professionals practice this way?

It is now February 2011 and 2 months since Laura died; our children's lives have been so horribly affected and our home will never be the same. Her last days were peaceful and pain free (thanks to hospice) but she had several months of repeated hospitalizations. Her encounters with the health system were substandard at best—poor communication, lack of compassion, inattention to basic hygiene, little information or participation in decisions was offered, leadership was unavailable, and, most disturbing, clinicians did not seem to care. The new healthcare law cannot fix these problems—they are fundamental aspects of the work that are usually not dealt with in the face of other seemingly important issues. I am so frustrated . . . .

Clinical processes such as ensuring the delivery of patient-centered care would have made this experience bearable. But numerous health systems fail to appreciate that simple, relationship-centered attitudes and actions used in clinical care (relational capacity) and concurrent ongoing practice improvement may in fact help them naturally self-advance.

In 2011, Chassin and Loeb reported that in spite of the external regulations, limited reimbursement, workforce issues, and the intricate knowledge required for safe, quality care, some health systems are consistently performing reliably at high levels. A common denominator of such organizations is that they lived their core values, or as Boehmer (2009) suggested, they aligned their fundamental nature with the management of healthcare. This includes understanding and continuously improving processes of care, that is, *how* care is delivered. The same holds true today. Health systems can generate sustained value by bolstering the distinct while mutually reinforcing attributes: relational capacity and practice improvement (Figure 9.2).

Relational aspects of professional practice that impact performance at the organizational level have been theorized and well documented by Gittell (2002, 2009, 2016). Labeled *relational coordination,* she suggests that the interdependent nature of interactions among health professionals is optimized when healthcare teams share purpose and knowledge and

FIGURE 9.2 Dual integration of relational capacity and practice improvement in self-advancing systems.

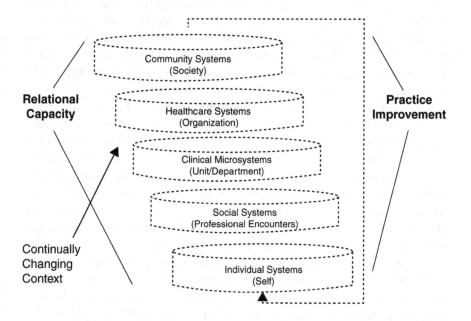

exhibit mutual respect that together maximize effective coordination of work. At the organizational level, relational coordination can be fostered through selective hiring of employees, measuring and rewarding team performance, resolving cross-disciplinary conflicts proactively, investing in frontline leadership, developing cross-disciplinary care pathways, broadening participation in interdisciplinary patient rounds, and developing shared information systems (Gittell, 2009, 2016; Gittell, Seidner, & Wimbush, 2010).

The human relational perspective of healthcare, when acknowledged and made explicit as the center of work, includes relationships not only with patients and families but also with other health professionals, oneself, and the communities served.

Organizations that attend to the complex interactions in their systems "see" more interconnections in the moment, enable quick adjustments, stay attuned to unfolding relationships longer, are better able to "marry" needs with experience and expertise, and use relationships to solve problems before they spread (or the converse, disseminate solutions to encourage their spread).

Likewise, in self-advancing systems, health professionals (knowledge workers) see their roles as simultaneously practicing and continuously improving the practice. They and their leadership understand that focus on the *process* is key to advancement and they continuously attend to its rearrangement, revision, and co-creation. The modes of learning about practice are informal, involve relationships, include patients and families, and are sensitive to failures in other organizations (see Chapter 8). For example, accidents on airplanes or bankruptcies in large companies provide opportunities for learning about hidden flaws that can be applied to healthcare or assumptions in health systems. Opportunities for practice improvement are often found in routine processes or situations that confront first-line workers versus quality and safety analysts. First-line workers (those delivering health services—i.e., health professionals) share goals, socialize new members, divide the work, make decisions, create protocols, and learn together. Their focus on the processes of care emphasizes the interdependencies among individuals or departments, better identifies how errors are started, reminds us of the benefits and consequences of certain practice changes, and considers the patient and family. Finally, high-performing organizations emphasize accuracy or use of fact (data) in practice improvement, constantly communicate (not just periodically), accept responsibility for mistakes, and do not allow self-serving defensive postures (American Council on Education, 2012). Rather, they tap into the underlying professional practice model and defend that interpersonal skills are as important (maybe more important?) as technical skills.

From an organizational perspective, fully embracing the dual integration of relational capacity and practice improvement seems simple, but it requires deep changes in thinking, assumptions, and expectations. Leaders join with employees in relationships based on mutual caring and expect those same relationships to distinguish patient and health team member relationships. Healthcare providers view their work as both clinical and learning, simultaneously providing care while examining ways to improve it. Over time and through experimenting and adapting to practice improvements based on attention to real-time clinical processes, the collective system begins to accomplish growth naturally while empowering employees and patients alike. The chart in Figure 9.3 serves as a reference point for evaluating self-advancing systems. Starting from the upper left box, health systems where leaders and employees relate well (relational capacity) but do not regularly participate in practice improvement (as described in this book) lack the insight required to engage in practice improvement or are complacent in its importance. They might also be very focused on measuring performance outcomes, or be under-resourced. In the lower left box, both relational capacity

FIGURE 9.3 Reference point for evaluating self-advancing systems.

High RC/Low PI	High RC/High PI
Low RC/Low PI	Low RC/High PI

PI, practice improvement; RC, relational capacity.

and practice improvement are low, indicating that health professionals are very task oriented and prefer the status quo *or* they don't feel their contributions are recognized. Leadership has little idea about what is going on at the patient level and may perpetuate an overly hierarchical or functional system. Or leadership teeters on trying to please everyone, and in so doing, has strayed from the core aspect of the work. In the lower right box, relational capacity is low while practice improvement is higher. In this type of organization, practice improvement is seen as important, but departments don't relate well (some withhold information from each other), and there is a lot of competition between people and departments. Employees and some leaders don't feel comfortable outside of their own departments and some continue to advocate for outdated services (sacred cows). Individuals shift blame and deny accountability and view leadership as "in it for themselves." Finally, the upper right box holds the most promise for self-advancement because these systems relate highly (relational capacity) and continuously improve practice. Clinical practice is always patient centered, based on caring relationships. Characteristics of such systems include:

- A focus on the basics of safe, high-quality, complete and connected patient care
- Health professionals and leadership who work together in informal, collegial relationships
- Routine encouragement and recognition
- Abundant knowledge (learning)
- The patient as *always* part of the decision
- An awareness that outcomes are important, but not all-consuming
- Being present but mindful of the future
- Holding one another to world-class performance
- Small, self-sufficient functional units
- Continuous reevaluation
- Partnering with stakeholders
- Spending time at the bedside

FIGURE 9.4   Self-advancing health systems.

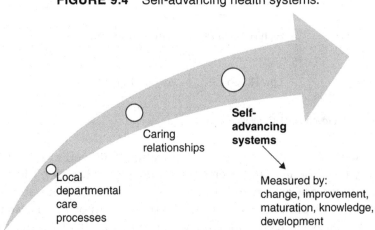

Fully embracing the dual integration of relational capacity and practice improvement, health systems are managing to grow, progress, expand, and, without focused attention on outcomes, deliver superior services with high-quality outcomes—that is, they self-advance (see Figure 9.4). Such advances optimize outcomes (providing the best, the ideal), which in turn offers value to patients and families, health professionals, and health systems. Caring relationships play a central role and, in fact, fuel self-advancing systems. Indeed, such systems are practicing in alignment with their values.

SUMMARY

The last concept in the QCM, self-advancing systems, is introduced and explained. It is viewed in a positive light, based on the underlying assumptions about humans and the power of relationships. Focusing on clinical processes as a means of self-advancement is stressed. What self-advancement means to patients and families is described in terms of their unique experiences of care and achievement of self-caring practices. For health professionals, self-advancement is facilitated through genuine caring relationships found in routine clinical practice. The suffering and joys that accompany clinical work can oftentimes provide profound opportunities for generating meaning and ultimately personal growth. Finally, the daily experience of patients and families is characterized as a reflection of a health system's well-being. Relational coordination is explained and the simultaneous integration of relational capacity and practice improvement is stressed as a means of aligning organizational practice with values.

Call to Action

Self-advancing health systems effectively use relational capacity and practice improvement to naturally progress, grow, learn, and expand. Embedded in clinical processes, self-advancing systems enhance patient outcomes and expose the meaning of health professionals' work. **Find** the meaning in your work by staying close to the patient and genuinely relating to those with whom you work.

REFLECTIVE QUESTIONS/APPLICATIONS

. . . for Students

1. Describe the concept of self-advancing systems.
2. Analyze your role in helping advance a health system.
3. How did you learn to relate to patients and families? Do you see this relationship as a source for learning or your own growth? How did the case study about the woman with cancer make you feel?
4. What does the phrase "Caring is not something we do after we finish the work or if you have time. Caring in nursing is part of the seamless whole" mean to you?
5. Explore the literature for high-reliability or high-performing health systems.
6. Read about relational coordination. What did you learn?

. . . for Professional Nurses in Clinical Practice

1. Describe how you personally find meaning in your work. Is this important? Why?
2. Do you know how to craft your job to provide meaning? Are you assertive in creating it?
3. Is your department self-advancing? How do you know?
4. Do you enjoy clinical work? Be honest. How could you better use this to find meaning in your work?
5. How often do you see outcomes data? Is it linked to specific processes of care? What nursing processes have you changed that have positively affected outcomes?

6. What have you learned about your own self-advancement as a result of reading this chapter?
7. Examine the list of "good, basic, complete nursing care" that is provided in this chapter. Is this occurring on your unit? How often do you assume responsibility for it?
8. What is your department's HCAHPS score? What ongoing practice improvements are you involved with that are designed to improve it?
9. Nurses report that relating to patients and families holds the most promise for finding meaning in their work. How do you relate to patients and families? Does it help?

. . . for Professional Nurses in Educational Practice

1. How do you teach about health systems? How does this differ in undergraduate and graduate programs?
2. Reflect on the need for relational coordination in high-performing organizations. How does this concept translate to the academic enterprise?
3. What can you do to help students focus on the importance of good, basic, complete nursing care?
4. How might you suggest increasing students' awareness of the meaning and joy associated with clinical work?
5. Provide some suggestions for exposing students to the concept of self-advancement.
6. As a health professions educator, do any potential research questions "pop out" at you as a result of reading this chapter? Be specific.

. . . for Professional Nurses in Leadership Practice

1. What is the state of advancement at your organization? How do you know?
2. How do you specifically hold yourself and your peers accountable for focusing on the real work of the organization?
3. Reflect on the quality improvement process in place at your institution. Does it focus exclusively on outcomes measurement? Are processes of care linked to specific outcomes? Are staff nurses involved in genuine practice improvements? Why or why not? What would it take to revise this?
4. How do you facilitate joint relational capacity and practice improvement at your organization?

5. Does your leadership team understand the organizational value of the fundamental clinical processes of good, basic, complete nursing care? If not, how will you help them understand?
6. In which health systems box of Figure 9.3 does your organization fall? If it is not already in the top right corner, what would it take to move it there?

PRACTICE ANALYSIS

At an academic medical center, pain and functional status of older adults, significant quality outcomes for this population, were observed as problematic. Pain always well controlled was reported by hospitalized older adults as occurring only 58% to 62% of the time (below the national average) and a pain management chart audit ($N = 92$) revealed that regular assessment and nursing knowledge of pain were missing or incorrect 70% of the time. Furthermore, functional decline among older adults was not routinely documented despite the national data that demonstrated the serious nature of this problem as it relates to older adult burden and increased costs. The average length of stay (LOS) for older adults was 5.4 days compared to 3.42 days for all other patients. Finally, only four of the eight domains on the HCAHPS Survey (patient experience of care) reached the 50th percentile for older adults.

In this acute care delivery system, multiple health professionals, organized in separate clinical departments and socialized by discipline, practiced independently. In fact, despite renewed interest in interprofessional collaborative practice (IPCP) education and training, translation of newly acquired behaviors into practice had been slow. Few structures supported it and, after training, health professionals typically reverted to old, traditional modalities of parallel practice. Real IPCP, although known by health professionals to be linked with improved patient outcomes, particularly among hospitalized older adults, was lacking. Health professionals indicated the need to collaborate, but changing long-established clinical workflow was challenging.

A small interprofessional group (two RNs, a clinical pharmacist, an attending physician, and a social worker) began to dialog about the patient population and its needs for improved outcomes. One interested member began to work on an idea of how IPCP could be integrated into the workflow. A model emerged that was patient centered, built upon existing interprofessional education already in existence at the health center, was progressive and comprehensive, and aimed to increase the number of health professionals practicing IPCP (the *process* of patient care).

Adopting this approach, the healthcare team would share the common purpose of improving outcomes for older adults and coordinate their work through structured working rounds and expanding the existing nursing performance improvement committee to include all health professionals and interested patients, providing a shared space for dialog about practice improvement. The group committed to try interprofessional rounds with a high degree of participation and use daily structured team checklists and patient input to evaluate and revise their real-time clinical processes. In addition, the re-formed nursing performance improvement committee refocused their work on actionable practice changes that might improve older adults' outcomes. Engaging the team of healthcare providers and patients to examine ways of improving practice was supported by regularly examining patient data looking for patterns, identifying contextual factors and practice patterns that may influence outcomes, and soliciting input from patients. After a couple of informal meetings, the whole group decided to pilot the new approach.

Two clinical units (that admitted most of the older adult population) agreed to implement the IPCP model for 2 months. It was expected that day-to-day activities would be characterized by mutuality, respect, engagement, transparency, accountability, ease, and other like features of cohesive, fully functioning teams, allowing for early recognition of abnormalities, deterrence of errors, more coordinated services, timely responses and anticipation of patient needs, and safe space to raise ideas. During the 2-month time frame, some issues related to leadership during rounds, active participation of members, integrating patients into the membership, and documentation of activities were raised and addressed. Based on the mutual respect and continued engagement of members, however, the innovative team held together and at the end of 2 months, older adult functional decline was reduced by 12%, pain control advanced to >80%, and HCAHPS scores improved slightly.

1. What features of self-advancing systems are evident in this case?
2. What did leaders do to support self-advancement in this situation?
3. How does this example demonstrate health professionals practicing in alignment with their professional values?

REFERENCES

American Council on Education. (2012). Assuring academic quality in the 21st century: Self-regulation in a new era. A Report of the ACE National Task Force on Institutional Accreditation. Retrieved from http://www.acenet.edu/newsroom/Documents/Accreditation-TaskForce-revised-070512.pdf

American Nurses Association. (n.d.). Healthy nurse, healthy nation. Retrieved from http://www.healthynursehealthynation.org

Berwick, D. (2016). *Eight ways to shift the power back to patients.* Twenty-eighth annual National Forum on Quality Improvement in Healthcare, concluding address. Institute for HealthCare Improvement. Retreived from https://www.hhnmag.com/articles/7916-don-berwick-offers-8-ways-to-shift-the-balance-of-power-back-to-patients

Boehmer, R. M. (2009). *Designing care: Aligning the nature and management of health care.* Boston, MA: Harvard Business Press.

Brooks-Carthon, J. M., Lasater, K., Rearden, J., Holland, S., & Sloane, D. M. (2016). Unmet nursing care linked to rehospitalizations among older black AMI patients: A cross-sectional study of US hospitals. *Medical Care, 54*(5), 457–465. doi:10.1097/MLR.0000000000000519

Cassel, E. J. (1982). The nature of suffering and the goals of medicine. *New England Journal of Medicine, 306*(11), 639–645. doi:10.1056/NEJM198203183061104

Cassel, E. J. (1992). The nature of suffering: Physical, psychological, social, and spiritual aspects. In P. L. Stark & J. P. McGovern (Eds.), *The hidden dimension of illness: Human suffering* (pp. 1–10). New York, NY: National League for Nursing Press.

Chassin, M., & Loeb, J. M. (2011). The ongoing quality improvement journey: Next stop, high reliability. *Health Affairs, 30*(4), 559–568. doi:10.1377/hlthaff.2011.0076

Curry, L. A., Spatz, E., Cherlin, E., Thompson, J. W., Berg, D., Ting, H. H., . . . Bradley, E. H. (2011). What distinguished top performing hospitals in acute myocardial infarction mortality rates? A qualitative study. *Annals of Internal Medicine, 154*, 384–390. doi:10.7326/0003-4819-154-6-201103150-00003

Donabedian, A. (1966). Evaluating the quality of medical care. *Milbank Memorial Fund Quarterly, 44*, 166–206. doi:10.1111/j.1468-0009.2005.00397.x

Doyle, C., Lennox, L., & Bell, D. (2013). A systematic review of evidence on the links between patient experience and clinical safety and effectiveness. *British Medical Journal Open, 3*(1), e001570. doi:10.1136/bmjopen-2012-001570

Gittell, J. H. (2002). Relationships between service providers and their impact on customers. *Journal of Service Research, 4*(4), 299–311. doi:10.1177/1094670502004004007

Gittell, J. H. (2009). *High performance healthcare: Using the power of relationships to achieve quality, efficiency and resilience.* New York, NY: McGraw-Hill.

Gittell, J. H. (2016). *Transforming relationships for high performance: The power of relational coordination.* Stanford, CA: Stanford University Press.

Gittell, J. H., Seidner, R., & Wimbush, J. (2010). A relational model of how high-performance work systems work. *Organization Science, 21*(2), 490–506. doi:10.1287/orsc.1090.0446

Goldstein, E., Farquhar, M., Crofton, C., Darby, C., & Garfinkel, S. (2005). Measuring hospital care from the patients' perspective: An overview of the CAHPS Hospital Survey development process. *Health Services Research, 40*(6 Pt. 2), 1977–1995. doi:10.1111/j.1475-6773.2005.00477.x

Institute for Healthcare Improvement. (2009). Improving the patient experience of inpatient care evidence. Retrieved from http://www.ihi.org/IHI/Topics/

PatientCenteredCare/PatientCenteredCareGeneral/EmergingContent/ Improvingthe PatientExperienceofInpatientCare.htm

Jha, A. K., Orav, E. J., Zheng, J., & Epstein, A .M. (2008). Patients' perception of hospital care in the United States. *New England Journal of Medicine, 359*(18), 1921–1931. doi:10.1056/NEJMsa0804116

Linetzky, B., Jiang, D., Funnell, M. M., Curtis, B. H., & Polonsky, W. H. (2017). Exploring the role of the patient–physician relationship on insulin adherence and clinical outcomes in type 2 diabetes: Insights from the MOSAIc study. *Journal of Diabetes, 9*(6), 596–605. doi:10.1111/1753-0407.12443

Oreskovich, M. R., Shanafelt, T., Dyrbye, L. N., Tan, L., Sotile, W., Satele, D., . . . Boone, S. (2014). The prevalence of substance use disorders in American physicians. *The American Journal on Addictions,* doi:10.1111/j.1521-0391.2014.12173.x

Pavlisch, C., & Hunt, R. (2012). An exploratory study about meaningful work in acute care. *Nursing Forum, 47*(2), 113–122. doi:10.1111/j.1744-6198.2012.00261.x

Press Ganey Associates, Inc. (2008). Return-on-investment: Reducing malpractice claims by improving patient satisfaction. White Paper, Press Ganey Associates, Inc. Retrieved from http://pressganey.com/cs/research_and_analysis/white_paper_registration2?id=/galleries/lead-generatingacute/Malpractice_Final_12-14-07.pdf&subject=Malpractice_paper

Sequist, T. D., Schneider, E. D., Anastario, M., Odigie, E. G., Marshall, R., Rogers, W. H., & Safran, D. G. (2008). Quality monitoring of physicians: Linking patients' experiences of care to clinical quality and outcomes. *Journal of General Internal Medicine, 23*(11), 1784–1790. doi:10.1007/s11606-008-0760-4

Song, S., Fonarow, G. C., Olson, D. M., Liang, L., Schulte, P. J., Hernandez, A. F., . . . Saver, J. L. (2016). Association of get with the guidelines-stroke program participation and clinical outcomes for Medicare beneficiaries with ischemic stroke. *Stroke, 47*(5), 1294–1302. doi:10.1161/STROKEAHA.115.011874

Steger, M. F. (2017). Creating meaning and purpose at work. In *The Wiley Blackwell handbook of the psychology of positivity and strengths-based approaches at work* (pp. 60–81). New York, NY: John Wiley & Sons.

United States Department of Health and Human Services. (1996). Understanding health information privacy. Retrieved from http://www.hhs.gov/ocr/privacy/hipaa/understanding/index.html

Weick, K. E. (1995). *Sensemaking in organizations.* Thousand Oaks, CA: Sage.

Weick, K. E., & Sutcliffe, K. M. (2015). *Managing the unexpected: sustained performance in a complex world.* New York, NY: John Wiley & Sons.

Wennberg, J. E., Bronner, K., Skinner, J. S., Fisher, E. S., & Goodman, D. C. (2009). Inpatient care intensity and patients' ratings of their hospital experiences. *Health Affairs, 28*(1), 103–112. doi:10.1377/hlthaff.28.1.103

West, C. P., Dyrbye, L. N., Rabatin, J. T., Call, T. G., Davidson, J. H., Multari, A., . . . Shanafelt, T. D. (2014). Intervention to promote physician well-being, job satisfaction, and professionalism: a randomized clinical trial. *JAMA Internal Medicine, 174*(4), 527–533. doi:10.1001/jamainternmed.2013.14387

III

LEADING AND LEARNING IN QUALITY-CARING HEALTH SYSTEMS

10

Leading Quality Caring

The main thing is to keep the main thing the main thing.
—Stephen R. Covey

THE CONTEXT OF CLINICAL PRACTICE

Health systems consist of a healthcare workforce (both employees and nonemployees), primary customers (patients and families with unique attributes), practice settings (and their varying characteristics), and suppliers (e.g., pharmaceutical companies and device manufacturers), and are associated with organizations responsible for workforce training (universities), research (funding agencies), reimbursement (insurance companies), and system oversight (accreditors). Within this complex network, there is enormous variation in terms of how the workforce delivers services. Take, for example, the present nursing workforce.

Although the registered nurse (RN) workforce is expected to grow from 2.7 million in 2014 to 3.2 million in 2024 (an increase of 16%), the need for 649,100 replacement nurses is projected during that same time period (American Association of Colleges of Nursing, 2017). Many nursing leaders are already reporting regional difficulties in recruiting and retaining new nurses as well as challenges engaging those nurses in the current workforce who are stressed, detached, and somewhat unsatisfied (personal conversations; Auerbach & Staiger, 2017). Furthermore, the current and impending retirement of nursing faculty is growing and represents a crucial national challenge given its potential impact on preparing future nurses (Fang & Kesten, 2017). Such conditions suggest that the modest increase in the nursing workforce in recent years will not be sufficient to meet the projected demand for professional nursing services, including the need for more nurse faculty, researchers, and primary care providers.

Moreover, in the current acute care environment, where most professional nurses are employed, the demand for highly developed cognitive, technological, and relationship skills associated with high-quality services delivered in a constantly changing context is taxing. Less and less time is spent by RNs in direct patient care, while many are working excessive hours to meet the demands. Meanwhile, the larger health system is dealing with uncertainties about future healthcare legislation, tax reforms, and continuing and unstable national security issues. All of these conditions affect how health services are provided.

Context in a health system is a multilayered construct that includes organizational culture and climate, leadership, interpersonal relationships, resources, patient and health provider characteristics, and workflow (how the work gets done). In nursing, "healthy work environments" has become the buzzword for an optimistic context that leaders are striving to cultivate and sustain. A healthy work environment has been defined as "a professional practice environment in which employees are skilled communicators and where face-to-face interactions are open, positive, and consistent with one's professional and ethical mandates" (Kupperschmidt, Kientz, Ward, & Reinholz, 2010) and is now seen as a shared responsibility of both leaders and those who follow. Yet unhealthy work environments continue to exist (Armmer, 2017) and are especially challenging for leadership and employees alike.

In a 2017 review article, Shirey reported the most desirable leadership attributes associated with healthy work environments included authenticity, having vision, and being empowering, approachable, and relational as opposed to being task focused (Shirey, 2017, p. 44). This view of leadership embraces the human connections and interdependencies in organizations: ongoing social relational processes of shared responsibility. These characteristics of *authentic* leadership (George, 2016) are optimized by leader self-awareness and self-regulation and the co-creation of meaning in the workforce (Waite, McKinney, Smith-Glasgow, & Meloy, 2014). Healthy work environments (a component of context) are increasingly tied to high-quality clinical outcomes; thus quality leadership at this dynamic time in history is particularly necessary.

LEADERSHIP AS A PRACTICE

Nursing as a practice responds to societal needs for health and wellness services, is based on ethical principles, and provides safe, quality care in accordance with disciplinary standards. Furthermore, nursing is holistic in that it considers the whole person and his or her environment. In the social realm, nursing's human-interactional capacity uniquely situates nurses to advance interactions, to reinforce relationships between health professionals and patients, to find solutions, and to foster positive experiences for patients and health professionals. Such actions are proactive, inclusive, and, oftentimes, innovative. Ethical principles guide this practice that is provided by competent individuals with advanced knowledge, skills, and attitudes. Patient–nurse relationships are the primary context of nurses' practice and, according to Kornhaber, Walsh, Duff, and Walker (2016), "have the capacity to transform and enrich patients' experiences" (p. 537). Empirically, they have been associated with improvements in patient satisfaction, adherence to treatment, quality of life, levels of anxiety and depression, and decreased healthcare costs (Kelley, Kraft-Todd, Schapira, Kossowsky, & Riess, 2014; Shay, Dumenci, Siminoff, Flocke, & Lafata, 2012; Step, Rose, Albert, Cheruvu, & Siminoff, 2009).

As leaders of nursing (and oftentimes nurses themselves), nursing administrators are guiding a practice whose first responsibility is to patients and families, that bears responsibility for providing competent, high-quality services, and that is uniquely qualified to advance relationships that improve the human experience. Appreciating, strengthening, and expanding these unique attributes of nursing practice is the first priority of nursing administration!

Yet, recently and in the spirit of patient-centered care, well-intentioned health systems' executives have adopted customer service models to promote better relationships between providers and patients. One example is the practice of scripting nurses' patient interactions. "Some administrators are ordering nurses to use particular phrases and to gush effusively to patients about both their hospital and their fellow nurses, and then evaluate them on how well they comply. An entire industry has sprouted, encouraging hospitals to waste precious dollars on expensive consultants claiming to provide scripts or other resources that boost satisfaction scores. Some institutions have even hired actors to rehearse the scripts with nurses" (Robbins, 2015, p. 220).

This approach does not, however, encompass real caring relationships that include mutual problem solving, human respect, attentive reassurance, encouragement, appreciation of unique meanings, fostering of a healing environment, attending to basic and affiliation needs—that is, the caring behaviors. Rather, in this customer service–oriented approach, the connections established between patients and health professionals are more removed and superficial. In the real world, customers are generally healthy individuals who are often purchasers of products or services. They are considered equal to or similar to the merchant. Patients, on the other hand, are generally unhealthy or seeking better health. In such a state, they are limited and vulnerable, often fearful and in pain, and somewhat confused (see Chapter 4). Furthermore, a critical knowledge gap exists between health professionals and patient/ families, creating further imbalance. Patients are seeking better health and relief from suffering and trust health professionals to keep them safe, ensure their dignity as worthy humans, effectively provide relief from discomfort, and inclusion in decision making. Using a customer service approach changes the fundamental nature of clinical practice from a moral, relational, and therapeutic practice to a prearranged, structured series of interactions and activities. In essence, the customer service–oriented approach, including forced scripting and other behaviors, may distract nurses even further from interacting in the authentic manner that characterizes caring patient relationships—the key to positive patient experiences.

Unlike retail services, healthcare involves a deeper level of human interaction with less predictable outcomes and in which multiple choices exist. "Nurses encounter patients in their most vulnerable moments, sharing an intimacy found in few other human relationships" (Chambliss, 1996, p. 1). Such intimacy is associated with self-disclosure, touch, emotions such as trust and empathy, and closeness (Kirk, 2007) and is a professional behavior (based on the professional code of conduct) nurses use to balance the private work they do to meet patient needs at the bedside with the more technological or scientific work they do. Intimacy is a "professional" behavior in that it is founded on deep values about the worth of humans and includes respecting another's privacy. It is a learned professional skill that develops over time. As one nurse put it: "Intimacy in nursing involves close personal relationships with patients (and families) that are simultaneously physical and emotional. Professional intimacy requires knowledge, strategies, and ethics" (personal conversation). Furthermore, intimacy is significant to patients and families and influences the patient experience (Faugier, 2006). This moral responsibility of nurses provides a safe, trustworthy, reliable, and secure foundation for therapeutic interactions.

> Genuine intimacy is integral to professional nursing practice and requires authentic engagement and advocacy on patients' behalf. Such care demands a closeness and relational quality that, without an organizing framework, can get lost in the workflow of endless priorities. The intimacy contained in the patient–nurse relationship is an expectation that shapes patients' experiences but becomes marginalized when delegated to caregivers who are trained only in task completion or when nurses themselves do not embrace its professional nature.

Consider this example:

A 45-year-old female was admitted to a large Magnet®-designated hospital for a spontaneous pneumothorax. With a chest tube in place, she had daily chest x-rays and was ordered a routine ECG as well. A male technician from another country approached the woman to perform the ECG. He could not speak the language well, but used a script to explain what he was going to do. He proceeded to open the woman's gown, exposing her fully. He placed the leads on her chest and began the ECG machine all the while assuming he was doing his job correctly. He did not close the curtains or safeguard the woman's privacy, but continued on as though nothing was amiss. Although the procedure only lasted about 8 minutes, the woman was extremely embarrassed and felt humiliated having a male technician who did not advocate for her basic human need for privacy, but rather considered his job so matter-of-factly—as a task or procedure that needed to get done—despite the obvious vulnerability of the patient.

A professional nurse would have understood the importance of this woman's privacy to her human worthiness and the overall hospital experience and would have safeguarded it while he or she performed an ECG. After all, it falls under the caring behavior human respect and is linked to human dignity! Despite the commercialistic or business-like approach to healthcare, nursing's fundamental commitment to persons in their care remains constant. This devotion to patients is the basis for nursing's codes of ethics and standards of practice (see Chapter 2) and is protected through various state practice acts.

> Thus nursing leadership is morally obligated to ensure that patients' privacy and confidentiality are protected by preserving the foundational caring patient–nurse relationship that gives nursing its identity, ensures ethical and legal services, and provides individual nurses with meaning.

The American Organization of Nurse Executives (AONE, 2015a, 2015b) competencies list numerous essential competencies for nurse leaders. They include to ensure compliance with the State Nurse Practice Act, State Board of Nursing regulations, regulatory agency standards and policies of the organization; to champion patient care; to ensure quality and nursing professionalism; to hold self and others accountable for actions and outcomes; to role model the perspective that patient care is the core of the organization's work; and to create an environment that facilitates the team to initiate actions that produce results. Setting expectations and holding each other accountable strike this author as particularly aligned with the characteristics of nursing practice (as described above). These competencies call for leaders who have the courage to "go against the grain" and intentionally focus on the fundamental work of the organization—quality patient care—as their number one priority. Appreciating and preserving the private, intimate, caring relationship between patients and nurses provides the opportunity to advance clinical practice (showcasing the value of nursing to the overall healthcare enterprise).

Interestingly, many of the AONE executive competencies use relationships as the method for getting this fundamental work done. For example:

> . . . build collaborative relationships, exhibit effective conflict resolution skills, create a trusting environment by following through on promises and concerns, establishing mechanisms to follow up on commitments, balancing the concerns of individuals with organizational goals and objectives, engaging staff and others in decision making, communicating in a way as to maintain credibility and relationships, establish an environment that values diversity (e.g., age, gender, race, religion, ethnicity, sexual orientation, culture) . . . are relationship-centered. (AONE, 2015a, 2015b)

RELATIONSHIP-CENTERED LEADERSHIP

Relationships (particularly those characterized as caring) provide an untapped resource for organizational advancement, growth, and/or renewal. Seen from this perspective, continuous interactions and relationship building form a paradigm for leadership that frames it as connected, interdependent, organic, alive, creative, and whole. It is from this standpoint that the health system continuously recreates itself. Moreover, as described in Chapter 9, the quality of relationships within health systems often counters the stresses and burdens of complexity and constant change.

Leadership centered on relationships as an essential competency acknowledges the interdependent nature of human beings and recognizes that self-advancement (individual and system) occurs naturally in complex systems but will spread more effectively and efficiently if leadership attends to relationships. The leader's role is to cultivate an ethos of inclusion, create safe space for genuine dialogue, facilitate information and ongoing learning, hold up professional standards, and allow health professionals to adapt their practice in ways that are meaningful to them. As Brene Brown (2017) states, "If leaders really want people to show up, speak out, take chances, and innovate, they have to create cultures where people feel safe—where their belonging is not threatened by speaking out and they are supported when they make the decision to brave the wilderness, stand alone, and speak truth" (p. 93). Such leadership sees the human person in the employee and vulnerability in the eyes of patients and families. It recognizes the inherent caring nature of health professionals and honors the special relationships they have with patients, families, and each other. Authentically caring for others provides leaders with the permission to give people direction, help them align with organizational goals, and provide the affirmative, positive energy to get the job done.

> **N**urse leaders who appreciate the caring relationships that nurses have with patients and families understand and work hard to preserve them; after all, these relationships provide the life lessons and ongoing renewal that inspire clinical nurses to continue their important work!

Most health systems leaders are aware of the importance of relationships—on balance, healthcare is built on relationships. But amid the hectic demands of day-to-day work, persistent crises, and the unyielding pressure to perform and innovate, leaders often act in ways that even they know are uninspiring or less than compassionate. The rationale or excuse given at the time is "They know I care," or "I don't have time," or "They are professionals—they can deal with it." The effect of such reasoning contributes to a downward spiral of interactions and patterns of behavior (avoidance, working to the job description) that diminish further relationships and eventually retard forward progression—self-advancement.

Yet nursing leadership occurs in context—the context of clinical work and the environment where it is delivered as well as in the interactions that shape the work. Relationships are central to these processes—attending to them with vigor (using social processes) stimulates openness, innovative solutions, and adaptation to change. With this perspective, leading is always a process of relating; creating meanings, sharing responsibilities, collective dialoguing, moving forward interdependently, co-evolving patterns all enhance the capacity of systems to advance. Leadership, then, occurs at the relationship level—not at the authority or supervisory level. As stated earlier in this chapter, relationally centered leaders were tied to healthy work environments (Shirey, 2017), an important ingredient for higher quality care (Lake et al., 2016; McHugh et al., 2016) and nurses' job satisfaction (Fallatah & Laschinger, 2016; Poghosyan, Liu, Shang, & D'Aunno, 2017).

A relationship-centered leader is a systems thinker who is authentic, empowers others, and considers caring relationships essential to strong, productive work teams. This type of leader also views decision making from a relationship-focused versus a power-based perspective. Using personal and disciplinary values, relationally oriented leaders examine how potential options will impact others. They are approachable, strive for harmony among their employees, and focus on interaction, conversations, and dialoguing while working to build consensus and trust. They also admit when they're wrong and seek constructive criticism.

Consider the following example as told to this author by Dawn Johnson RN, BSN, a nurse in the Indiana University nurse practitioner program:

One of the most amazing leaders I had the privilege to learn under was the vice principal at a special needs school where I worked with autistic children. She was authentic! She was intelligent, always available, knowledgeable about the children and the system. She navigated personalities above and below her with amazing grace and resolve. She loved the children, loved her job, and was confident in her role with no excuses. She would apologize when she was wrong and be outspoken when necessary. What I was most impressed with was when I first met her, she was on the ground holding a child in a basket hold, keeping him from banging his head against a concrete wall. She was not a big lady by any means and she was in her dress suit for a meeting. All the while, she was directing staff on removal of the other children. As soon as the child calmed down, she gave him a big hug and told him she loved him. He was big enough that he could have hurt her if she had not gotten the upper hand. It all happened very quickly. I thought to myself, now this is a lady I could follow to hell and back.

Or this example:

One night I was on fire watch in Afghanistan, which is late night watch while everyone else sleeps. I heard footsteps walking up to my post . . . it had to be 0100. I look up, and it's the battalion commander. I quickly stood up straight, and greeted him. He said "Relax, I wanted to come stand watch with you for a bit." This was amazing to me, as I didn't think he even knew my name—he oversaw approximately 1,000 Marines. He proceeded to ask me about my background and why I wanted to serve. I could tell that he really wanted to get an idea about who I was, and how I felt about the mission. He commended me often, and made me feel bigger than I was. He told me something that I will never forget . . . he said "Son, the best advice I can give you is as you advance in leadership, never ask someone to do something that you wouldn't do." He won me that night, as he let me know that I mattered, and I felt appreciated. (Benjamin Hanenkratt, RN, BSN, inpatient mental health nurse and former U.S. Marine)

These two examples give me chills as I think about how these authentic leaders are still influencing the lives of these young nurses!

Relationship-centered leaders engage in developmental discussions, are passionate about the work, lead by example, solicit input, make the time to dialogue and understand employees, facilitate "feeling cared for," and use employees' feedback to adjust processes and guide future decisions. Regularly interacting with employees (not just at evaluation time) to discuss what's working and what's not, and identifying new challenges and training opportunities, is key. Although we have more immediate access to information than ever before, it can never replace the real human connection of in-person recognition, communication, including listening, sharing, and coming to know each other. Such actions by leaders engage, empower, respect, build up, and reassure, providing the affirmative ("I matter") fuel necessary for co-creating success. This ongoing presence with employees (how authentic leaders spend their time) also enhances the leader's relationship skills—that is, relational capacity—a critical aspect of relationship-centered leadership and organizational advancement. And as Yoder-Wise (2017) espouses, leaders' presence improves with practice and reflection!

Working with interprofessional teams, nurse leaders must be able to translate the work of nursing into familiar terms and demonstrate how its work contributes to patient outcomes. Using a relational approach, nurse leaders can educate teams using evidence that describes interventions that enhance outcomes, or provide examples, such as reviewing specific patient cases or situations that may have personal meaning to team members, helping to ensure team-based, patient-centered care that optimizes value (Moss, Seifert, & O'Sullivan, 2016). Nurse leaders who obtain advanced knowledge or broaden their experiences outside of nursing can better influence organizational colleagues as well.

At the heart of relationship-centered leadership is a different employer–employee relationship that de-emphasizes status (e.g., dress, offices, power) and reemphasizes teamwork and innovation by providing interesting work in healthy environments. Such leaders stay present to self and others and remain steadfast during crises and periods of doubt. Doing so requires leaders who lead from within, that is, halting the "thinking and doing" mode long enough to reflect, become aware, "to be," and cultivate the self. As an executive practice, relationship-centered leadership requires the capacity to care for self, comprising one's physical health—including diet and exercise, adequate sleep, and the social and emotional self. Nurse leaders at all levels need time for renewal to continuously remain in relationship mode.

Executive nurse leaders stimulate a culture of caring in an organization and maintain the focus on caring relationships, which demonstrates its high priority. Creating unity of purpose, setting high expectations, and consistently reminding employees why they are there influences positive interactions that fuel advancement. Even during times of conflict, staying "in relationship" by keeping an open mind and continuing to dialogue leads to deeper connections that over time may bring about resolution of the conflict. They also provide the critically necessary appreciative and transparent infrastructure needed for effective middle management.

Department-level leaders are pivotal to the success of relationship-centered caring.

Reinforcing the purpose (what we are here for) and translating that purpose to the bedside through caring relationships sets the tone of a department. Through visible, hands-on leadership, department-level leaders look for and encourage the small practice improvements that health professionals construct. Acting as resources to frontline health professionals and peers, they actively respond to questions, provide feedback, and help employees find meaning in their work. Maintaining a constant focus on the centrality of caring to patient outcomes, department-level leaders encourage staff members to contribute; over time, more individuals interact and become engaged, leading to larger changes.

The department-level leader who is self-aware brings staff members together, keeps them informed, and helps them learn about and use

TABLE 10.1   Benefits and Challenges of Relationship-Centered Leadership

Benefits	Challenges
Engaged employees	Maintaining purpose/momentum
Less conflict	Uncomfortable/sometimes painful encounters
Professionalism	Holding others accountable
Healthy work environments	Unpredictable situations
Teamwork	Effective communication
Refine leadership skills	Balancing separateness and engagement
Source of pride	Placing professional practice first
Positive patient experiences	Time-consuming tasks
Self-caring employees	Resourcing strategically

caring relationships while simultaneously encouraging them to innovate. See Table 10.1 for the benefits and challenges of relationship-centered leadership. Department-level leaders have a central position within the leadership hierarchy of healthcare that reinforces their "broker" roles in creating cultures of caring. Ultimately, such middle-level leadership is a valuable resource in steering health systems toward self-advancement.

IMPLEMENTING AND EVALUATING RELATIONSHIP-CENTERED PROFESSIONAL PRACTICE MODELS

Much confusion exists concerning professional practice models (PPMs), nursing theory, shared governance, nursing councils, and the like. Quite simply, PPMs provide the infrastructure for professional nursing practice. Hoffart and Woods (1996) first described five components of a PPM: values, professional relationships, a patient care delivery model, a management approach, and compensation and rewards. Over time, this has evolved to:

- Professional values
- A framework that specifies the relationships, roles, and boundaries of nursing practice
- A patient care delivery system
- Governance
- A system of recognition and rewards

Thus, a PPM "is a multicomponent system that serves as a guidepost for nursing and fosters the alignment of nursing practice with organizational priorities and professional values" (Duffy, 2016, p. 4). More specifically, when practicing under such a model, nurses are viewed as autonomous, competent health professionals who apply evidence to their care, exercise clinical and organizational judgment, use safe and ethical methods, and improve themselves through peer evaluation. Additionally, their practice is collaborative, ensuring comprehensive, coordinated services. In essence, a PPM provides a comprehensive foundation for clinical practice that theoretically enhances patient, nurse, and system outcomes—self-advancing systems. And nursing leaders provide the impetus, resources, and guidance required to select and integrate such models into health systems.

With the underlying philosophical beliefs (assumptions) clearly articulated and the concepts defined, the Quality-Caring Model (QCM) has provided the foundation for nursing practice that honors the holistic nature of humans and the caring relationships essential for high-quality outcomes in many organizations (see Appendix B). Because the QCM views independent and collaborative caring relationships as the primary responsibility of professional nurses, and "feeling cared for" as a crucial intermediate outcome sensitive to nursing, organizing how nursing work gets done in health systems flows more easily.

> Using a theoretical model to design how work is accomplished is challenging because it may change work roles, how decisions are made, staffing and scheduling approaches, and reporting relationships.

Yet addressing the roles and responsibilities of nurses and those who support them, communication mechanisms, resources, and the environment are foundational to nursing leadership roles. Specifying aspects such as how nursing work is assigned, planning care, implementing and evaluating care, responsibility for care completion (reporting relationships), appropriate staff mix, responsible numbers of staff, how members communicate, what the environment looks like, and so on helps to facilitate workflow and limit conflict. For example, when addressing communication mechanisms, shift report should be considered from the standpoint of who should be there, what is discussed, where it is discussed, how it is discussed, and who remains responsible on the unit during report times. The underlying QCM, as this example highlights, provides the necessary foundation for the actual nursing report. Similarly, when discussing resources, if caring relationships are the essence of the underlying model, translating this to numbers, skill mix, and scheduling practices is crucial. Clearly articulating the alignment of aspects of care with the major concepts of the theoretical model can often be accomplished through an organizing diagram (see Figure 12.1). Thus fully integrating a PPM is a long and arduous process that is best accomplished in a shared fashion with leadership, staff nurses, clinical experts, and others who are involved with nursing on a daily basis.

After careful consideration of how the work gets done using a relational PPM, an implementation schedule and an evaluation plan that are carefully designed will help assure its operationalization. Essential components to such a strategy include preliminary education, selection of indicators of success, implementation schedule, ongoing education and support, and the evaluation method. Education that draws on the underlying nursing philosophy and theoretical model as the rationale for change is valuable. But ongoing demonstrations, coaching, regular feedback, repeated learning boosters, and accountability mechanisms are key to integration (Duffy, 2016). Indicators of success should reflect patient, nurse, and system metrics that are grouped into an "indicator set." This set of indicators should clearly reflect the model outcomes and, to be practical, be few in number (fewer than 10). Although this describes a quantitative approach to evaluation, using qualitative methods is also acceptable. Better yet, a combination of both approaches may provide the best evidence of success.

Although there is no one approach to an implementation schedule for a newly designed patient care delivery system, some examples include the following:

- Whole-systems implementation—select a start date and all departments implement together
- One unit at a time
- Several implementation units "demonstrate" the patient care delivery system for several weeks (preferably 12 or more), offer opinions about its feasibility, revise as needed, and then proceed to the rest of the organization
- Select patient populations (high risk or low risk, depending on desire) and trial the new system

The schedule chosen should reflect the best fit for the organization and allow for adequate staff nurse involvement. During the initial implementation phase, it is necessary to build in supports in the form of education, leadership presence, unit-level champions, expert practitioners, and recognition to keep the momentum going and build confidence in the new system. Finally, the evaluation method, clearly thought through before implementation, serves as the organization's way to judge success. Just as there are multiple implementation schedules, there are multiple evaluation methods. Examples include:

- Pre- and post evaluation of key indicators
- Longitudinal evaluation of key indicators
- Comparison of key indicators between implementation and non-implementation units
- Combination of methods

The method chosen is not as important as whether it gets done, so assigning the evaluation component to a responsible individual (preferably someone with advanced research skills) who understands the importance of rigorous assessment and who can disseminate results both internally and externally in an easy-to-understand fashion is an important priority. Results should be shared with staff nurses, so their voice guides ongoing improvement.

Just as a patient care delivery system forms the infrastructure for caring professional practice, a shared leadership system, or governance model, is necessary for decision making. Because nurse work is knowledge work, RNs increasingly have information to share, desire input, and want to make an impact on healthcare organizations. "Shared leadership occurs when all members of a team are fully engaged in the leadership of the team and are not hesitant to influence and guide their fellow team members in an effort to maximize the potential of the team as a whole" (Pearce, 2004, p. 48). This definition connotes mutuality, equality, inclusion, and a sense of comfort between staff and leadership whereby both perspectives are acknowledged and decisions are made jointly in the best interest of the patient. Groups of RNs organized around key dimensions (such as practice, education, research, professional development), typically called councils, can have a great influence on the success of a nursing department. Designing these teams, including the purpose, resources, membership, and procedures, along with facilitating the boundaries of the teams, is best co-shared between staff and leadership. Sharing power in this manner strengthens individuals' capabilities and cultivates an environment where employees feel free to take charge. It is vitally important to provide clarity regarding the boundaries of decision-making power (e.g., personnel record may be off limits) and not to "second guess" their decisions. Using caring relationships as the basis for design and facilitation stimulates systems thinking, engagement, creativity, and empowerment. It ensures preservation of human dignity and maximizes motivation and, ultimately, success. Likewise, establishing alliances with community partners, schools of nursing, and others can be best served by caring relationships.

USING THE QCM TO LEAD

Exemplary nursing leadership is "relationship-oriented and understands the wisdom of actively involving others and investing in partnerships, trustworthy cooperative relationships and team-building" (Forrester, 2016, p. 14). It includes planning, organizing, staffing, directing, and controlling caring relationships with those staff nurses in areas of responsibility, other leaders in the organization, stakeholders such as physicians and external partners (e.g., schools of nursing, accrediting organizations), and particularly patients and families. Holding these relationships close and actively working to strengthen them through inclusion and connection—essentially, hardwiring caring—is the secret to small changes that eventually allow larger self-advancing systems to emerge.

Although the caring behaviors are most often applied in direct patient care (see Chapter 5), examining them in a leadership context is helpful for they can also serve as guides for administrative professional practice. In fact, the caring behaviors are analogous to many contemporary leadership terms (see Table 10.2). For example, mutual problem solving is a caring behavior that facilitates decision making. As leaders provide information, help staff members see the bigger picture, explore alternatives, brainstorm together, and validate perceptions, they provide a safe atmosphere for planning a course of action together.

> Leaders who accept feedback from staff and use it to make decisions convey caring. Implicit in performing this way is comfort "in relationship": an open, engaging stance and reciprocal, shared dialogue. An example of this caring behavior would be engaging staff in planning, organizing, directing, and evaluating (controlling) a new patient care delivery system.

Attentive reassurance—being physically present often with an optimistic outlook—is nurturing to employees and conveys the leader's recognition. Noticing and listening to nurses, acknowledging changes

TABLE 10.2 Comparison of Caring Behaviors, Leadership Functions, and Relevant Leadership Behaviors

Caring Behaviors	Traditional Leadership Function(s)	Contemporary Leadership Function(s)	Relevant Leadership Behaviors
Mutual problem solving	Planning Organizing Directing Staffing Controlling	Shared visioning Evidence-based practice Shared leadership Reframing Conflict management Budget development Variance analysis Performance improvement	Brainstorming Soliciting feedback Providing information Educating Engaging Clarify and validate Practice improvement
Attentive reassurance	Directing	Action inquiry Appreciative inquiry Circular leadership Recognition programs Management by walking around (MBWA)	Availability Optimistic/convey possibilities Authentic presence Notice, recognize Maintain belief in employees Use of humor and celebrations Temporarily postpone action
Human respect	Planning Organizing Directing Staffing Controlling		Acceptance, value Recognition of rights, responsibilities, ethics, standards, legalities Patients first Call people by name Eye contact

Encouraging manner	Directing Staffing Controlling	Evaluation/performance appraisal Empowerment Human resource management Remuneration and rewards	Encouraging demeanor Enthusiastic Provide support and training Congruent verbal and nonverbal communication See patterns Build relational capacity
Appreciation of unique meanings	Planning Organizing Directing Staffing Controlling	Systems thinking Meaning in work	Appreciate frames of reference Point out meaning in the work Acknowledge the subjective Preserve the uniqueness of the patient–nurse relationship
Facilitating a healing environment	Planning Organizing Directing Staffing	Behavioral interviewing Hiring and selection process Human resource management Remuneration and rewards Evaluation/performance appraisal Safe staffing Organizational culture Culture of safety	Respect privacy and confidentiality Create a unit culture of caring Foster teamwork Design manageable workflow Safe environment
Basic human needs	Directing Staffing		Attend to personal and employee's physical, emotional health Recognize higher level needs—achievement, self-esteem
Affiliation needs	Directing Staffing	Work–life balance Membership in professional organizations	Responsive to belonging needs

or improvements and their caring behaviors, or a gentle affirmative touch shows nurses that they matter and builds confidence in the system. Using appropriate humor to lighten stressful situations and taking the time to appreciate someone's effort can be transforming. Of course, practicing this caring behavior requires frequent interaction, so regular rounding, assistance with certain patient care activities, or joint projects can provide the means to enact this behavior. Called "management by walking around" (MBWA) many years ago by Peters and Waterman (1982), put in plain words this factor implies "being there" and with a hope-filled attitude.

Human respect conveys the worth of the unique person who is an employee, a health professional, a stakeholder, another leader, or a patient. Not only does it signify value for the person but in this case it creates an appreciation for the contribution of the individual. Remembering and calling employees by name and conversing about appropriate personal issues (such as children's sports, birthday celebrations, or marriages), using eye contact, and allowing safe space for dialogue can remind employees that they are inherently worthy and valuable to the organization. Upholding rights and responsibilities in an ethical manner, expecting high standards, and appropriately following legal statutes convey unconditional acceptance and high regard for patients and families as well as employees.

Using an encouraging manner when interacting both verbally and nonverbally provides support for nurses that can lead to empowerment and risk-taking. Pointing out the good along with the challenging behaviors, especially during formal disciplining, helps others learn and advance in their roles. For nurses who take risks on behalf of patients or the organization, formal recognition is appropriate. For those who offer to chair a council or lead a meeting, being there with them especially for the first meeting promotes the confidence required to volunteer the next time. An example of this behavior occurs when a nurse who has never written an abstract or proposal for a professional conference volunteers to do it but stipulates that he or she has never done it before. Supporting him or her through the writing process, artfully critiquing the work, and offering praise where appropriate are supportive behaviors that encourage the employee to finish the task.

Appreciating the unique context of employees recognizes the importance of culture, past and current experiences, and other unique meanings that impact the work life of the employee. Attuning to these meanings and allowing them to influence decisions at times are affirming for the individual. For example, a nurse from a different culture might be allowed to explain the origin of a certain nursing action that is pertinent to his or her culture. Followed by discussion and a search of the literature, this action might be adopted for use, upholding this individual's personal worldview.

Facilitating a healing environment is one of the most important leadership roles that may be tied to RN job satisfaction and patient outcomes. Such an environment includes the surroundings in which nurses work, including their privacy and safety. It also includes the organizational culture or the norms and behaviors that characterize a patient care department. Relationship-centered cultures enhance one's sense of worth and encourage one to take risks. They focus on frequent interaction, open communication, and flexibility. Making sure that the body, mind, and spirit are in optimal condition for patient care is a role of the leader that often is tied to resources. Yet a healthy work environment includes regular periods of relaxation, available and healthy food choices, special quiet places for reflection and renewal, and uplifting continuing education. The leader who is focused on a caring–healing–protective environment will arrange the resources to support these activities. Making sure the night shift gets access to decent food is an example. This gesture relieves many who work nights from the hassle of "ordering out" or eating from machines. Other examples of healing environments include the many quiet rooms or peaceful artwork that now can be found in healthcare organizations as well as professional continuing education focused on relaxation and mindfulness practices.

Attending to basic human needs, such as not only those described above but also those higher level needs for group activities and self-esteem, keeps us connected to one another and generates the confidence so necessary for safe, effective practice. Finally, affiliation needs recognize humans' need for belonging and honors the extended family of employees, other leaders, and stakeholders and includes them in celebrations and other work initiatives. Their special needs can also be noticed in staffing and scheduling practices.

In summary, leadership practice that is based on caring relationships requires leaders who live the caring behaviors and use the unique network of relationships that define health systems to energize staff, stakeholders, and other leaders. Interestingly, using the caring behaviors in leadership practice provides a living model of relevant behaviors for health professionals to emulate! By integrating professional practice with the mission of the organization and holding each other accountable, health systems leaders elevate the unique patient–health professional relationship as the most fundamental aspect of professional work. Helping to develop caring knowledge, behaviors, and attitudes and making decisions based on a caring ethic/philosophy are facilitated through a PPM that clearly delineates roles and responsibilities. Using the caring behaviors as a guide for leaders is congruent with expectations of employees, sustaining passion for the work, and expert care to the vulnerable persons who deserve safe and quality healthcare.

SUMMARY

The context of clinical practice varies and currently is challenged by disengaged employees, high stress, and demanding work schedules in a constantly changing external environment. Nursing leaders, in their support of health professionals, have a moral obligation to uphold the professions' ethical standards, including the intimate caring relationship so necessary for high-quality care. With performance pressures rising and other external forces mounting, nursing leaders often forget that caring relationships serve to ground decisions in their practice and can be tapped as resources for advancement. Leadership based on caring relationships acknowledges the connections among humans and upholds the special relationship nurses have with patients and families. In fact, caring leaders set the tone for health professionals, generate confidence in their staff, and shape the infrastructure that supports them. Use of the caring behaviors personally and with others energizes organizations and their employees toward self-advancement. Relationship-centered PPMs provide the infrastructure needed for caring professional nursing practice and are comprised of five components: professional values, a theoretical framework, a patient care delivery system, a governance structure, and a process for recognition and rewards. Implementing and evaluating PPMs is a long and sometimes grueling process that is best planned and executed by a multilevel group of nurses. Finally, the caring behaviors provide leaders with specific approaches and behaviors to effectively ensure caring relationships are at the center of health professionals' work.

Call to Action

Health systems, comprised of people who live and work in relationship, are living systems that are complex, dynamic, and vary in context. Sustaining caring relationships energizes employees, stakeholders, other leaders, and the health systems and influences their ability to be self-caring. **Get up, walk around,** and **engage** to appreciate the contributions being made. Protecting the caring relationships that professional nurses cultivate with patients and families is a responsibility of nurse leaders. At the end of the

(continued)

(continued)

day, it is the patient–nurse caring relationship that provides the inspiration that drives staff nurses to continue their important work! **Safeguard** patient–nurse relationships. A caring-based PPM provides the infrastructure to operationalize caring professional practice. **Review** the patient care delivery system and shared leadership structures at your organization. Living the caring factors enables nurse leaders to make better use of the unique network of relationships that define health systems. **Cultivate** caring relationships.

REFLECTIVE QUESTIONS/APPLICATIONS

... for Students

1. Describe the term *healthy work environment*. Do you see it in your clinical courses?
2. Explain relationship-centered leadership. Contrast this term with other forms of leadership. Provide some examples of relationship-centered leadership.
3. Complete a review of the literature on the linkage between patient–nurse relationships and patient outcomes. Summarize your findings. On the basis of the findings, how do you recommend professional nurses spend their time?
4. Explain each of the components of a PPM. How do these components provide the structure for nursing practice?
5. Interview a nursing leader. Ask specific questions related to relationships and how they are leveraged in his or her leadership style. Characterize this leader's form of leadership.

... for Professional Nurses in Clinical Practice

1. Reflect on a leader who greatly influenced your work life. Who was it, what did he or she do, how did he or she do it, when did he or she do it, where did he or she do it?
2. Does your health system have a PPM? What does it say? Where is it kept? Is it used? Has it been evaluated?
3. Do nurses in your health system regularly interact with first-line leaders? How about executive-level leaders?
4. What caring behaviors does your nurse leader display? How often? Does it make a difference to you?

... for Professional Nurses in Educational Practice

1. Design a case study around the concept of relationship-centered leadership.
2. Critique the discussion of relationship-centered leadership presented in this chapter. Is relationship-centered leadership evident at your university?
3. What teaching/learning strategies do you think will best guide graduate students to apply the caring behaviors to leadership practice?
4. Are the development, implementation, and evaluation of PPMs part of your curriculum? Why or why not? What would it take to include it?

... for Professional Nurses in Leadership Practice

1. As a leader of a caring profession, relate how you care for yourself. How do you relieve/cope with job stress? Who can you point to that listens to your concerns about work-related matters?
2. When was the last time you enjoyed an evening out with friends? What practices do you routinely perform to help you feel a sense of harmony with yourself and your work life? How do you care for your body, your mind, and your spirit?
3. Examine your calendar for the past month. Where did you spend most of your work time? What does this say about what you value? What do your actions reveal about your fundamental beliefs about caring relationships? How might your actions affect the results you are getting?
4. Create a calendar for self-care that includes time for physical, reflective, and expressive practices. Be specific, including dates, times, frequency. Now *do it*!
5. Think about the patient care delivery system at your institution. Is it relationship centered? Is caring for self and others a predominant theme? Using the QCM, design a patient care delivery system that fits with the system's mission and addresses RN roles and responsibilities (what will they be held responsible and accountable for), resources (what staffing, scheduling is necessary), communication (how will RNs communicate with each other and the healthcare team), and the environment (what is necessary to create a healthy work setting for patients and staff)?
6. Draw a diagram depicting the congruence between the QCM and the patient care delivery system developed in number 5.

7. Discuss approximately how much time nurses spend "in relation-ship" at your organization. What activities do nurses perform that interfere with time spent "in relationship"? Offer some innovative ways to eliminate or decrease these activities so more time can be spent "in relationship" with patients and families.
8. Explain the approach of nursing leadership to professional nursing care at your institution. What is their involvement? How do they ensure nursing care is performed in accordance with professional standards?
9. How does shared leadership promote "what's best for the patient"?

PRACTICE ANALYSIS

A departmental-level nurse manager who is smart, ambitious, and com-mitted moved quickly from staff nurse to charge nurse to nurse manager. She had a stellar clinical track record but was recently reported by the staff nurses as not being "present or engaged." In fact, staff nurses character-ized her as not only distracted but also domineering and fast-paced, while other managers were worried about how she was representing nursing in the organization. So her immediate supervisor, the Director of Medical Nursing, took her aside (in the middle of the evaluation year) and sat with her to relay needed feedback. Together, the director and the departmental manager reflected on the gap between how others viewed her and how she viewed herself as leader. The middle manager acknowledged her fast-paced approach and nonverbal reactions. She also reported feeling stressed and "drained out," but remained energetic in meeting system outcomes.

Accepting this feedback was difficult for the nurse manager, who prided herself on excellence, and she seemed to be ambivalent and a little defensive about it. But the director pursued and together they developed a plan for behavior change. It included:

- Reminders for "big picture" framing
- Recognizing anxieties
- Slowing down long enough in tense situations to pay attention to physical sensations
- Practicing mindfulness
- Reorganizing routines for high energy
- Relaxation techniques

The departmental nurse manager practiced these techniques over the next 2 months and has integrated many of them into her routine. She is more aware now, taking her time to engage colleagues and ask questions rather than doing, doing, doing. She takes the time to "sense" the tone of the unit prior to taking action and, in so doing, has built more genuine connections with her employees. In essence, she has learned that authentic leadership requires internal guidance.

1. How did the nursing director's behavior prompt the departmental nurse leader's behavior change? Or did it?
2. How might the nursing director guarantee lasting or sustained behavior change in the departmental nurse leader?
3. Why do you think the departmental nurse leader accepted the guidance of the nursing director?

REFERENCES

American Association of Colleges of Nursing. (2017). Nursing shortage fact sheet. Retrieved from http://www.aacn.nche.edu/media-relations/fact-sheets/nursing-shortage

American Organization of Nurse Executives. (2015a). Nurse executive leader competencies. Retrieved from http://www.aone.org/resources/nec.pdf

American Organization of Nurse Executives. (2015b). Nurse manager competencies. Retrieved from http://www.aone.org/resources/nurse-manager-competencies.pdf

Armmer, F. (2017). An inductive discussion of the interrelationships between nursing shortage, horizontal violence, generational diversity, and healthy work environments. *Administrative Sciences, 7*(4), 34. doi:10.3390/admsci7040034

Auerbach, D. I., & Staiger, D. O. (2017). How fast will the registered nurse workforce grow through 2030? Projections in nine regions of the country. *Nursing Outlook, 65*(1), 116–122. doi:10.1016/j.outlook.2016.07.004

Brown, B. (2017). *Braving the wilderness: The quest for true belonging and the courage to stand alone.* New York, NY: Random House.

Chambliss, D. (1996). *Beyond caring: Hospitals, nurses, and the social organization of ethics.* Chicago, IL: University of Chicago Press.

Duffy, J. (2016). *Professional practice models in nursing: Successful health system integration.* New York, NY: Springer Publishing.

Fallatah, F., & Laschinger, H. K. (2016). The influence of authentic leadership and supportive professional practice environments on new graduate nurses' job satisfaction. *Journal of Research in Nursing, 21*(2), 125–136. doi:10.1177/1744987115624135

Fang, D., & Kesten, K. (2017). Retirements and succession of nursing faculty in 2016–2025. *Nursing Outlook, 65*(5), 633–642. doi:10.1016/j.outlook.2017.03.003

Faugier, J. (2006). Intimacy in nursing. *Nursing Standard, 20*(52), 20–22. doi:10.7748/ns.20.52.20.s25

Forrester, D. A. (2016). *Exemplary nursing leadership. Nursing's greatest leaders: A history of activism.* New York, NY: Springer.

George, B. (2016). The rise of true north leaders. *Leader to Leader, 2016*(79), 30–35. doi:10.1002/ltl.20215

Hoffart, N., & Woods, C. Q. (1996). Elements of a nursing professional practice model. *Journal of Professional Nursing, 12*(6), 354–364. doi:10.1016/S8755-7223(96)80083-4

Kelley, J. M., Kraft-Todd, G., Schapira, L., Kossowsky, J., & Riess, H. (2014). The influence of the patient-clinician relationship on healthcare outcomes: A systematic review and meta-analysis of randomized controlled trials. *PLoS One, 9*(4), e94207. doi:10.1371/journal.pone.0094207

Kirk, T. W. (2007). Beyond empathy: Clinical intimacy in nursing practice. *Nursing Philosophy, 8*(4), 233–243. doi:10.1111/j.1466-769X.2007.00318.x

Kornhaber, R., Walsh, K., Duff, J., & Walker, K. (2016). Enhancing adult therapeutic interpersonal relationships in the acute health care setting: An integrative review. *Journal of Multidisciplinary Healthcare, 9*, 537–546. doi:10.2147/JMDH.S116957

Kupperschmidt, B., Kientz, E., Ward, J., & Reinholz, B. (2010). A healthy work environment: It begins with you. *OJIN: The Online Journal of Issues in Nursing, 15*(1), Manuscript 3. doi:10.3912/OJIN.Vol15No01Man03

Lake, E. T., Hallowell, S. G., Kutney-Lee, A., Hatfield, L. A., Del Guidice, M., Boxer, B. A., . . . Aiken, L. H. (2016). Higher quality of care and patient safety associated with better NICU work environments. *Journal of Nursing Care Quality, 31*(1), 24–32. doi:10.1097/NCQ.0000000000000146

McHugh, M. D., Rochman, M. F., Sloane, D. M., Berg, R. A., Mancini, M. E., Nadkarni, V. M., . . . American Heart Association's Get With The Guidelines-Resuscitation Investigators. (2016). Better nurse staffing and nurse work environments associated with increased survival of in-hospital cardiac arrest patients. *Medical Care, 54*(1), 74–80. doi:10.1097/MLR.0000000000000456

Moss, E., Seifert, C. P., & O'Sullivan, A., (2016). Registered nurses as interprofessional collaborative partners: Creating value-based outcomes. *OJIN: The Online Journal of Issues in Nursing, 21*(3), 4. doi:10.3912/OJIN.Vol21No03Man04

Pearce, C. L. (2004). The future of leadership: Combining vertical and shared leadership to transform knowledge work. *Academy of Management Executive, 18*(1), 47–57. doi:10.5465/AME.2004.12690298

Peters, T. J., & Waterman, R. H. (1982). *In search of excellence: Lessons from America's best run companies.* New York, NY: Harper and Row.

Poghosyan, L., Liu, J., Shang, J., & D'Aunno, T. (2017). Practice environments and job satisfaction and turnover intentions of nurse practitioners: Implications for primary care workforce capacity. *Health Care Management Review, 42*(2), 162–171. doi:10.1097/HMR.0000000000000094

Robbins, A. (2015). *The nurses: A year of secrets, drama, and miracles with the heroes of the Hospital.* New York, NY: Workman Publishing.

Shay, L. A., Dumenci, L., Siminoff, L. A., Flocke, S. A., & Lafata, J. E. (2012). Factors associated with patient reports of positive physician relational communication. *Patient Educational Counseling, 89*(1), 96–101. doi:10.1016/j.pec.2012.04.003

Shirey, M. R. (2017). Leadership practices for healthy work environments. *Nursing Management, 48*(5), 42–50. doi:10.1097/01.NUMA.0000515796.79720.e6

Step, M. M., Rose, J. H., Albert, J. M., Cheruvu, V. K., & Siminoff, L. A. (2009). Modeling patient-centered communication: Oncologist relational communication and patient communication involvement in breast cancer adjuvant therapy decision-making. *Patient Education and Counseling, 77*(3), 369–378. doi:10.1016/j.pec.2009.09.010

Waite, R., McKinney, N., Smith-Glasgow, M. E., & Meloy, F. (2014). The embodiment of authentic leadership. *Journal of Professional Nursing, 30*(4), 282–291. doi:10.1016/j.profnurs.2013.11.004

Yoder-Wise, P. S. (2017). The essence of presence and how it enhances a leader's value. *Nurse Leader, 15*(3), 174–178. doi:10.1016/j.mnl.2017.01.001

11

Learning Quality Caring

Let us tenderly and kindly cherish, therefore, the means of knowledge. Let us dare to read, think, speak, and write . . . everything in life should be done with reflection.
—John Adams

NURSING PRACTICE

A practice involves the performance of specific activities or behaviors, but also includes conceptual (theoretical) and unique viewpoints or approaches. Practices usually conform to certain standards and thus can be performed well or poorly (e.g., one who regularly practices yoga can do it properly, satisfactorily, skillfully, or badly, inadequately). In nursing, biopsychosociocultural concepts are learned and then used to behaviorally and cognitively assess, plan, implement, and evaluate that practice. We also use those same concepts to communicate about the practice so that over time, familiar language about the practice evolves, making it meaningful and even regulating its conduct.

In 2004, the American Association of Colleges of Nursing (AACN) defined nursing practice as "any form of nursing intervention that influences health care outcomes for individuals or populations, including the direct care of individual patients, management of care for individuals and populations, administration of nursing and health care organizations, and the development and implementation of health policy" (AACN,

2004, p. 3). As a professional practice, nursing is founded on ethical standards and has specific social/public responsibilities (see Chapters 2 and 10). As a caring practice, it is undergirded in an ethic manifested by "understanding and being with the patient person and preserving the patient's personhood and dignity in the midst of depersonalized health care" (Benner & Lazenby, 2017, p. x). Nursing's specialized knowledge, skills (behaviors), and attitudes ultimately converge in the clinical setting with professional actions or behaviors that uphold human worthiness and contribute to the health of individuals and groups.

This union of knowledge, skills, and professional behaviors is much like a performing art, similar to playing the piano. Music theory must be understood, psychomotor exercises with scales and chords repetitively carried out to perfect the practitioner's technique, and musical pieces rehearsed over and over again in order to culminate in a beautiful performance. The value of music as a social good by the musician underlies his or her performance. Nursing practice is similar. It has discipline-specific knowledge that must be comprehended, psychomotor techniques that must be perfected, and professional behaviors undergirded by disciplinary values. It is dynamic and contextual, demanding an awareness of the self, others, and the larger systems in which it is performed.

Most importantly, good nursing practice focuses on the patient's experience, including the delivery of patient-centered care; it protects patients from harm; it is interprofessional; it is *always* professional; it integrates being and doing; it is evidence based; it uses high-level reasoning skills; and it has a contextual component. Good nursing practice requires a curious nature that slowly and continuously reflects upon questions such as "What am I observing about this patient and family?" "What am I learning about me?" "What am I learning about nursing?" Listening for answers to these questions over time helps one discern what is relevant or salient about clinical situations and gain the ability to respond accordingly.

Yet most prelicensure educational programs still educate according to old rules that fail to consider learning how to embody good nursing practice. Today's prelicensure nursing students are pressured to learn everything there is to know about the sciences; disease and pathophysiology; treatments, including medications and specific interventions; technical and interpersonal skills; safety precautions; interprofessional teamwork; leadership and delegation; evidence appraisal; and increasingly difficult cognitive applications in shorter periods of time compared to their counterparts in the social sciences, the arts, or business. Many clinical courses are separated from their associated didactic counterparts and are of short duration—that is, fewer than 6 hr/d or for a few short weeks. The objective seems to be exposure to multiple clinical and learning situations, leaving little time for deeper thinking, reflection, and focused application (necessary for a developing practice).

At the graduate level, most students are working (many full time) while simultaneously supporting families. Many courses are taught "online," and although this format accommodates students' schedules, it may not leave enough time for dialoguing together to learn from each other's experiences. In addition, many courses conducted in person continue to be teacher-driven lectures without many opportunities to think about and apply what is learned in the real context of advanced clinical practice. There continues to be concerns about the differences and similarities between doctor of nursing practice (DNP) and doctor of philosophy in nursing (PhD) programs in terms of outcomes, course content, and rigor. *Both* undergraduate and master's nursing programs continue to teach the rigorous process of research versus the *use* of research for clinical care, leaving many graduates with a negative attitude toward research and perceptions that evidence-based practice is unrealistic in the practice setting (Melnyk, Fineout-Overholt, Gallagher-Ford, & Kaplan, 2012).

Nursing faculty are getting older (AACN, 2017) and have demanding work lives, balancing teaching with research and service activities. Newer faculty members are being hired with limited teaching preparation and little understanding of their tripartite role. The continued low salaries, ongoing retirements, faculty vacancies, and increasing student demand have created burdens for nursing faculty members that limit in-person interaction time. Student–teacher relationships are also compromised by the hectic lives of faculty members and their busy students, complicated by the obvious separation of senior-level faculty (many of whom are established researchers who have a lot to offer students) from clinical course work. Thus, a serious practice–education gap exists that threatens professional practice.

To further complicate the situation, those relationships between busy faculty members and students represent lost opportunities to form and cultivate the necessary caring relationships that allow for ongoing role formation (i.e., learning about the *real* practice of nursing). In fact, positive learning outcomes have been linked to the quality of the student–teacher relationship (Gramling & Nugent, 1998; Mikkonen, Kyngäs, & Kääriäinen, 2015; Pullen, Murray, & McGee, 2001; Wubbels, Brekelmans, Mainhard, den Brok, & van Tartwijk, 2016). Caring relationships between faculty members and students are occasions to be nurses *together*, understand patients' perspectives, mutually consider the context of patient situations, decide on a course of action and associated priority setting, think about the rationale or evidence base for actions, and, together, evaluate performance.

> **B**eing attuned to students' needs, reassuring them of their abilities, supporting them through hard times, being receptive to suggestions and feedback, understanding their family and peer groups' pressures (being there), and sometimes doing for—such as specific helping behaviors that enable and empower students to be more self-reliant or successful—are examples of caring student–teacher relationships.

Consider the following:

A busy 39-year-old DNP student who worked as a nurse practitioner (NP) in an outpatient facility was in her final course, working on completing her DNP project. In addition to her full-time job as an NP, this student had multiple personal issues—she was a recent divorcee and a mother of two—and was barely getting by, doing most of her assignments rushed at the last minute. Although the project was already under way with data collection completed, the remaining data analysis, interpretation, and formal written and poster presentations were going to demand lots of thought time. As her faculty member for the course and project director, a professor sat down with her and in a very firm but caring manner relayed her concern that the student may not finish on time. She listened as the student told her about her problems and suggested that the student extend her time in the program in order to complete the DNP project well. The student, however, resisted the idea as she could not afford to pay another semester's fees. She begged the professor to work with her to get the project completed. The professor, knowing the student, didn't think there was much hope to complete the project during the final semester, but after listening to the student, she agreed to work with her for a few weeks to give the student the benefit of the doubt that she could do the work.

    She sat with the student and together they made a detailed plan for completion with weekly assignments. The student was told that she would need to work hard, spend time thinking and brainstorming, be receptive to feedback, and turn in her assignments on time. The professor agreed to quick turnaround times for providing feedback and "being there" for

*ongoing support. Although the professor was quite busy teaching two
other courses, directing dissertations, and conducting her own research,
she kept her commitments to this student despite the time it took to read
and reread multiple drafts. There were times during the semester when the
professor had to impose strict time frames, give uncomfortable feedback
about the work, and ask the student to redo sections of her paper multiple
times. The poster required five revisions before it was in good enough shape
to present! Each time, the professor provided some guidelines about how
to do the revisions but required the student to do the work. The professor
provided the student with websites, assistance with interpreting data,
and implications for practice, each time asking the student "What do you
think about . . . ?" A few times throughout the semester the professor had
her doubts about the student's ability to complete the project on time. But
the student was committed to completion, worked very hard, and in the
end, she did successfully complete the project on time, surprising and
delighting the professor.*

*In the course evaluation, the student wrote, "Dr. XXX was the best
thing that happened to me. She knew exactly what I needed and pushed me
to succeed. I couldn't have done it without her. Her caring wisdom guided
me to project completion." The professor was pleasantly surprised at the
evaluation because she had pushed the student hard, provided some very
detailed and hard-to-take feedback, and never received much in the form of
reaction from the student during the process.*

*The professor did, however, integrate "being with and doing for" by
being attuned to the student's need for structure and setting priorities, by
demanding times for dialogue in person, by providing frequent, detailed
feedback, by showing the student how to interpret data so that it has meaning for advanced practice nursing, and helping the student present data
in a way that others could understand. In the end the student was proud
of her project, learned how to be more self-confident and resourceful, and
discovered much about how to contribute to the* real *practice of nursing.*

NURSING EDUCATION AS A PRACTICE

Just as clinical nursing and nursing leadership is a practice, nursing
education is viewed as a practice that unfolds each day as faculty
members repetitively extend their knowledge, skills, and attitudes
through specific actions (in classrooms, online, in chat rooms, and
in the clinical setting). It is a creative practice that influences others
with the actions that are displayed, the shared ideas that are communicated, the skills that are employed, and the values and beliefs about
nursing that are transmitted overtly and covertly. Nursing educators

are called to uphold the ethical principles and standards of nursing as well as those of education.

A s educators of nurses, nursing faculty members are shaping a clinical practice whose first responsibility is to patients and families, that bears responsibility for competent and quality services, and that is uniquely qualified to advance relationships that improve the human experience. Facilitating the lifelong development of these responsibilities inherent in the clinical practice of nursing is a priority of nursing educators!

The National League for Nursing's (NLN, 2017) *Core Competencies for Academic Nurse Educators* lists several proficiencies that speak to the most fundamental obligations of nurse educators. For example, nurse educators are called to:

. . . recognize their responsibility for helping students develop as nurses and integrate the values and behaviors expected of those who fulfill that role. (NLN, 2017)

There are many other competencies, yet the one listed above describes how proficient academic educators are responsible for facilitating passionate professionalism, caring relationships, accountability, and ongoing self-advancement in students. Cultivating such knowledge, skills, and attitudes in students sets the tone for a *professional* career (and resulting clinical practice) that is responsive, caring, and continuously advancing. Nursing education is an exceptional form of nursing practice with specialized knowledge, skills, and abilities that profoundly impact the future of nurses, nursing, and health systems.

LEARNING HOW TO CARE

Most health professional students learn a lot about assessing patients, diagnosing health problems, pathophysiology, chemistry, and microbiology, and have specialized skills ranging from taking blood pressure to appraising scientific publications. Fewer have been patients. Lacking this experience, young health professional students may not fully appreciate what it feels like to be in chronic pain, wait endlessly in doctors' offices or emergency rooms while taking precious time off from work, hear conflicting advice from several different health professionals, take multiple pills (with countless side effects) or assess one's blood daily, have emergency medication on hand at all times, or deal with impossible billing personnel.

> **Y**et comprehending the human person's experience of health and illness, including the adjustment to a new illness, changes in social roles and family responsibilities, and the many personal losses inherent in illness, is necessary to adequately respond to health needs. A deep understanding of these experiences grounds health professionals in providing expert care.

Nevertheless, a focus on biological systems, diseases, or patient populations is what typically organizes the thoughts of health professionals, and it starts in educational programs, continues during clinical courses, and, most often, is the basis for state licensing examinations.

In schools of nursing, for example, students complete the familiar medical–surgical, family (obstetric and pediatrics), mental health, and community health clinical rotations, are assigned to patients in the clinical site, and terminate their relationships with them when the assignment is over or the patient gets transferred. Many times, nursing students spend a little time in specialty areas (e.g., the operating room or interventional radiology) and have no relationship with patients, but rather just observe. Why do we center clinical learning on geographic areas versus the health and illness trajectories of patients and their families? How does this form of learning prepare students for seeing the bigger picture, including the complexities of illness, the system, and various treatment regimens? How does it foster professionalism? How does it help students learn how to initiate, cultivate, and sustain caring relationships while at the same time perform highly technical procedures and make important judgments?

In a descriptive study of what "users" (patients) seek from healthcare, Wen and Tucker (2015) found that although technical competence and willingness to seek information were expected, even more important was who listens to them, who is caring and compassionate, and who explains well. When people are asked about their healthcare experiences, they often speak about the desire for a caring professional relationship with a physician or healthcare provider.

> Focusing on the health experience of patients through mutually relating and helping students adopt interventions that are meaningful to patients and families may be more beneficial than completing checklists of procedures or skills that do not impart patient-centered care. Such a focus, however, requires drastic new learning strategies, a renewed emphasis on the clinical aspect of learning (including revamping and elevating clinical courses), and a revised evaluation structure.

Although caring relationships are implicit in nursing education and occur over time, making them explicit in terms of course objectives or program outcomes, tying them to cognitive and behavioral domains of learning, and following their development over the course of a program may help bridge the practice–education gap. Moreover, as the body of nursing knowledge is ever expanding, it is not possible to teach "everything."

> Thus rethinking which cognitive, psychomotor, and affective concepts are enduring principles foundational to nursing practice and exposing students to them in depth may be a more effective and efficient way to learn the *real* practice of nursing.

To better meet the needs of patients and families, therefore, conceptualizing which major concepts are *necessary, and therefore primary,* for expert professional nursing practice. Once these are known (or made explicit), designing a curriculum around them such that they are learned in depth and over time and evaluated for competency at graduation may foster easier translations to the clinical setting. One of those concepts is caring.

The profession of nursing has considered caring relationships fundamental to good practice. It is often cited as one of the central concepts in nursing curricula and is frequently "taught" through faculty role modeling or embedded in classes on therapeutic communication and is often assessed in clinical practicums. Caring relationships are critical to patient-centered care, have been linked to improved patient outcomes (Epstein & Street, 2011), and are considered critical to meaningful nurse work (Duffy, 2013). One would deduce that a concept considered so crucial to a practice would be extensively taught by highly competent experts, in a rigorous manner, with multiple ways of assessing its achievement!

Still, prelicensure students are often exposed to caring relationships as interpersonal behaviors in mental health courses or therapeutic communication content and graduate students have even limited exposure, since it is presumed that graduated nurses already have the requisite knowledge, attitudes, and skills to care. Thus, the teaching and learning of caring relationships is fraught with discrepancies, at a time when the ongoing needs of health systems and patients for nurses with the relational knowledge, skills, and values that comprise inclusion, interaction, connection, collaboration, teamwork, communication, big-picture thinking, and reflective awareness have never been greater!

In reality, nurses perform what they know and value "in relationship"; likewise, learning about nursing occurs "in relationship" (between students and faculty members, among groups of students, between students and self, or between students and preceptors [clinical role models]). Why not use this medium to teach students "how to care (and therefore, to nurse)?"

> Understanding nursing as a practice with its inherent relational performance as the goal is fundamental to learning how to care. Appreciating that an ongoing shared relationship between a patient (and family) and nurse is needed to achieve deep levels of caring where patients can trust, be comforted, become empowered, engage, and feel understood is significant to the practice. Understanding the development of caring competence as a process that builds over time and often involves struggle, discovery, repetition, encouragement and optimism, humility, and spirituality (Purnell, 2009, p. 115) is paramount. And rediscovering the meaning of nursing "in a highly technological classroom, re-grounding it in a caring paradigm within that classroom, and transmitting this knowledge of caring to millennial students for use in their profession" (Bonaduce & Quigley, 2011, p. 158) emphasizes its significance.

Transforming the learning environment (both didactic and clinical) to one that is authentic, connected to the real world, supportive, and mutually beneficial (in terms of learning) helps students share meanings, elicit relevant data, listen, notice cues, establish rapport, and develop mutually caring interactions that may increase caring capacity from admission to graduation. Monitoring such progression or evolving caring capacity is a faculty responsibility. Furthermore, sustaining caring relationships with students may be considered a moral responsibility of nurse educators so that caring interactions as the basis for professional practice can be affirmed and operationalized, facilitating students' internalization of the concept (Adamski, Parsons, & Hooper, 2009). It is worth remembering here that, as suggested by Inui (2003), students in the health professions learn from the informal or hidden curriculum (what they see us do); thus professional caring may be learned (whether we intend it or not) by what students perceive that faculty do with respect to clinical practice or by how they behave in learning situations. Within this relational context, then, the specialized knowledge, behaviors, and attitudes associated with expert clinical practice are learned.

CARING PEDAGOGIES

Pedagogy refers to the art of teaching that encompasses specific methods, strategies, and instructional technologies. A caring pedagogy utilizes the caring factors (see Chapter 4) to create an environment of engagement and inclusion that is genuine and student centered. *Caring*, as one of the core values of professional nursing, is honored, given high regard, and lived out through the behaviors of faculty members and staff in a school or work environment. In other words, teaching caring begins with faculty members themselves who create a "caring milieu," facilitate the learning of caring by noticing and pointing out "caring moments," and then share in caring relationships.

> Faculty members who continuously reflect on the nature of nursing, the experience of learning, and integrate the caring core of nursing with their words and actions set the tone for a school and become powerful role models for students.

Caring pedagogy emphasizes relationships as primary and implies that both subjective and objective components of learning are valued and used to adequately develop and evaluate the knowledge base. Simply put, caring knowledge is partially learned in the classroom (or online) through innovative teaching strategies, followed up in the simulation laboratory, and evidenced as performance in clinical courses. For example, a classroom or online activity directed at understanding caring collaborative relationships (among health professionals) may involve readings, reflective questions, discussion forums, and a culminating dialogue that includes elements of the affective domain. In the simulation lab, a difficult scenario involving deep conflict among a physician, a nurse, and a respiratory therapist concerning the course of treatment for a ventilator-dependent patient could be presented to an interdisciplinary group. The students would be directed to work with the team and patient in making a safe and quality health decision about ongoing treatment. Behaviors such as focusing, active listening, clarification, assertiveness, gathering of facts, readiness to engage, acceptance of feedback, optimism, confidence, deep breathing, congruence between verbal and nonverbal message, and use of humor might be observed by peers and faculty members to assess the student's skill in relating to others, including the patient's view, use of the caring factors, and ultimately collaborating in decision making. Finally, in associated clinical courses, faculty members could expect students to engage in and even lead such collaborative discussions with those in other disciplines. Using this method of learning, the emphasis is on the collaborative nature of decision making (including the patient/family) versus the respiratory disease or ventilator (yet this was implicit). The concept central to the profession in this case (caring, patient-centered, collaborative relationships) remained foremost in the minds of students; cognitive, psychomotor, and affective domains were all apparent, and students were exposed to the concept multiple times with gradually increasing expectations of performance.

Likewise, evaluation of learning should examine deep understanding versus superficial knowledge of core concepts. Thus, competency is developed. Using the traditional domains of learning (Bloom, 1956), cognitive, psychomotor, and affective caring knowledge is gained by learner-centered activities/experiences that facilitate depth, connection, and context. The faculty member's role is to design, facilitate, and evaluate the learning experiences in the context of relationship.

The caring behaviors provide the groundwork for student–teacher relationships and create the context for learning. *Mutual problem solving* assists students in understanding how to approach and think about clinical situations. Providing some information, reframing students' perceptions, brainstorming together, and using back-and-forth active discourse with appropriate feedback, faculty members help shape students' comprehension of specific content. The faculty member caringly uses the relationship as the basis for learning by engaging and encouraging student-led participation. In a study of dental students, instructor characteristics such as "checking-in" with students and an interactive style, characteristics of the learning process (focus on the "big picture"), modeling and demonstrations, opportunities to apply new knowledge, high-quality feedback, focus, specificity and relevance, peer interactions, and the learning environment impacted students' perceptions of effective learning experiences (Victoroff & Hogan, 2006). In medicine, a consensus conference in England identified that in addition to specific medical knowledge, learner-centeredness, interpersonal and communication skills, professionalism and role modeling, practice-based reflection, and systems-based practice were necessary competencies for physician educators (Srinivasan et al., 2011). In nursing, a descriptive study conducted in Kurdistan concluded that the majority of participant students emphasized the importance of treating students, clients, and colleagues with respect, being eager for guiding students and managing their problems, and establishing effective communication with students (Valiee, Moridi, Khaledi, & Garibi, 2016). In addition, many of the most effective teaching strategies demonstrated by clinical instructors in this study were reported as examples of caring behaviors by students:

- Providing students with verbal and nonverbal encouragement for promoting their learning
- Encouraging students to strive for gaining knowledge and skills
- Motivating students to think about the possible answers to questions and possible solutions to problems
- Encouraging students to think, ask, and opine
- Being a good role model in dealing with clients and colleagues
- Treating students, clients, and colleagues with respect
- Having patience for addressing students' questions and problems
- Creating an appropriate learning environment
- Providing students with feedback about their performance
- Striving to promote students' independence and self-confidence

Attentive reassurance requires availability on the part of the teacher along with a positive outlook on student performance. Availability of faculty is always an issue for students and faculty because demanding work lives and lifestyles often interfere. It is important for faculty members to take a look at how often and in what ways they allow students access to them.

Office hours may not be enough, especially for online students who often do not come to campus. Multiple ways to ensure regular access to faculty are paramount; likewise, faculty members who make a point to initiate conversations (using various means) are considered important to students (Leners & Sitzman, 2006). Paying attention to students' progress requires faculty members to slow down enough to listen and notice students' behaviors. In a phenomenological study of caring in nursing education, Coyle-Rogers and Cramer (2005) highlighted how educators "cared enough to recognize in the student a need for supportive assistance" (p. 164). Noticing behaviors in students, particularly those that are of a caring nature, and following up with recognition are important aspects of this caring factor. Likewise, noticing behaviors that threaten patients' safety and remediating early is crucial. Failing students, in particular, need special time and an open and confident stand. Occasionally students will fail; faculty members who offer students other hopeful futures (suggest alternative courses or careers) can help students find meaning and strength in the process.

Human respect, or honoring the inherent worth of individuals and accepting them unconditionally, is a fundamental caring factor that conveys that people matter. All individuals want to feel significant, so when faculty members acknowledge students by name, use eye contact, maintain appropriate nonverbal behaviors, and remember that students are members of families and larger communities that they value, students learn the importance of human dignity. Approaching patients and families in clinical areas this way also conveys the importance of this factor.

Using an *encouraging manner* refers to the demeanor of the faculty member. It consists of the congruence between verbal and nonverbal messages, showing enthusiasm for student activities, cheering for students, attending and supporting student functions, and providing appropriate positive feedback. This last behavior is frequently missed as faculty members often assess examinations (particularly multiple-choice tests) and scholarly papers looking for mistakes or weaknesses in the student's work. Taking an alternative approach, choosing essay-type or other more reflective evaluation methods, and assessing them for strengths, pointing out the good aspects of students' work, takes more time but promotes confidence and builds independence.

Appreciating the unique meanings or what is important to students is a caring factor that requires intention on the part of nursing faculty. This factor honors the individuality of each student and his or her background, culture, and life experiences. At the graduate level, using the varied nursing experiences of students in seminar discussions recognizes the expertise of students and enhances learning. Directing attention to students or staying student centered is a purposeful behavior that is especially difficult when faculty members have large class sizes or online courses. Yet recognizing the unique frame of reference of students, acknowledging their subjective perceptions, and using these to devise meaningful learning experiences avoid speculation and enhance further interactions.

Creating and maintaining a caring, healing environment in schools of nursing or care delivery environments is a vital role for faculty administrators; individual faculty members are co-creators of that environment as they go about interacting with students, staff, and other faculty members. Surroundings that are conducive to learning are comforting to students and may reduce their anxiety. Such actions as maintaining a safe and confidential student lounge, providing adequate lighting, reducing noise, keeping safety a priority, resolving conflicts or disputes early, and bringing together experts or resources that augment classroom activities provide students with a caring milieu that enhances learning. The organizational culture or tone of the school, including the teamwork among faculty and staff, the vibrancy of employees, certain behavioral norms, and traditions add to the circumstances surrounding learning and have an impact on student performance. For example, faculty members in one school of nursing host a journal club once a month. By hosting this scholarly activity, faculty members demonstrate the importance of research by taking the time to coach a student leader who chooses and distributes an article and leads the discussion. The faculty member advises the student in the process and provides a safe space for dialogue. Another example is the emphasis that clinical faculty place on the safety culture of the school and/or a patient care unit. A caring faculty member will consistently scan the environment for risks, attend to them, and provide safe space to discuss, inquire about, and share concerns. Maintaining student confidentiality is important to future interactions and creates one of the conditions necessary for high-quality learning.

Meeting students' *basic human needs* is a caring factor that, on the face of it, doesn't seem pertinent to young, healthy persons. Yet, as individuals, physical, safety, social/relational, and self-esteem needs are important. It is critical that faculty members remember that basic human needs provide the motivation for behavior (Maslow, 1943). Adequate fluid and nutrition, rest and sleep, and exercise are physical needs that remain important during the educational process. Maintaining social relationships such as including students in group activities preserves belonging needs, whereas a sense of security provides order. In clinical situations, making sure students get to lunch or dinner, are recognized for their achievements, and are not manipulated by employees meets basic human needs. Helping students learn to meet these needs through self-caring activities such as specific health promotion activities contributes to the students' future caring capacity.

Keeping in mind that students have *affiliation needs* and belong to larger family and community groups is also caring in nature. When faculty members allow students to remain engaged in these groups through specific behaviors (e.g., allowing a student in a community health course to complete a project for her own community), students may find more significance in their assignments and acquire more in-depth knowledge. Using the full range of caring factors provides quality learning experiences that may have profound consequences in student learning outcomes.

CLINICAL LEARNING: INTEGRATING COGNITIVE, PSYCHOMOTOR, AND AFFECTIVE DOMAINS

Within the framework of the Quality-Caring Model© (QCM), the cognitive and psychomotor learning domains are rather easy to articulate. However, the need to translate this learning into clinical practice is the ultimate goal of learning a practice; thus the affective domain, or the feelings, emotions, values, beliefs, and attitudes of students must be integrated with the cognitive and psychomotor activities in the performance of nursing. For example, assuming responsibility for a patient's discharge planning occurs through the interplay of cognitive and psychomotor activities that manifest in a distinct series of caring interventions. As a student engages in the clinical setting with patients, families, and other health professionals, the affective domain of learning is manifest in the motivation, attitudes, perceptions, and values surrounding the performance of clinical practice (see Figure 11.1). Over time, new perspectives of clinical practice (and maybe some revisions of it) arise and are internalized.

FIGURE 11.1   Contribution of three learning domains to discharge planning.

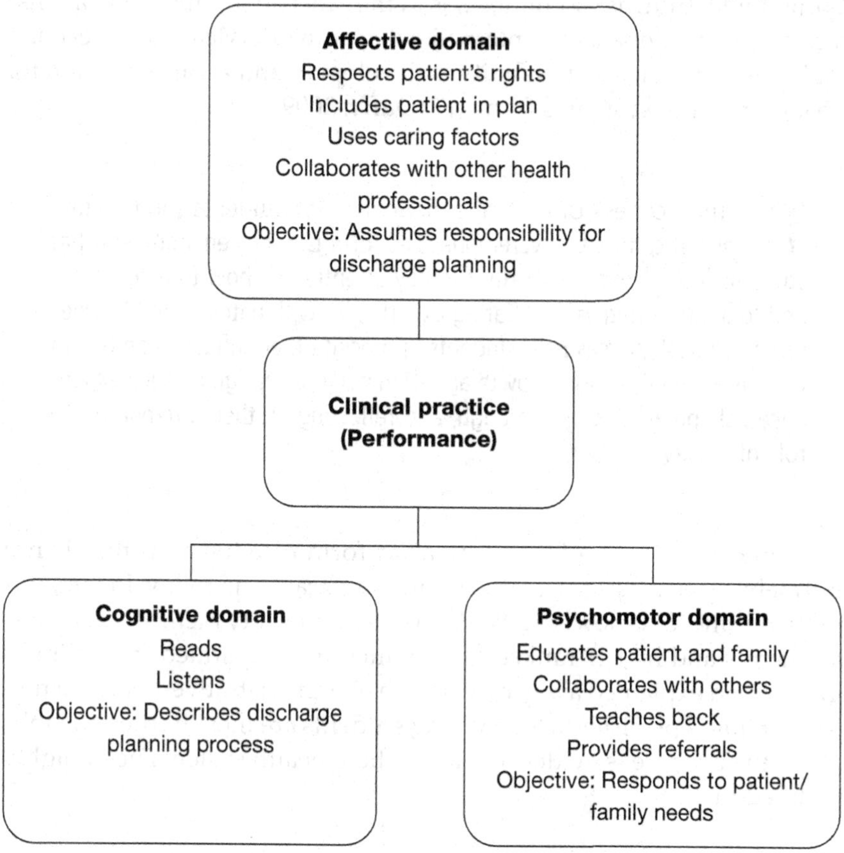

Affective domain
Respects patient's rights
Includes patient in plan
Uses caring factors
Collaborates with other health
professionals
Objective: Assumes responsibility for
discharge planning

**Clinical practice
(Performance)**

Cognitive domain
Reads
Listens
Objective: Describes discharge
planning process

Psychomotor domain
Educates patient and family
Collaborates with others
Teaches back
Provides referrals
Objective: Responds to patient/
family needs

> The affective dimension of learning is best supported in a learner-centered environment with full use of the caring behaviors, observed and evaluated in the clinical setting by expert practitioners and reinforced through reflection. Reflection, an essential activity of self-caring and a fundamental relationship of the QCM, helps one see more clearly how life experiences shape thoughts and behaviors.

Expecting students to be self-aware, lifelong learners is an outcome of most nursing programs that can be integrated throughout nursing curricula and at all levels. Integrating the patient's perspective, including his or her feedback, helps students integrate all domains of learning while keeping the patient at the center, progressively enhancing students' caring behaviors.

As affective learning is most apparent in clinical settings where caring relationships are easily observed, acknowledging the importance of this setting for learning is essential. "It is in the practice setting where a sense of caring professionalism is internalized, teamwork is learned, safety and quality is ensured, accountability is developed, and an appreciation for the larger health system is formed" (Duffy, 2009, p. 137).

> Thus the richness of clinical experiences for students (and faculty members) cannot be overemphasized for it is in this environment that students learn what is important to pay attention to, how to react safely, and to adopt caring values. Caring experiences with patients and families during clinical courses help students appreciate their influence on health outcomes and their own growth as caring persons. Designing such experiences, shepherding them through, and reflecting on them afterward is a role of faculty members.

Clinical education is an advanced form of education that is not routinely given a rightful status in nursing academia today. In fact, it is pretty routine to see lower-ranked or part-time faculty members as course instructors and higher-ranked faculty members separated from clinical practice and explained away by research or administrative-related activities. Yet this is precisely where young students are most impressionable, where the practice is evidenced, and where health systems need highly qualified nurses!

Health professional faculty members who are separated from clinical practice are missing out on the opportunity to align education with real-world clinical practice, emphasize enduring concepts that are central to their discipline, influence employees to advance their education, participate in ongoing clinical research, and renew their own passion for their chosen profession.

Despite course and program revisions, the structure of prelicensure nursing clinical education remains constrained by older models, role strain among faculty, limited sites and opportunities, and the limited involvement of senior faculty. Yet healthcare information, patients, interventions, and payment models are rapidly changing, requiring new graduates to rapidly transition from students to practicing nurses. To meet these challenges, pilot studies, nurse residency programs, and dedicated education units have begun; yet the evidence related to these is sparse. One area of promise is the cultivation of strong academic–practice partnerships that share resources, provide research opportunities, increase the availability of clinical preceptors, facilitate the transfer of knowledge from the classroom to the clinical setting, increase student and staff satisfaction, and improve patient outcomes (Dobalian et al, 2014; Keough, Arciero, & Connolly, 2015; Needleman, Bowman, Wyte-Lake, & Dobalian, 2014; Pearson, Wyte-Lake, Bowman, Needleman, & Dobalian, 2015; Smith, Lutenbacher, & McClure, 2015; Snyder, Milbrath, Gardner, Meade, & McGarvey, 2015).

Although this is a good first step, schools of nursing are struggling to revise their curricula, including this crucial clinical aspect, in light of faculty shortages and expected retirements, fewer clinical placements, and changing student characteristics. And, at present, the organization, sequencing, and time spent in clinical courses for the most part remains stagnant, with senior-level faculty separated from clinical practice and student experiences still based on exposure to multiple diseases/patient populations.

Radical change is needed, however, to meet the demand for nurses who can relate in a caring manner, engage in real-time practice improvement, collaborate with others to ensure safe, quality outcomes, and honor patient experiences. Some general recommendations include the following:

- Design learning experiences that foster caring relationships (with self, patients and families, other health professionals, and the community served)
- Facilitate learning about disease and illness through *patient connections*—case studies, rounding, patient and family "guests" in the classroom

(continued)

(continued)

- *Use caring relationships over the course of a chronic illness or health event* (pregnancy and child-rearing or palliation and death) versus a specific clinical setting or a specific timeframe to facilitate learning
- Provide ongoing feedback about performance (practice) through observation, strength-based evaluations (Bouskila-Yam & Kluger, 2011), and *expect practice revision in real time*
- Reconceptualize both the clinical faculty role and more senior faculty roles, *elevating the status of clinical teaching*
- Dialogue about the wisdom of innovative models where students from all levels and associated faculty *work together in partnership with health system employees* to provide care for small groups of patients and families—assume assigned roles allowing students to learn how different functions facilitate patient outcomes in health systems
- Consider clinical education centers where interprofessional faculty members can design and evaluate the feasibility of innovative clinical learning ideas
- Use existing partnerships between academia and service to better *integrate clinical learning with provision of services*

Clinical education is a vital faculty assignment that offers the opportunity to role model, invite thinking, create safe space for exploration, evaluate effectiveness of various teaching methods, and stay close to the patient. In an integrative review, a synthesis of 37 articles found that the ability to develop interpersonal relationships was the most valuable skill for effective clinical instruction (Collier, 2017). Facilitating student learning while honoring patients and families by asking questions such as "What is happening in this relationship?" or "What seems to be important to this patient?" or "How can I engage this patient and family?" places caring relationships at the center of clinical learning, better preparing today's students for the realities of *real* clinical practice. There is no greater privilege.

THE IMPORTANCE OF A REVISED NURSING CURRICULUM

Since the publication of "Educating Nurses: A Call for Radical Reform," a Carnegie Foundation study that examined the state of nursing education, presented results and offered recommendations in light of changing nursing practice and health systems (Benner, Sutphen, Leonard, & Day, 2010), nurse educators have continued to dialog about curricular revision. The four major recommendations in this report were:

1. Emphasize teaching for a sense of salience, situated cognition, and action in particular situations—facilitate the use of knowledge and skills in clinical settings
2. Integrate clinical and classroom learning—decrease the divide between the two
3. Emphasize clinical reasoning and multiple ways of knowing (including scientific)
4. Focus on formation—changes in identity and self-understanding toward professionalism.

In 2018, how many of these recommendations have really been implemented? How many have been thoroughly evaluated? Besides the summary report, *The Future of Nursing: Leading Change, Advancing Health* (Institute of Medicine, 2010; see Chapter 1), what will it take to generate curricular change to meet the demand for a transformed health system?

Today's practice environment requires a new kind of nurse (a systems thinker, i.e., someone not bound by procedures and tasks), one who draws on knowledge (research, evidence-based practice, performance improvement), incorporates knowledge of self, and, most importantly, possesses relational knowledge. Such characteristics call for mature professional nurses who understand nursing science, the natural sciences, social sciences, technology, and the humanities *and*:

- Can set priorities
- Know how to respond to changing conditions
- Recognize the patient/family as the decision maker
- Protect patients and families from harm
- Relate in a caring manner
- Identify self as a health professional and practices in accordance with ethical standards
- Can lead
- Are able to access information and use evidence as the basis for practice
- Can engage patients, families, and health professionals
- Contribute to policy development and implementation
- Can gather and use data to make decisions
- Regularly evaluate self (including self-reflection and the development of clinical wisdom) and revise practice
- Are able to care for self
- Understand and are proud of their contribution to the nation's health

These professional characteristics require a new, revised educational system that works in tandem with service to support learning across the life span. Strong leadership, mutual collaboration, and using data to assess outcomes, all in the context of professionalism and accountability, provides the basis for such curricular change.

Nursing educators must respond by designing curricula that are focused on nursing's enduring concepts, that are more experiential—that is, they must elevate clinical courses or remake them to provide strong learning experiences centered on patients and families and with emphasis on evidence and multiple opportunities for feedback on key nursing concepts.

Moreover, they must also change didactic courses to include active learning approaches, such as case methods with innovative questioning techniques, ongoing coaching and role modeling to keep students engaged and help them understand the importance of various clinical situations as well as the bigger picture. Implementing simulations based on nursing's enduring concepts and increasingly providing depth throughout the curriculum, providing *real* leadership opportunities, not observation of leadership, and requiring multiple interprofessional clinical experiences will strengthen students' experiences of the real world. Applying professionalism through one's own demeanor throughout the curriculum, designing and using a system of ongoing inquiry at the university so that students internalize the value of lifelong learning and use of evidence (e.g., regular journal clubs, grand rounds, improvement, and research), renewing and elevating pre- and postclinical conferences, and redesigning how students are evaluated adds depth to the learning experience that hopefully will translate to the practice environment.

Such recommendations give both nursing faculty and educational leaders heartburn! With the faculty shortage looming, educational revision of this magnitude carries many risks. Yet the health system requires fully educated professional nurses who can practice in the real world. Nurses in educational practice and their leaders must rise to this challenge. Accepting that students cannot learn everything, and selecting those concepts that best drive professional practice, is a first step. Designing curricula geared toward teaching these concepts in depth, using both revised didactic and multiple clinical experiences, will add value. It will be important not to teach to a particular textbook or test but rather use multiple readings from the current literature, real case studies, and group dialogue to help students really understand versus memorize. Evaluation techniques must move away from primarily using multiple-choice tests; although these serve their purpose, they don't easily allow for application of knowledge, responding to changes, clinical reasoning, or assessment of the affective domain—all essential for professional practice.

Nursing faculty must align with current clinical practice and be able to move easily between practice and academia to build relationships with service partners and other health professionals. This ensures quality experiences for students. An example of this is true joint appointments where faculty members serve their health system partners in specific roles so as to better understand the current requirements of staff nurses (e.g., Magnet® criteria, National Database of Nursing Quality Indicators® [NDNQI], and Centers for Medicare and Medicaid Services indicators), enabling staff and advanced practice nurses to more effectively participate in clinical teaching and learning. For the article "Evidence-Based Nursing Leadership: Evaluation of a Joint Academic-Service Journal Club," Duffy and colleagues (Duffy, Thompson, Hobbs, Neimeyer-Hackett, & Elpers, 2011) evaluated a leadership journal club that involved a faculty member and a nursing leadership group meeting monthly to appraise the leadership literature in an effort to enhance leadership decision making. Both groups were involved in goal setting, evaluation, and eventual publication of this activity. Likewise, in a practice improvement project, a group of staff nurses met over a period of 1 year with a nursing faculty member to redesign a nursing shift report. The faculty member facilitated the development of an intervention, a proposal for funding, and a publication. Staff nurses learned how to review the literature, develop a nursing intervention for feasibility, and the rigors of publication and presentation. One of the staff nurses has since applied and was admitted to a master's program, an unintended benefit, and a publication is in process. Mutual goal setting, collaborating on research and/or practice improvement projects, joint teaching and learning activities, and ongoing evaluation all provide relationship-building opportunities that translate into better learning experiences for students.

Present and future nursing faculty must be clinically credible—aware of and knowledgeable about current clinical practice; adept at a wide range of technology, practice improvement, and research approaches; possess relational capacity; be able to role model caring relationships; provide academic progression models that engage students and practicing nurses; facilitate and seek grant proposals and funding streams; and convey passion for the practice of nursing.

EVALUATING CARING RELATIONSHIPS

Assuring Individual Caring Capacity

Caring capacity is a complex phenomenon referring to an individual's expertise and ability to engage in caring relationships. As such, its measurement is daunting and requires multiple approaches. It is best accomplished through formative and summative approaches that help prepare health professionals "to be" as well as "to do" work in their respective disciplines. Attending to all three domains of learning (with an emphasis on the affective domain) is essential (e.g., an increase in knowledge, for example, does not ensure adequate performance of caring behaviors or internalization of caring values in the practice setting). Despite the fact that graduates of nursing programs are expected to initiate, cultivate, and sustain caring relationships with themselves, their patients, members of the healthcare team, and the community served (Duffy, 2013), caring competency in nursing is rarely measured summatively in the academic setting and even less so in the practice environment (Duffy, Kooken, Wolverton, & Weaver, 2012).

Starting with the QCM and its assumptions, concepts, and definitions, however, a set of specific caring objectives encompassing all domains of learning can be developed that increase in complexity over the course of a curriculum. For example, while a sophomore student might "establish caring relationships with patients and families," a senior student may "independently monitor and modify their caring relationships with patients and families." Multiple evaluation techniques, such as written essays, critical analyses, concept mapping, role playing, peer review, simulations followed by reflective analysis, taped observations of behaviors, and patient feedback administered over time versus the traditional multiple-choice testing approach, allow for more comprehensive evaluation of developing caring capacity. At graduation, caring competency should be summatively assessed; multiple approaches (e.g., actual measurement tools from the students' perspective, peers' perspectives, patients' perspectives, and faculty evaluations; final reflections, portfolio) are available for this, but the key is that it is completed and used to revise curricula. Such a rigorous summative evaluation approach provides a comprehensive perspective of overall caring ability and assures faculty that students are prepared for practice.

After graduation and in the clinical setting, assessing the caring capacity of staff nurses can be done using a novice-to-expert approach (Benner, 1984) in which multiple perspectives (self, patient, supervisor, and peers) provide evidence of progression. Evaluation of caring capacity from the patient's perspective offers unique insights into how patients view professional nursing practice and can assist nurses to better understand how to improve their practice. For example, Duffy and Brewer (2011) used a collaborative quality improvement approach with 12 hospitals to assess patients' perceptions of nurse caring and provided feedback for use in practice revision. On a more individual level, Duffy et al. (2012) pilot tested the feasibility of assessing hospitalized older adults' perceptions of nurse caring using an electronic format during hospitalization. Using a mobile device, 86 older adults provided feedback on RNs' caring relationships. The study demonstrated feasibility and is intended to be applied in a larger intervention study to provide data for real-time practice improvement. Using the wisdom of multiple sources and perspectives to provide this important feedback is a generative approach that is less threatening to individual nurses and allows for patient participation.

Feedback from patients in both academia and the clinical setting keeps the focus on patients and can be used creatively to:

- Encourage more open dialogue about caring professional practice
- Reinforce the importance of caring processes (or factors)
- Reflect back to students and/or staff how significant their practice is to patient outcomes
- Identify strengths and areas for development
- Raise awareness of faculty and nurse leaders of how the curriculum or the practice environment might be influencing caring practice

Much more research is needed to determine whether these approaches will improve nursing students' and practicing nurses' caring capacity.

Program Evaluation Using the QCM

Formative and summative evaluation of concepts considered central to a program's curriculum and based on that program's philosophy and objectives provides important evidence of the program's success. Such evaluation helps meet the mandate of producing competent clinicians who can fulfill practice expectations. One such practice expectation is caring relationships. In an educational environment that uses caring as one of several enduring nursing concepts and teaches it in depth across all curricular levels, it would follow that a quality program evaluation would encompass caring-based performance indicators. A framework for program evaluation helps guide the assessment process. To that end, an adaptation of the QCM for program evaluation could provide such a foundation. For example, identification of student and faculty variables that contribute to learning processes and outcomes could be included under the concept *humans in relationship*. Relationship-centered professional encounters in an adapted QCM for program evaluation might include those student–faculty, faculty–faculty, and faculty–practice partner relationships that are established, nurtured, and sustained through the curricular processes, such as curriculum and instruction, research, and service, that comprise the work of nursing faculty. In a student-centered environment, the independent relationship between students and faculty is primary and includes values, attitudes, and behaviors that faculty members carry out in partnership with students during the learning process. Such relationships undergird and facilitate student learning, leading to specific educational outcomes.

Collaborative relationships include those activities and responsibilities that nursing faculty members share with other faculty members, administrative personnel, and practice partners throughout a university system. Meetings, task forces, and coordinating activities among university departments represent many disciplines working together in collaborative relationships that ultimately lead to shared educational outcomes. For example, a nursing department and an informatics department may work together to design a novel nursing intervention and pursue funding for research. Such work is collaborative and enriches quality educational outcomes.

The third major component of the QCM, "feeling cared for," is an intermediate outcome that is the immediate result of the educational process. "When one feels 'cared for,' a sense of security develops making it easier to learn, change behaviors, and take risks" (Duffy & Hoskins, 2003, p. 83). Students who feel cared for while in the learning environment have reported less anxiety and more skill acquisition (Pullen et al., 2001). "Feeling cared for" in students and faculty leads to similar outcomes as those in patients—feeling safe, empowered, respected, listened to, encouraged, connected—that ultimately result in self-advancement.

A self-advancing educational system reflects forward progress that enhances the systems' well-being. It evolves naturally without external control, provided attention is paid to the relational components of the model.

Self-advancing educational systems can be evaluated through empirical indicators (summative learning outcomes, faculty productivity, system utilization, and resources used) and are used to provide ongoing evidence for process changes.

With a foundational model as a guide, a program's evaluation plan should reflect the faculty's decisions about responsibility, frequency of assessment, specific measurements, and acceptable criteria. Multiple perspectives applied formatively over the course of the curriculum culminating in end-of-program summative evaluation are recommended. In this case, assessing those relationships inherent in educational processes and relational learning outcomes is crucial. Assuring caring competence from the perspective of the student, the faculty, and, most important, the recipients of caring (patients) is worthy. Patients' perceptions of student nurse caring capacity better assesses whether students are actually conveying caring to patients and families. To prevent faculty and patient burden, a limited number of these evaluations is recommended at key points in a program. Using valid and reliable instruments, faculty can design how students will best select patients and administer the instrument. Scores from such evaluations should be shared with students and used by faculty (along with the other evaluations) to provide feedback about performance and make judgments about the effectiveness of the curriculum in preparing caring graduates.

Although subjective, student self-reports of nurse caring can provide a baseline assessment at program entry and then be followed annually (or more frequently) to determine improvement. This allows for trending by program level and over time. Clinical evaluation tools that include both subjective and objective measures of nurse caring that are consistent across the program can be used from a faculty perspective to assess students' progress in caring competence. Such measures can be as simple as one item with higher scores expected as students progress in the program or composed of multiple items that are summed for a total score. Faculty evaluation of students' caring competencies can then be easily assessed in each clinical course and compared across the program.

Creating caring environments during the educational process and role modeling caring relationships seem to raise awareness and facilitate learning. Assessing students' perceptions of faculty caring can yield important data about the structure and processes of an educational program. The Caring Assessment Tool-Educational Version (CAT-edu) is an example of an instrument used to evaluate this variable (Duffy, 2007). Students can complete this assessment at the end of their program and results can be used by faculty members to revise their interactions with future students. Although this discussion has centered on quantitative program evaluation, using qualitative approaches such as reflective journaling, narratives, portfolios, focus groups, and other methods adds valuable information to the quantitative assessment. Finally, correlating model components (and their subconcepts), such as student demographics or faculty credentials with specific learning outcomes, provides data that can be used to adjust learning outcomes and generate policy revision. In addition, ongoing feedback and revisions are consistent with educational practice improvement.

SUMMARY

This chapter focused on teaching and learning the practice of nursing. In particular, nursing practice was likened to a performance integrating "being" and "doing" simultaneously. Learning how to care was described as a repetitive process that occurs over time and in a context requiring relational learning strategies, renewing emphasis on the clinical courses, and revising how one evaluates learning. Student-centered caring pedagogies using the caring processes (or factors) and encouraging openness, risk-taking, and engagement facilitate the design of meaningful learning experiences that contribute to self-advancement (positive learning outcomes). Incorporating aspects of these factors into learning objectives across the curriculum best integrates the concept of caring as the key ingredient in professional practice. Emphasizing the affective domain of learning, or the integration of cognitive and psychomotor activities in the performance of nursing, is key to quality clinical education. Best evidenced in clinical courses, nursing faculty have multiple opportunities to role model, facilitating student learning while honoring patients and families. The importance of a revised curriculum to meet complex health systems' needs for professional nurses is stressed, with recommendations for curricula and faculty members. Finally, assessing developing caring capacity throughout educational programs, at graduation, and within the practice environment is discussed. Using the revised Quality-Caring Model for Educational Program Evaluation as a guide, schools of nursing can incorporate caring assessments formatively and summatively to ensure that this important and enduring concept is embedded in both the curriculum and the environment, and students' progress is followed.

Call to Action

S tudent–faculty caring relationships combined with rich experiential learning in the clinical setting are the best possible ways to help students learn professional caring. *Evaluate* your relationships with students. Using the context of caring relationships to design and implement learning experiences assists nursing students to understand complex phenomena. Faculty members who connect caring nursing situations to the larger whole enable graduates to adjust to the complex healthcare system and transfer their knowledge to a variety of nursing situations. *Increase* the amount of time you spend with students this week. The performance of nursing is best demonstrated during clinical education. In the clinical situation, faculty members have the opportunity to encourage opinions, shape ideas, establish a secure system for inquiry, and assess the usefulness of their teaching. *Sign up* for a clinical course. Noticing students' attitudes and actions, actively listening to verbal and behavioral cues, and showing interest in their work is necessary to gauge student progress. It requires faculty members to remain unhurried, focused, and deliberate enough to pay attention. *Acknowledge* the strengths of students' work.

Professional nurses are better able to advance their practice (and resulting caring capacity) when they receive information from the patient's perspective. Such detail offers unique insight directly from the source and suggests specific ways to improve. *Rewrite* your last lecture to include the patient's perspective. In the context of caring relationships, nursing faculty members have the responsibility to design, facilitate, and evaluate learning experiences that positively impact student learning and enhance patient outcomes. *Revise* your student evaluation method(s) to enhance student learning. Important information about an educational organization and its curriculum can be obtained by assessing students' perceptions of faculty caring. *Use* a valid and reliable tool to measure students' perceptions of faculty caring upon graduation.

REFLECTIVE QUESTIONS/APPLICATIONS

. . . for Students

1. Discuss what it means to be a practice discipline.
2. How did you learn "to care"? How do you keep this knowledge current?

3. What reflective learning activities are you engaged in? How would you evaluate and/or revise them?
4. Critique the idea of learning nursing's enduring concepts in depth versus learning a little bit about "everything."
5. Think about being ill in a hospital with a chronic disease. How do you feel when you must wait 1.5 hours in a cold hall for a chest x-ray? How would you react to conflicting advice from three different physicians? How would you keep your 12 different medications straight?
6. Have you encountered faculty incivility? Analyze the circumstances and the consequences to your practice.
7. What about student incivility? What have you seen? What could you do to alleviate it?

. . . for Professional Nurses in Clinical Practice

1. Do you engage in student learning activities—as a preceptor, clinical instructor? Do you see how affective learning brings together knowledge and psychomotor skills? What will you do to foster this domain?
2. Analyze the education–practice gap. How would you recommend it be narrowed?
3. What is your stand on "caring can be learned"? Why?
4. Are you surprised to hear that patients reported that caring relationships with nurses and patient-centeredness was a need? Why or why not?

. . . for Professional Nurses in Educational Practice

1. Does your educational program still use the traditional four clinical courses? Are they separated from didactic content? How much clinical time do students get? Are they experiencing *real* nursing practice?
2. Appraise the phrase *caring pedagogies.* How is it operationalized in your curriculum?
3. Appraise the phrase "Clinical education is an advanced form of education that is not routinely given a rightful status in nursing academia." What challenges or conflicts does this imply?
4. List baccalaureate and graduate student demands that limit authentic relationships in the educational environment. How could these be eased or the environment revised to enhance relationship building?

5. What caring and non-caring faculty behaviors do you observe at your institution?

6. Analyze the core concepts that undergird your curriculum. Are they enduring? How are they learned in depth and advanced over the program? What evaluation methods do you use to ensure profound understanding of these concepts?

7. What innovative strategies can you identify to ensure the three domains of learning related to caring are threaded throughout your curriculum?

8. How would you implement a 360-degree student evaluation program in your curriculum?

9. Reflect on your role as a faculty member. How do you role model caring? What self-caring practices do you regularly carry out? Are you certain that meaningful (i.e., breadth and depth of the content) learning occurs in your classroom? What ways can you identify to integrate caring pedagogies into your teaching style? How can you better integrate didactic and clinical learning?

10. Make a list of the caring factors and describe how you enact them in relationships with baccalaureate and graduate students. Do they differ based on level? Should they?

11. Consider an online course with graduate students. Develop at least three learning objectives each for the cognitive, psychomotor, and affective domains that include caring relationships with patients. How would you ensure by your interactions with students that caring was conveyed?

12. Consider a course that you currently teach. For a student-centered course, design a caring learning experience that includes five small (three to five students) groups each with its own activity that blends into one larger caring concept.

13. What ideas do you have to help baccalaureate students develop deep meaning in the caring relationships they have with patients and families? How would you implement them? What practice experiences could best provide opportunities for students to know and connect with patients and families?

14. What strategies might you use with graduate students to help them develop deep meaning regarding the caring relationships they should cultivate with the healthcare team? How would you implement them?

15. What type of faculty members can best utilize caring pedagogies? Are there some who can't? What are the characteristics of those who are successful?

16. Describe how you are able to transfer humanness from the simulation lab to the clinical area.
17. Is your educational program currently in the process of revising its curriculum? How many of the recommendations from this chapter have you incorporated? Be honest.
18. How do you assure caring capacity in your students?
19. Does your program use a conceptual framework to guide evaluation? How could you influence that?
20. How do you partner with clinical service?

. . . for Professional Nurses in Leadership Practice

1. Do you agree that a curriculum change is in order?
2. How does the new graduate experience at your institution affect caring professional practice?
3. What continuing education activities at your institution promote caring professional practice?
4. Are nurse caring behaviors integrated into the required annual competencies at your institution? Could they be integrated? How would you go about revising them?
5. How do you partner with schools of nursing? What competencies in new graduates do you expect? Have they been discussed and agreed to?

PRACTICE ANALYSIS

After multiple attempts at teaching nurses the value of high-quality patient experiences at a large community hospital, the nurse educators were frustrated. Over the last 2 years they had developed online learning modules, in-class lectures, and annual competency assessments to help RNs improve their practice. These learning activities were required and over 85% of the hospital RNs had attended at least one of the above classes. But patient experience scores had not improved. They concluded that simply having the knowledge and skills does not ensure that the behavior will be performed.

During a series of discussions with a faculty member at a local nursing school, they decided to turn their attention to RNs' values and attitudes about patient experiences in an effort to change behavior. As a first step, the educators exposed the nurses to the value of positive patient experiences using video clips of real patients, stories, and brainstorming techniques to raise awareness. Then they asked each RN to reflect in writing on the story or video clip. Secondly, a cased-based exercise was used to engage the RNs in active review of a real situation. Evaluation of this activity included active participation and the co-creation of an ideal patient experience diagram. In the next class, role playing was used based on a real case and during debriefing the educators observed the RNs for voluntary expressions of the value of positive patient experiences commitments to change. At the next class, RNs were asked to write how their learnings up to this point were being translated into their clinical practice. The educators reviewed the written reflections and provided pointed feedback that showed the link between any new practice behaviors and the new value of positive patient experiences.

Continued observation of the RNs on the clinical units by the educators was completed looking for evidence of "advocating" for positive patient experiences. Reinforcement and advanced facilitation techniques (e.g., coaching, conflict management) for consistent performance were provided on the clinical unit with real patients by the educators. Finally, tracking the RNs' behaviors over time to continue their development through self-assessments at the annual performance review were conducted. In this review, the self-assessment was again tied to the value of positive patient experiences and linkages to other important patient outcomes were pointed out. Encouragement and positive rewards as well as opportunities for sharing their newfound expertise were offered.

1. What did the educators do differently after they met with the university professor?
2. What did the clinical aspect of this learning experience accomplish?
3. How do you think RNs would adapt to this form of learning? Why?
4. What do you think the educators should do related to evaluating this learning experience?

REFERENCES

Adamski, M., Parsons, V., & Hooper, C. (2009). Internalizing the concept of CARING: An examination of student perceptions when nurses share their stories. *Nursing Education Perspectives, 30*(6), 358–361. doi:10.1097/HNP.0b013e3181dd47bc

American Association of Colleges of Nursing. (2004). AACN position statement on the practice doctorate in nursing. Retrieved from http://www.aacn.nche .edu/publications/position/DNPpositionstatement.pdf

American Association of Colleges of Nursing. (2017). Nursing shortage fact sheet. Retrieved from http://www.aacn.nche.edu/media-relations/fact-sheets/ nursing-shortage

Benner, P. (1984). *From novice to expert: Excellence and power in clinical nursing practice* (Commemorative ed.). Old Tappan, NJ: Addison Wesley.

Benner, P., & Lazenby, M. (2017). *Caring matters most: The ethical significance of nursing* (p. x). New York, NY: Oxford University Press.

Benner, P., Sutphen, M., Leonard, V., & Day, L. (2010). *Educating nurses: A call for radical transformation.* San Francisco, CA: Jossey-Bass, Higher and Adult Education Series.

Bloom, B. S. (Ed.). (1956). *Taxonomy of educational objectives, the classification of educational goals—Handbook I: Cognitive domain.* New York, NY: McKay.

Bonaduce, J., & Quigley, B. (2011). Florence's Candle: Educating the millennial nursing student. *Nursing Forum, 46*(3), 157–159. doi:10.1111/j.1744-6198.2010.00186.x

Bouskila-Yam, O., & Kluger, A. N. (2011). Strength-based performance appraisal and goal setting. *Human Resource Management Review, 21*(2), 137–147. doi:10.1016/j.hrmr.2010.09.001

Collier, A. D. (2017). Characteristics of an effective nursing clinical instructor: The state of the science. *Journal of Clinical Nursing, 27*(1–2), 363–374. doi:10.1111/jocn.13931

Coyle-Rogers, P., & Cramer, M. (2005). The phenomenon of caring: The perspectives of nurse educators. *Journal for Nurses in Staff Development, 21*(4), 160–170. doi:10.1097/00124645-200507000-00007

Dobalian, A., Bowman, C., Wyte-Lake, T., Pearson, M., Dougherty, M., & Needleman, J. (2014). The critical elements of effective academic-practice partnerships: A framework derived from the Department of Veterans Affairs Nursing Academy. *BMC Nursing, 13*(1),183. doi:10.1186/s12912-014-0036-8

Duffy, J. (2007). Caring assessment tools. In J. Watson (Ed.), *Instruments for assessing and measuring caring in nursing and health sciences* (2nd ed.). New York, NY: Springer Publishing.

Duffy, J. (2009). *Quality caring in nursing and health systems: Applying theory to clinical practice, education, and leadership.* New York, NY: Springer Publishing.

Duffy, J. (2013). *Quality caring in nursing and health systems: Implications for clinicians, educators, and leaders.* New York, NY: Springer Publishing.

Duffy, J. & Brewer, B. (2011). Feasibility of a multi-institution collaborative to improve patient–nurse relationship quality. *Journal of Nursing Administration, 41*(2), 78–83. doi:10.1097/NNA.0b013e3182059463

Duffy, J., Hobbs, T., Elpers, S., & Neimeyer, N. (2011). Evidence-based nursing leadership: Evaluation of a joint academic–service journal club. *Journal of Nursing Administration, 41*(10), 1–6. doi:10.1097/NNA.0b013e31822edda6

Duffy, J., & Hoskins, L. (2003). The Quality-Caring Model©: Blending dual paradigms. *Advances in Nursing Science, 26*(1), 77–88. doi:10.1097/00012272-200301000-00010

Duffy, J., Kooken, W., Wolverton, C., & Weaver, M. (2012). Evaluating patient-centered care: Feasibility of electronic data collection in hospitalized older adults. *Journal of Nursing Care Quality, 27*(4), 307–315. doi:10.1097/NCQ.0b013e31825ba9d4

Epstein, R. M., & Street, R. L. (2011). The value and values of patient-centered care. *Annals of Family Medicine, 9*(2), 100–103. doi:10.1370/afm.1239

Gramling, L., & Nugent, K. (1998). Teaching caring within the context of health. *Nurse Educator, 23*(2), 47–51. doi:10.1097/00006223-199803000-00018

Institute of Medicine. (2010). *The future of nursing: Leading change, advancing health.* Washington, DC: National Academies Press.

Inui, T. (2003). *A flag in the wind: Educating for professionalism in medicine.* Washington, DC: Association of American Medical Colleges.

Keough, L., Arciero, S., & Connolly, M. (2015). Informing innovative models of nurse practitioner education: A formative qualitative study. *Journal of Nursing Education and Practice, 5*(5), 88–91. doi:10.5430/jnep.v5n5p88

Leners, D. W., & Sitzman, K. (2006). Graduate student perceptions: Feeling the passion of caring online. *Nursing Education Perspective, 27*(6), 315–319.

Maslow, A. H. (1943). A theory of motivation. *Psychological Review, 50,* 370–396. doi:10.1037/h0054346

Melnyk, B. M., Fineout-Overholt, E., Gallagher-Ford, L., & Kaplan, L. (2012). The state of evidence-based practice in U.S. nurses: Critical implications for nurse leaders and educators. *Journal of Nursing Administration, 42*(9), 410–417. doi:10.1097/NNA.0b013e3182664e0a

Mikkonen, K., Kyngäs, H., & Kääriäinen, M. (2015). Nursing students' experiences of the empathy of their teachers: A qualitative study. *Advances in Health Sciences Education, 20*(3), 669–682. doi:10.1007/s10459-014-9554-0

National League for Nursing. (2017). Core competencies for academic nurse educators. Retrieved from http://www.nln.org/professional-development-programs/competencies-for-nursing-education/nurse-educator-core-competency

Needleman, J., Bowman, C., Wyte-Lake, T., & Dobalian, A. (2014). Faculty recruitment and engagement in academic-practice partnerships. *Nursing Education Perspectives, 35*(6), 372–379. doi:10.5480/13-1234

Pearson, M., Wyte-Lake, T., Bowman, C., Needleman, J., & Dobalian, A. (2015). Assessing the impact of academic-practice partnerships on nursing staff. *BioMedCentral, 14*(28), 1–9. doi:10.1186/s12912-015-0085-70

Pullen, R., Murray, P., & McGee, K. (2001). Care groups: A model to mentor novice nursing students. *Nursing Educator, 26*(6), 283–288. doi:10.1097/00006223-200111000-00014

Purnell, M. J. (2009). Gleaning wisdom in the research on caring. *Nursing Science Quarterly, 22*(2), 109–115. doi:10.1177/0894318409332777

Smith, K. M., Lutenbacher, M., & McClure, N. (2015). Leveraging resources to improve clinical outcomes and teach transitional care through development of academic-clinical partnerships. *Nurse Educator, 40*(6), 303–307. doi:10.1097/NNE.0000000000000166

Snyder, A., Milbrath, G., Gardner, T., Meade, P., & McGarvey, E. (2015). An academic and free clinic partnership to develop a sustainable rural training and clinical practice site for the education of undergraduate and advanced practice nurses. *Journal of Nursing Education and Practice, 5*(4), 7–12. doi:10.5430/jnep.v5n4p7

Srinivasan, M., Li, S. T., Meyers, F. J., Pratt, D. D., Collins, J. B., Braddock, C., . . . Hilty, D. M. (2011). Teaching as a competency: Competencies for medical educators. *Academic Medicine, 86*(10), 1211–1220. doi:10.1097/ ACM.0b013e31822c5b9a

Valiee, S., Moridi, G., Khaledi, S., & Garibi, F. (2016). Nursing students' perspectives on clinical instructors' effective teaching strategies: A descriptive study. *Nurse Education in Practice, 16*(1), 258–262. doi:10.1016/j.nepr.2015.09.009

Victoroff, K. A., & Hogan, S. (2006). Students' perceptions of effective learning experiences in dental school: A qualitative study using a critical incident technique. *Journal of Dental Education, 70*(2), 124–132. Retrieved from http:// www.jdentaled.org/content/70/2/124.full

Wen, L. S., & Tucker, S. (2015). What do people want from their health care? A qualitative study. *Journal of Participatory Medicine, 7*, e10. Retrieved from http://www.jopm.org

Wubbels, T., Brekelmans, J. M. G., Mainhard, T., den Brok, P., & van Tartwijk, J. (2016). Teacher-student relationships and student achievement. In K. R. Wentzel & G. B. Ramani (Eds.), *Handbook of social influences in school contexts: Social-emotional, motivation, and cognitive outcomes* (pp. 127–145). New York, NY: Routledge.

12

The Value of Quality Caring

Strive not to be a success, but rather to be of value.
—Albert Einstein

ENVISIONING THE FUTURE: TEN YEARS, FIFTY YEARS, AND BEYOND

Futurists speculate on how people will live, work, die, be educated, pay for, and experience healthcare 50 to 60 years from now—and in some cases, in the next few years. For example, from the perspective of a cardiologist, Chazal (2017) recognized how precision medicine, rapid diagnostics, breakthrough interventions, biomarkers, nanotechnology, gene and stem cell therapies, and three-dimensional printing will significantly affect peoples' lives. From an economic and regulation perspective, recent and continuing healthcare reform efforts will demand health systems and health professionals deliver care differently, specifically in relation to increasing value and preventing or reversing disease. From a nursing perspective, contemporary care delivery systems, data-informed decision making, more engaged patients and families, rapidly changing technology, and a shifting workforce will require higher and more sophisticated levels of knowledge and optimum flexibility. From the patient perspective, expectations for individualized care delivered by health teams that actually talk to each other, active roles in decision making in regard to health parameters, treatment options, and financing alternatives, virtual visits and electronic communications, all provided within a framework of patient-centeredness, will significantly affect healthcare delivery and the work of all health professionals.

Others see the future as expanding global connectivity via expansive cloud computing, redefined employment trends with more self-employed persons, use of "smart" products focused on personal wellness that have the ability to sense, process, report, and take corrective action, drastically different higher education systems. Yet no one can predict the future with certainty. In general, however, individuals tend to underestimate advancements and their advent. For example, from the time the first edition of this book was published until now (9 years), several of the original projections have already come true. Real-time virtual meetings and animated emojis are already available, distance learning dominates graduate education programs, and technological advances in healthcare such as smartphone diagnostics, virtual doctor's visits, and transparent, integrated, electronic information systems connect hospitals, physician offices, and outpatient clinics. And, as has been the case for many years, healthcare costs continue to dominate the discussions around healthcare and will continue to do so.

> Health expenditures in the United States grew 5.8% to $3.2 trillion in 2015, or $9,990 per person, and accounted for 17.8% of gross domestic product (GDP). Medicare spending grew 4.5% to $646.2 billion in 2015 and Medicaid spending grew 9.7% to $545.1 billion in 2015. Private health insurance spending grew 7.2% to $1,072.1 billion in 2015 while out of pocket spending grew 2.6% to $338.1 billion in 2015. Hospital expenditures grew 5.6% to $1,036.1 billion and physician and clinical services expenditures grew 6.3% to $634.9 billion in 2015 and prescription drug spending increased 9.0% to $324.6 billion in 2015, slower than the 12.4% growth in 2014. Finally, national health spending is projected to grow at an average rate of 5.6 percent per year for 2016–2025, and 4.7 percent per year on a per capita basis. (Centers for Medicare and Medicaid Services [CMS], 2017b).

There remains much disagreement among policy makers, healthcare providers, and the American public about the best way to address healthcare costs. Despite the enactment of the Affordable Care Act (ACA), 28 million Americans still remain *without* health insurance, increased premiums occurred for many, and reduced access to preferred providers has frustrated some members of the public (Kantarjian, 2017).

The projected advances and challenges simultaneously affecting healthcare highlight the growing complexity of an integrated, interactive, interdependent, and global system that requires a more sophisticated workforce—one that understands the significance of big-picture thinking, whose practice is based on knowledge, multiple and oftentimes competing connections, and that values relationships as the basis for actions and decision making. This new healthcare system is rapidly emerging, and the shift to sweeping transformation is already occurring.

In fact, as the American health care system continues to evolve, hospitals and emergency departments are battling the opioid epidemic, more older adults leave hospitals in functional decline, too many 30-day readmissions occur, the American public weighs more on average (Steelman & Westman, 2016), and health systems continue to struggle to reduce errors in care while simultaneously delivering real patient-centered care. Most importantly, health systems are battling the increased demand and range of services required as expanded access and more baby boomers, who are rapidly turning 65, are expected to live longer and require more health services. And the persistent challenges inherent in professional nursing (e.g., the workforce, the workflow, and the workload) continue to plague hard-working professional nurses—and their leaders and educators. However, yesterday's solutions will not repair today's burgeoning health problems.

The future of healthcare—and the quality of patient care—depend upon health professionals participating with the right leadership, and the right openness, training and education for the development of skills that are flexible and adaptable to new models of care.

The Centers for Medicare and Medicaid Services' accountable care organizations, medical homes, and innovation center encourage and test novel health care payment and service delivery models.

(CMS, 2017a, 2018). Combined with CMS's already established reimbursement system based on hospital-acquired conditions and publicly reported outcomes, nursing and other health professionals are experiencing dramatic change.

Luckily, recent nursing graduates are more authentic and tech savvy than previous generations (Weirich, 2017). Most grew up with handheld technology and understood its inner functions before they entered the workforce, giving them skills that are crucial in healthcare today. They also have ambition, embrace change, are innovative, and have a desire to keep learning, but are uncomfortable with rigid organizational structures and get turned off by information silos. They expect rapid progression, recognition, a varied and interesting career, and encouraging, constant feedback, and will move on quickly if their expectations are not met (Price Waterhouse Coopers, 2017). Such expectations require very different workplaces—those focused on employee and customer needs.

In fact, the millennial generation of nurses (1980–2002), has surpassed Gen Xers as the largest generation in the U.S. labor force (Fry, 2015) and they hold many of the qualities needed by health systems today. Working with this talented group of nursing professionals is a privilege, *provided they are empowered to lead health systems where caring relationships dominate.*

The real challenge facing the nursing profession is ensuring that the core processes of mutual problem solving, human respect, attentive reassurance, encouraging manner, appreciation of unique meanings, facilitating a healing environment, and ensuring basic and affiliation needs remain central to all aspects of nursing practice. A practice profession that *uses* the knowledge of relationships as the basis for its work understands the nature of humans as they exist in relationship to others and their communities. And a practice profession that acknowledges and acts in accordance with its implicit knowledge is able to progress and advance itself.

RENEWED AND REVITALIZED QUALITY CARING

Health professionals well understand the benefits of caring relationships, but oftentimes seem timid about fully actualizing them.

> **C**aring relationships are fundamental to patients, health professionals, and health systems' advancement—they provide the context for health behaviors, offer health professionals meaningful work, and are vital for safe, quality patient outcomes.

Given that all health professionals learn about, provide care within, and are expected to participate in caring relationships, the fact that they are not fully actualized is a great irony. The ability to deliver safe, high-quality services, collaborate, engage, continuously learn and be innovative, and ultimately advance, depends on caring relationships. In fact, caring relationships are the basis for patient-centered care and health professionals' own work-life satisfaction. The theorized results of caring relationships—feeling cared for and ultimately self-advancement—become obvious when we examine those health systems and health professionals who are choosing to embrace caring relationships as the basis for their work.

As Margaret Wheatley (2017), a world-renowned leadership consultant, declared, those who "choose who they want to be" are present to others, committed to serving patients and families, embrace and create new possibilities and ways of being, are brave (in this case, willing to face the chaos and uncertainty characterizing this time of transformation), and caring enough to lead individuals toward a greater understanding of who they are as human persons make a difference. These are courageous health professionals and systems who understand that caring relationships elevate healthcare from a commodity that can be nicely packaged and paid for to an ethical, human partnership based on professional ethics, joint knowledge of the other, and ongoing accountability.

One might ask, "How can high-caring organizations—those with better relational capacity, energy, and joy—operate with high caring in such an uncertain, metric-focused world?" The answer lies in their grasp of caring relationships as the fuel that propels self-advancing systems. As such, these organizations continuously work on faithfully integrating quality caring throughout the system. Examples are presented in the following paragraphs that represent both academic and community health systems, larger and smaller (in terms of numbers of beds), urban and rural, diverse and homogeneous, and with differing patient populations. Their choice to continue the focus on caring relationships is gaining momentum in health systems—transforming lives, clinical practice, leadership practice, and

educational practice. They represent clinical, collaborative, and administrative cases.

- At Lowell General Hospital (LGH) in Lowell, Massachusetts, a
  Magnet®-designated hospital that has been using the Quality-Caring
  Model© (QCM) for at least 3 years, multiple examples exist of caring
  relationships as the center of practice. Interestingly, most are designed
  and implemented by staff nurses themselves. One example of how
  caring relationships are integrated throughout the system at Lowell
  General occurred when a group of educators were reviewing the
  preceptor program. Although education regarding the QCM had
  occurred early on, it was not a focus of preceptor training. Seeing this
  as a deterrent to full integration, the Nursing Education Department
  added tenets of the model to preceptor training in order to facilitate
  utility of the model with new nurses at the bedside. After mapping
  the caring behaviors from their professional practice model to the
  organizational promises of complete, connected care, nurse orientees
  were able to demonstrate that preceptors were more knowledgeable and better able to integrate the QCM in their various learning
  activities. This project was disseminated via a poster presentation at
  a regional meeting. In fact, this health system designed a diagram
  depicting how preceptors use the caring behaviors to facilitate pre-
  ceptee outcomes. (See Figure 12.1.)
- At South Florida State College School of Nursing, faculty members
  have used the QCM to guide curriculum for several years. To advance and extend the model's reach outside the school of nursing,
  more than 150 nurses, students, and university administrators
  attended an all-day conference to celebrate what was in place and
  to stimulate further application of the model, both in the university and the community it serves. The dean, Dr. Michelle Heston,
  received funding and then reached out to a partner hospital, the
  theorist, and faculty from other schools to develop the day-long
  event. Results published in the school newspaper showed that
  attendees' were profoundly impacted by the knowledge gained
  and were eager to incorporate it into their careers.
  At St. Barnabas Medical Center in Livingston, New Jersey, development of nursing leaders for quality caring was evaluated through
  the use of the Caring Assessment Tool-admin version. In this study,
  an educational intervention was developed, implemented, and then
  evaluated through the pre–post-test method. The intervention was
  implemented by the Chief Nursing Officer and Vice President of
  Patient Care Services and Innovation herself and results are pending.

- At Lakeland Regional Medical Center, an 851 not-for-profit hospital in Florida, leaders and health professionals across the system researched, read, discussed, examined themselves as individuals and team members and discovered key motivators to bring out the best every day—for themselves, their colleagues, the community, and, most of all, for patients and their families. Out of this extensive work, the QCM made a significant impression on the team. What resonated most was the relationship-centered focus of the model, which was inspiring because it put into words what the team strongly believed to be the best way to provide care. Then the team acted. Leaders from human resources, public relations, information technology, nursing, clinical services, support services, and financial services participated in focus groups in order to craft a compelling message. Then they gave of their time, their passion, and they educated and role modeled. Out of this work was born the Lakeland Regional Health Promises.

  These statements shaped and continue to shape the organization's culture:

  We Promise . . .
  to treasure all people as uniquely created
  to nurture, educate, and guide with integrity
  to inspire each and every one of us to do our very best

  The Promises are prominently displayed on the system's walls, within the elevators, and are exhibited in its people. Accordingly, they are at the heart of caretaking, decision making, and in everyday interactions.
- At the Massachusetts Department of Health and Human Services Sexual Assault Nurse Examiner (SANE) program, a national nursing telemedicine center was established to serve victims of sexual assault. Over the past 3 years, the National TeleNursing Center has evolved from a vision to a functioning center, with a team of expert SANEs "choosing" to provide 24/7 consultation to licensed providers across the country as they care for adults and adolescents who have recently experienced a sexual assault (Massachusetts Department of Health and Human Services, 2017). As does its parent organization, the International Association of Forensic Nurses, the National TeleNursing Center uses the QCM to provide real-time guidance and support to victims as well as to health professionals, mostly nurses, as they collaborate to enhance the capacity to assist crime victims and to provide

leadership that promotes justice and healing for all victims. Using videoconferencing technology, 150 SANE-certified nurses in Massachusetts respond to hospitals in six regions of the country and, after patient consent, facilitate up to 6 hours of care. As of this writing, the program has provided over 67 consults with 106 patient victims nationwide.

FIGURE 12.1   Integrating the Quality-Caring Model into preceptor training.

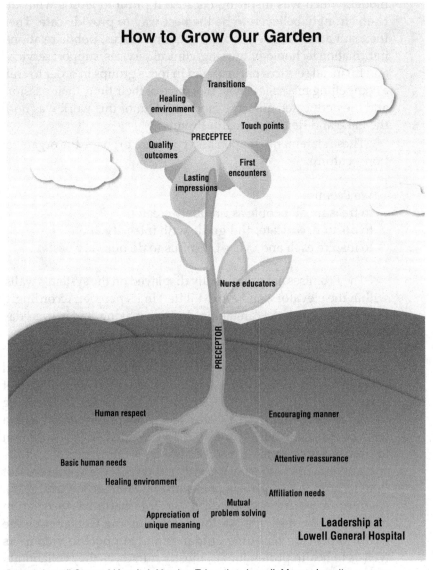

Source: Lowell General Hospital, Nursing Education, Lowell, Massachusetts.

As demonstrated by these courageous health systems that have chosen "who they want to be" (Wheatley, 2017) by holding caring relationships at the center of practice, others may be reassured and find strength and encouragement during this challenging time. These caring leaders are creating a critical mass of health professionals that are dramatically affecting the work of clinical practice and the course of patient care. As a whole, these health systems have been visited and observed by others to learn what they are doing differently. And in the interconnected world we currently live in, their influence may be larger than they even think. Health systems that have chosen to embrace caring relationships are benefiting in multiple ways: reduced adverse outcomes, positive patient experiences, better and faster communication and collaboration, and patient and staff engagement.

> Caring relationships are fast becoming a new asset in healthcare—they are critical for patient-centered care, high-functioning teams, engaged patients and employees, and the best-quality outcomes.

QUALITY CARING IN ACTION

Nurses in Clinical Practice

A more mature nursing workforce is emerging today—one whose members are true knowledge workers—that is, practicing to their fullest by leading health systems to respond in caring ways to patient and family needs. These professionals are experts in and use caring relationships as the basis of their work. To do this, they simultaneously make use of both inner and outer resources to provide strength and renewal. In other words, they can replenish themselves or are self-caring. The dominant biomedical, task-oriented, shift-focused approach of today is being transformed in the moment to an alert, confident, engaged professional workforce that is true to its nature, *caring*. Not only does this group have relational capacity, it embodies it—in other words, these nurses work in congruence with their knowledge base and values.

> Professional nurses are using their time "in relationship" with patients and families, other health team members, and themselves to promote feeling cared for. They focus on the person rather than on the disease and have an appreciation for the larger system in which they work. They are responsible yet flexible, see possibilities, and strive for self-improvement by accepting feedback and continuously learning.

Such maturity is not related to age but to a willingness to take the essence of nursing, along with current knowledge, and recreate a practice that is meaningful, a basis for pride, and that positively impacts patient outcomes.

Consider the following advice as expressed by a clinical nurse for other nurses:

> *We have all learned many clinical and technical skills as we journeyed through nursing school and our careers. Did you even imagine that the critical one would be relational? It is the lifeline between nurses, doctors, and patients and families. Although it may not be conveyed verbally, many times fear is the emotion that most patients experience as they encounter the health system. Fear is defined as that unpleasant emotion caused by the belief that someone or something is dangerous, likely to cause pain, or is a threat. It provokes feelings of anxiety concerning the outcomes of something or the safety and well-being of someone. I want to share my own personal story as I experienced the vital importance of verbal and nonverbal interactions that took place through the course of my husband's illness:*
>
> *Four years ago, my husband was admitted to the hospital after a traumatic experience. I had just begun nursing school and although I knew the basics, there was so much that I did not know at the time. It was during our month-long stay that I remember the impact of caring during a particular bedside shift report that took place. We had never spent any amount of time in this setting except for the joyful birth of our children. We were filled with the unknown, not only about my husband's prognosis but also the hospital setting, what would happen, and the uncertainty of or if he would ever get home again. As nurses, we are so accustomed to our work environment and what we do that I don't think we realize, for many people, the hospital is a scary place, an unknown territory, and is usually experienced due to uncertain circumstances and occurrences, and possible outcomes that are filled with intense fear. We looked forward every day for that period of time when the nurse would come in and share the plan for the day, reiterate what had transpired the previous days, inquire as to our concerns, check that equipment was operating properly, and notify us who would be responsible for my husband during the next shift. This small interaction and connection with those that were caring for my husband provided confirmation, reassurance, and an understanding of what was expected of us, as well as what we could expect. It reiterated that everyone was on the same page. We could discuss our concerns, ask questions, and witness the passion of nursing as we met with each of you. We really needed that interaction as we began yet another day facing the unknown.*
>
> *It was during my absence and during a bedside report that it was noted that my husband was in respiratory distress and transferred once again to the intensive care unit. If you had not come in to do bedside report, he would not have received the higher level of care necessary on such a timely basis. In the early hours of the morning, as a nurse sat with him and provided coffee and*

companionship during her hourly rounds, he was able to communicate his fears as well as enjoy a lighthearted conversation during his sleepless nights. As he progressed and moved on toward rehab, he experienced a pulmonary embolism. My husband never made it home again. I will never forget those of you who participated and joined us in his care and shared with us your time, expertise, advice, and caring during this difficult time. Who knew that at the age of 56 his final days on this earth would be spent in a hospital setting?

As a bedside nurse now, I truly believe in the difference those few moments spent "being with" patients and families can make, and the lasting impact it can have. We never have enough time to do our jobs, and it may seem to be unnecessary or inconvenient to do it, but I want to let you know how crucial it is for patients and, yes, their families. I recall my husband's comments during our stay: "I can't believe that these people who don't even know me, complete strangers, would care about me so much." The love, respect, and attention he received during those last days truly made a difference in his life and mine. So, remember to include your patients in their plan of care, check on them frequently, keep them safe, and develop your relationship with them. It has been said that although people may not remember what you said or what you did, they will remember how you made them feel. There is not a better time than the initial encounter to relay the true purpose of nursing, "caring for individuals and their families to improve their quality of life," even if it is for a short period of time!

(Patricia Marchessault, RN, Winchester, VA)

The professional caring delivered to this family generated relaxation, security, knowledge, a sense of comfort, and hope for an easier time. The patient's wife, although a beginning nurse, needed this reassurance and still remains appreciative of the caring received 4 years later! The nurses expertly practiced the caring factors by placing this family first; expecting *them* to participate, integrating *being* with *doing*, and maintaining a purposeful, inclusive manner. In so doing, they met the needs of the patient and his wife.

Nurses in turn gain from such experiences in terms of their own learning, and the personal significance that is generated from the work. By genuinely caring, nurses in clinical practice experience many life lessons.

Nurses, as one of several health professionals, forge collaborative relationships with other health team members for the benefit of patients and families and actively incorporate evidence from quality improvement and research activities into their practice. In many places, the clinical nurse of today is an admired and essential member of the healthcare workforce and is included in important healthcare decisions.

Recently, a nurse relayed this story:

Mr. Carey was a 52-year-old male with chronic lymphocytic leukemia (CLL). He was post two bone marrow transplants (one autologous and one allogeneic) and one round of chemo and was in the process of a second round of chemo. He was admitted to a large suburban Magnet-designated hospital on an evening in May with herpes zoster (shingles) of his left arm starting at the axilla and continuing to his fingers. He had been suffering with this for over 3 weeks. Tonight the pain was unbearable and he was also experiencing brief episodes of shortness of breath. His wife of 8 years had been supportive of his treatment, traveling with him cross-country twice for the bone marrow transplants. Lately, however, she was irritated by an increasing use of narcotics to ease the pain and wanted to pursue more aggressive treatment. It was in this spirit that the two appeared on the oncology unit. After the admission process, Mr. Carey had his blood drawn, was offered pain medication, and Mrs. Carey stayed with him for an hour before going home. The next morning, Mrs. Carey became irritated after the oncologist elected to stop Mr. Carey's chemo—he recognized it as the cause of increasing herpes and was not convinced it would actually prolong Mr. Carey's life. (Mr. Carey and the oncologist had discussed this together and made a joint decision.) Mrs. Carey demanded to talk to the doctor who she felt wasn't doing everything possible for her husband. The nurses assigned to Mr. Carey interacted with the couple and provided pain control, but did not address the conflict in treatment. The oncologist finally showed up at 8 p.m. at which time he took Mrs. Carey aside and discussed with her the poor prognosis of Mr. Carey, reinforcing to her that "there was no hope." Mrs. Carey went into a tailspin trying to process the fact that her 52-year-old husband would die despite all the agony he had been through during two transplantations and she did not agree to the planned course of action.

Meanwhile, Mr. Carey was fully conscious and agreed to the physician's assessment and recommendations. The situation became tense on the unit first between the couple and then between the wife and the nursing staff. (By this time the oncologist had left.) Mrs. Carey continued to demand treatment. The night shift nurses came on and Mr. Carey's assigned nurse was one with about 8 years of experience. She assessed the situation and understood that the wife was not ready to accept the prognosis of her husband and possibly had misconceptions of the therapeutic value of further treatment, whereas Mr. Carey had accepted his condition. Once Mr. Carey was settled and she had assessed her other three patients, the nurse asked the charge nurse to look after her other patients and she invited Mrs. Carey to sit with her in a private room to talk. She listened as Mrs. Carey recounted the long and unpleasant months posttransplantation only to have the cancer come back twice. She stayed as Mrs. Carey spoke of her frustration, isolation, and money lost during Mr. Carey's failed treatment. The nurse's nonverbal behaviors were encouraging and unhurried. Then she took Mr. Carey's chart and gently went through it with Mrs. Carey and used the laptop computer in the room to provide the current guidelines for CLL treatment to her. Mrs. Carey gradually began to comprehend that the oncologist was following current guidelines—even more so—and her attitude softened. The nurse, who was conscious of the time that had passed while her other patients were waiting, provided Mrs. Carey with a cup of tea and said she would return in an hour. Upon her return, she found Mrs. Carey sitting with her husband and talking softly with him. The following evening, she checked in with Mrs. Carey and reflected to herself, "Now I understand how to interact with my brother-in-law who is dealing with his father's colon cancer diagnosis."

Although this is an ideal situation, the nurse could have acted otherwise. Instead, she *chose* the power of a caring relationship to help this family member process a poor prognosis. She took responsibility and demonstrated an ethic of caring that is consistent with the profession. In so doing, she alleviated some of Mrs. Carey's suffering (and Mr. Carey's too), generated a sense of security in the process, and instilled hope for their ongoing relationship. She learned some life lessons in the process. As Swanson (2008) once stated, she was "being a nurse" versus "doing nursing."

On a typical day most of us have opportunities for caring—instances in which we are able to build, cultivate, or extend caring relationships. Our response in those times often has a disproportionate impact:

A young nurse (this author) was scheduled to work on Christmas day (her favorite of all holy days). She purposefully chose the evening shift because she had young children and wanted to spend Christmas morning with them as they opened their presents. She was angry she had to work—after all, her entire family was gathering for a big meal and her children wanted to play with her. But she trudged on in to the coronary care unit (CCU) where she was employed. She was assigned one patient with a myocardial infarction (MI) and the first admission. It was quiet for a while and she kept ruminating with her colleagues about why nurses always had to work holidays and weekends while other professionals were at home, having fun. Her anger increased, and she was in the midst of deciding whether she wanted to continue working on this unit when a new admission was called up from the emergency department (ED). He was a 56-year-old man, from out of town, visiting his daughter and newborn baby granddaughter. He had chest pain and shortness of breath, was brought by ambulance to the hospital and it was determined by ECG that he was suffering an anterior wall MI. He was stabilized in the ED and brought to the CCU on a monitor with multiple intravenous drips and an oxygen mask. He arrived pale, blood pressure was 92/50, heart rate 110, with minimal chest pain (he had morphine in the ED). The young nurse assessed him, made him comfortable, and got orders from the resident on call, all the while deliberating about her employment situation. She was not aware that his wife and daughter were in the waiting room. Within 20 minutes, the patient's heart rhythm started to decrease and he felt "queasy." When the resident arrived, it was obvious that the patient needed a pacemaker and the nurse became even more distressed that on Christmas evening she had to spend her time in a fluoroscopy room (with no window)—it meant she couldn't call and say good night to her children!

Wheeling the patient to the fluoroscopy room, the nurse saw the patient's wife and daughter in the waiting room. They were distraught—no one had interacted with them since the ED and now they saw their husband/father on a gurney going somewhere. The nurse stopped and let them know what was going on and allowed them a couple of seconds to talk to the patient. Because of his condition, they had to move fast, so she rolled him into the room. As she settled the patient on the table, he told her that he and his wife had made the trip to visit his daughter to see their new granddaughter on Christmas. He was so excited about the baby, describing her in detail. Tears appeared in his eyes as he realized that he was in a very precarious situation . . .

The nurse touched his arm gently and began explaining the procedure. She donned a mask and made sure the resident had his on, adjusted the monitor and all his invasive lines, and assisted the physician with the insertion, all the while monitoring the patient's vital signs—it was 5 p.m.

An hour passed and the pacemaker was in, but just would not capture (it did not generate a rhythm) and the patient's heart rhythm (Mobitz II, AV block) continued with dropped beats and a rate ranging between 48 and 55, with a BP of 90/50. The nurse went to see the family and explained what was happening and that the physician was working hard to get the pacemaker working. They thanked her. She then went to the nurses' station and asked a colleague to call the chaplain to sit with them while she went back to the fluoro room. They worked on the patient for another hour and still no pacing. Meanwhile, the patient was alert and oriented and softly speaking about his trip and the baby. He asked to see his wife and daughter and the nurse allowed the wife and daughter in the room for about 15 minutes. They appeared to have a wonderful, loving relationship.

Gradually, the patient's blood pressure started dropping, so additional meds were added to his IV (intravenous medication). The nurse smiled at him over her mask and he held her hand tightly. Occasionally the nurse remembered her children at home on Christmas, but she knew her husband was taking care of them and they were snuggled in their beds—now all her attention was on this patient and his Christmas night. It was now 8:15 p.m., the cardiac fellow had been called in, the pacemaker was still failing to capture, the patient's blood pressure continued to drop, and it was apparent that his prognosis was very poor. The nurse then reflected on how she had had a beautiful Christmas morning, while this man was dying on Christmas night, after only spending a few hours with his beloved new granddaughter. How lucky she was. She held onto his hand under the sheets, looked at him over her mask, and he returned the look—somehow they both knew his fate. The two physicians were conversing about the pacemaker and the drugs while the patient and nurse were communicating silently about the meaning of this Christmas night! After multiple attempts at the pacemaker, the patient lost consciousness, arrested, and despite a full code, he died— it was 8:40 p.m. The two physicians, who were also angry that they were called away from their Christmas dinners, left, leaving the nurse to interact with the family.

She went to the waiting room to find them sitting, softly crying with a priest in attendance—the young resident had given them the news and then gone home. When the nurse entered, they immediately stood up and hugged her. Then they spoke about the patient—his quirks, his love, and his humor. The daughter mentioned how happy she was that he got to see his granddaughter and his wife remarked about their long marriage. The young nurse was sad—after all, they had not saved him—and it was Christ-mas. She thought, "Every Christmas from now on, they will remember this sad, sad day." The nurse could not contain her emotions and she cried too, thinking again of her own family. After she cleaned up the patient, the family visited him, and were getting ready to go home around 9:30 p.m., when the wife said, "Thank you so much for caring for him, this was the greatest of Christmas gifts, his last hours were not alone, he spent them with an angel."

Although it has been 39 years since this incident, this nurse can remember it like yesterday—the details, the emotions, the smells, the faces. And every Christmas since that night, the new grandpa, his wife, and daughter remind her of the real meaning of Christmas. The nurse's response to this patient and family have had a lifelong impact on *her*, as similar situations do for so many nurses and other health professionals. *Clinical practice is the place where health professionals find meaning and renewal.*

Leadership

Nurse executives are challenged daily to *deliver superior services in healthy work environments at the lowest possible cost.* Balancing organizational costs with the human caring processes required for superior patient outcomes and healthy work environments, however, depends on relational exper-tise. Moreover, that expertise must generate "feeling cared for" in others to drive self-advancement; in other words, the quality of relationships nurse executives use must be of a caring nature.

Health systems using the QCM have nurse leaders who extend caring to others first, building their relational capacity and disseminating the benefits. Such leaders inspire by example, mutually relating in caring ways that generate energy and even joy. Extending authentic caring works with patients and families—we have empirical data to support this. So, why can't these same results apply to employees and other stakeholders?

> Caring leaders make it easy for employees to relax, do their best work, enjoy themselves on the job, engage in innovation, and maybe even share economic benefits.

Wouldn't it be interesting, for example, to compare absenteeism, presenteeism, and productivity in health systems with relationally oriented leaders versus those who are not?

It is the job of leadership to extend caring as it engages and motivates others. Such leaders' actions have almost a ripple effect that snowballs throughout the organization, ultimately affecting the culture.

> Leaders who are observed in caring relationships with patients and families and with other stakeholders both in and outside the health system uphold the ethical principles and standards on which healthcare is based, demonstrating that healthcare is *not* just a service but, rather, a professional, accountable, highly regarded series of professional actions that benefit society. Likewise, when leaders display caring relationships with employees, they are actively reminding them of their value to the system and creating the conditions for reciprocation.

Several nurse leaders who are experts in caring relationships in an organization oftentimes inadvertently create cultures of caring characterized by expert professional practice in an open, inclusive atmosphere that demonstrates its value (through evidence) to the health and well-being of the community served. In this way, nursing's powerful impact on persons' lives is visible, documented, and celebrated. In an interesting ethnography, Grundy and Malone (2017) provide an explanation for nurses' continuing invisibility in health systems. As the largest proportion of health professionals who are "situated at the hub of multidisciplinary teams and focused on the prevention and management of increasingly common and costly chronic diseases" (p. E29), many nurses prefer to use their influence covertly in order to avoid conflict while maintaining their long-held insider knowledge. While this may work in individual situations, unfortunately in the wider world, nursing still is considered a cost that has limited tangible value in health systems. Quality caring leaders are able to transcend this challenge by demonstrating how the patient–nurse relationship (or the community–nurse relationship), in essence, the processes of nursing, impact organizational performance, effectiveness, efficiency, and outcomes of care.

What keeps nursing administrators up at night are the continuing problems of adverse events, productivity, staffing and retention, workflow, professionalism, and the leadership abilities of first-line managers, to name a few. The cost implications of nursing-related adverse outcomes portray nursing not only as a health system expense but, at times, a liability. Individual nurse factors (such as experience and credentials), patient treatment–related factors, missed or incomplete care (Kalisch, Tschannen, Lee, & Friese, 2011; Lucero, Lake, & Aiken, 2010), and environmental factors such as physical facilities, workflow, and staffing (Oppel & Young, 2017; Stalpers, de Brouwer, Kaljouw, & Schuurmans, 2015) are implicated in adverse outcomes. Increasingly, nurse presenteeism, or being present at work but not fully productive (because of a variety of factors; Lack, 2011), is becoming noteworthy as a variable associated with poorer nursing-sensitive quality indicators. Letvak, Ruhm, and Gupta (2012) first reported nurse presenteeism (related to musculoskeletal disorders and depression) was associated with increases in medication errors and patient falls, and with lower self-reported quality of care, ultimately raising costs of care. Furthermore, some of the highest rates of presenteeism were found among healthcare workers, resulting in lost productivity, patient safety concerns, and long-term health consequences (Rhodes & Collins, 2014).

Although the real cost and adverse outcome burden of presenteeism in health professionals are not known, one can conjecture about some of its causes. For example, today's health systems are workplaces that have encountered serious change over the last two decades, and employees themselves have altered their work styles. The increase in households with sick children or older adults, fear of "calling in sick," working more than one job (especially as 12-hour shifts have increased the number of available days off), and care demands at work are examples of situations that might affect an individual's productivity and engagement while at work. Nursing administrators thus must be concerned not only with attendance (staffing numbers) but with the contributions and productivity (particularly, the ability to engage in caring relationships) of their workforce.

Clinical workflow, or how care processes are organized, sequenced, and performed *for patient-centered care*, is a national priority. Consider how hospital nurses *continue* to use their time during a shift. First, they spend about 1 hour receiving report from the previous shift—oftentimes this is not comprehensive or relationship-enhancing. Next, they organize themselves according to the various tasks—assessments, medication administration, and treatments that need completion. Then, as they proceed down the list of tasks, they check off tasks one by one making sure that the electronic health record (EHR) is updated. Oftentimes, updating the EHR takes tremendous amounts of time. Finally, nurses report to the oncoming nurse. One or two disruptions or emergencies can throw the entire checklist off, necessitating overtime in order to complete the list. This process has not changed for over 40 years, with the exception of the EHR. But, during this 8- to 12-hour period, one of the patients received a cancer diagnosis, another remained in pain, another patient required a complex dressing change after his daughter was told that she would not be able to take him home with her, and a physician on the staff just found out his daughter was admitted to the psych ward for bulimia. In the busyness of completing the checklist, how aware were the nurses on this unit of the complexities of their patients' or coworkers' lives? Or for that matter, their own stomachs or bladders? How well does ensuring the completion of a series of important tasks contribute to patient-centeredness or enhance the patient experience?

Patients and families desire information, reassurance, acceptance, support, commitment, kindness, acknowledgment, competence, mutual decision making, vigilance, comfort, security, family engagement, and their basic human needs met (Duffy, 2009). They want to be treated as if they were a close relative of the care provider; they want to matter. And don't we all? Nurses consistently say they want to relate more to their patients and work with other nurses who perform the same way. In other words, professional nurses desire a more relationship-centric environment.

Designing care delivery models that are patient centered while integrating health information technology (HIT) requires careful, reflective analysis of the work of professional nursing, identification of key role dimensions, and tough decisions about how the work will be accomplished. Included in this analysis must be the fundamental understanding that professional nursing incorporates *both being* with and *doing for* in an integrated fashion. Thus, the use of a theory-guided model to redesign patient care delivery can help provide the foundation for workflow redesign.

One approach to achieving a relationship-centric patient care delivery system is the use of a diagram that depicts the relationships between theoretical concepts and components of the patient care delivery system, that is, conceptual–operational linkages (see Figure 12.2). Such an illustration aids in ensuring accurate operationalization of the model.

Difficult decisions will need to be made *in the best interest of patients and families* while considering nursing workflow. For example, what will be the major components of RN work? Who will support RN work? What human and environmental resources will be required and how will they be scheduled and assigned to optimize patient-centered care? What means of communication will enhance RN work?

As caring relationships are tied to intermediate and terminal health outcomes for both patients and health professionals (see Chapter 7), nursing administrators are faced with balancing the competing needs of patients for human caring with the economic complexities of the current system. Yet the value of nursing lies in its caring core. Leaders who can demonstrate a return on investment for the caring behaviors of professional nurses are needed. Evidence such as increased safety (for both patients and the healthcare workforce); enhanced patient experiences; faster and better attainment of clinical outcomes; long-term health outcomes such as reduced 30-day readmissions, functional status, and return to work; nurse retention; and improved mental and physical health of the workforce are needed to show how health professionals influence the performance of a healthcare system (self-advancing systems). Leaders who are able to pull together an expert nursing workforce that incorporates the caring factors in their work create health experiences that are safe, comfortable, optimistic, and preserve the wholeness of persons. In other words, dramatically restructuring professional nurse work such that specific knowledge, actions, and attitudes are delivered in a patient-defined context is increasingly tied to good leader behaviors. Inspiring staff by including them in important decisions (see Table 12.1 for leadership behaviors), visiting frequently with patients and families (the customer), cultivating meaningful caring relationships with healthcare colleagues, and teaching and learning how to improve nursing practice builds a lasting legacy for the next generation of nurses.

In fact, creating a legacy of caring so that others will continue to provide patient-centered care and new nurse leaders with similar knowledge, skills, and attitudes is invigorating. Periodically asking "Am I doing what enhances self-advancement? Am I preserving the essence of nursing? Am I really practicing self-caring?" provides consistent reinforcement and inner confidence.

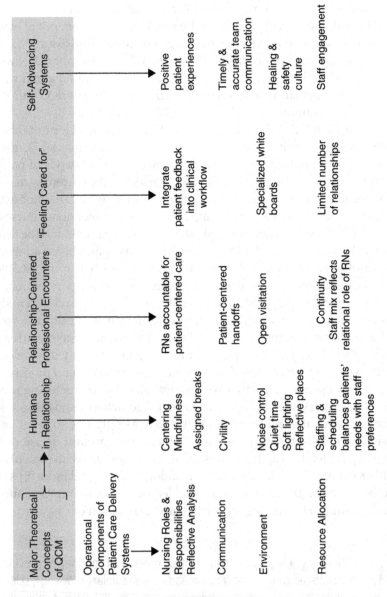

FIGURE 12.2   Conceptual–operational linkages.

QCM, Quality-Caring Model.

TABLE 12.1 Executive Leadership Behaviors Associated with First-Line Managers

Listen and understand concerns

Provide constructive and consistent feedback

If there is a disagreement, don't claim the manager is wrong

Acknowledge strengths

Look for positive intentions

Challenge first-line managers

Support first-line managers' growth and development

Leaders who know how to determine what is important versus what is urgent will have the energy and resilience to cope with the daily emergencies so prevalent in health systems. Often solving symptoms (or urgent problems) feels satisfying, but is only an easy substitute for attending to the real, underlying foundation of the profession. This mode of attending to the urgent often drives out the important, limiting leaders' effectiveness in sustaining cultures of caring.

Sustaining professionalism in complex and dynamically changing health systems demands no tolerance for aggressive, disruptive, or inappropriate behaviors. Expecting caring relationships at all levels as the foundation for clinical practice requires relationship-centered leadership with skills in consensus building, conflict resolution, and maintaining a workforce focused on the patient and family.

> Although knowledge and technical skills are crucial to health professionals, it is the *manner* in which they are used that comprises professionalism. The humanistic qualities inherent in caring relationships are equally important and must be upheld by leadership.

Most would argue that the ethical values of excellence or competence, accountability, integrity, respect for others, duty, and workplace civility are components of professionalism in nursing. These qualities apply not only to relationships with patients and families but to those relationships among medical professionals, specialties, and professional organizations.

Ethical values and resulting practices are the foundation upon which moral actions in professional practice are based (LaSala & Bjarnoson, 2010). Being able to recognize, respond to, and report (if necessary) unethical practices or failure to provide complete, quality nursing care is an obligation of professionalism. Leaders who value and attend to caring relationships create safe environments where others are not fearful when sharing concerns or reporting unethical behavior. They accept constructive criticism so others learn how to demonstrate respect when delivering uncomfortable news or naming conflicting situations. By making professionalism an explicit objective or goal so that it remains in full view for all to see and continuously evaluate, nurse leaders sustain a culture of openness where civility remains the norm. Displaying the code of ethics in a public space and acting with moral courage enables nurses and other health professionals to commit to patient-centered care, question practices, and sustain the professionalism that guides their practice.

Lastly, maintaining a team of first-line leaders who value and focus primarily on high-quality nursing care, including caring relationships with patients and families and other health professionals, is central to patient-centered care. Today's nurse leaders are responsible for large workforces and deal with complex, life-threatening patient situations every day. Additionally, they are responsible for legal, regulatory, budgetary, human and other resources, and safety standards in their units. So, on the one hand, they are responsible for quality patient care, and on the other, they are asked to prepare reports, attend meetings, attain advanced education, attend to facilities, and reconcile the budget. The nurse leader position is vital but often under-recognized and under-respected for its ability to influence health system outcomes (Edmonson, 2010). Compared to counterparts in other professions, first-line nurse leaders often have more employees, larger spans of control, less real authority, and more stress (Shirey, McDaniel, Ebright, Fisher, & Doebbling, 2010).

> Yet the connection between the work of nurse leaders and the mission of health systems (quality patient care) is often unclear. Reinforcing this connection daily is key to self-advancing systems.

Creating safe, open microsystems (nursing units) that successfully safeguard patients and families and guarantee quality outcomes, preserving the integrity of professional nursing, and containing organizational costs are the roles of the first-line nurse leader—a large order indeed! This important work requires global awareness; analytical and sophisticated research and evaluation capacity; expert interpersonal relationship skills; self-caring ability; advanced knowledge of nursing, including nursing theory and professional practice models; the ability to collaborate, share successes, and acknowledge failures; and most importantly, the ability to express caring. Frequent contact by nurse executives (and others in the C-suite) in the actual practice setting helps top leadership appreciate the realities of the clinical practice environment, including leader needs. Creating safe space for frank dialogue and open, flexible communication; fostering self-caring practices in first-line leaders; expressing caring often, through internal and external recognition; and, most importantly, taking a hard look at the role to ensure that attention to quality patient care is the number one priority are essential. To build teams capable of leading in a quality caring practice environment, some nurse executives are using a coaching approach, have created dedicated self-caring meetings, participate in book clubs, attend off-campus gatherings once a month to work on mutual goals and support each other, order *only* "healthy" foods during gatherings, partner with universities to provide "internal" consulting or assistance with leadership evidence-based practice, participate in annual nursing renewal ceremonies, and designate innovation or demonstration units. Expecting and ensuring that future front-line nurse leaders have the knowledge, skills, and values necessary to keep the focus on caring relationships means making hard decisions about what the preparation is for the role, who is hired, how persons will be on-boarded, evaluated and rewarded, and who will be retained.

> Value-based health systems demand high-quality relationships, true patient-centeredness, and optimism. This suggests attention to making others "feel cared for," establishing partnerships and collaboration, empowering and engaging patients and families, and offering hope—for progress, new possibilities, and discovery. Each of these principles hinges on relationships.

Nursing leaders who embrace caring relationships "chose who they want to be . . ." and make the hard decisions required for radical and lasting value.

Education

Building a workforce of professional nurses who are competent; accountable; engaged; practice the caring factors; continuously monitor and perfect relationships with self, patients and families, other health professionals, and the community served; and who look for opportunities to improve clinical practice requires educational programs that adequately prepare them for this role. Although many nursing faculty are busy evaluating and revising their curricula in order to meet the mandates of current healthcare reform, concerns exists that *real, profound* revision of nursing education may not take place (personal conversations with faculty members).

mmediate needs for more experiential and reflective learning, including increased time in practice, attention to pre- and postclinical conferences, the use of real situations in interprofessional classrooms or simulation laboratories, and increased use of evidence as the basis for practice is needed. Such learning requires the expertise of senior faculty members, comfort with open dialogue, student-led discussions, multidisciplinary classrooms, closeness to the practice environment, ongoing and rigorous faculty development, and awareness of the characteristics of today's health professional students.

In a typical health professions course today, the composition of the class might include an occasional baby boomer and a large number of generation X, generation Y, and millennial students who are of varying ages, diverse in terms of gender, race, and ethnicity, and for the most part are tech savvy. Many students are working, commuting, and raising families. Each of the represented generations of students has its own unique set of characteristics that have been shaped by the values, trends, behaviors, and events in place in society at that time. These generational characteristics create vast opportunities to learn, but the differences can also create challenges for faculty.

Using a caring approach of shared learning, educators will need to value caring relationships as essential to health and be committed to the development of caring knowledge in themselves and their students. To promote a growing awareness of self, students need to be exposed to nursing early in their freshman year and build on the life experiences and characteristics they bring to the program. A focus on personal knowing or balancing inner and external knowledge is paramount. The days of planned content delivered in lecture format with set course scheduling may not always be the best way to learn and be caring! Caring experiences with patients and families during clinical courses help students appreciate their value to healthcare outcomes and their own growth as a caring person. Designing such experiences is a role of the faculty. Crucial to such experiences is asking probing questions while in practice that stimulate students to think about their experiences with patients and families. Questions such as "What relationships are emerging?" "What is the quality of the relationships?" "What seems important to the relationship?" and "What are the potential consequences of the observed relationships?" provide opportunities for much more introspection.

Helping students learn the caring factors through study, simulations, and role modeling creates situations in which students can test their interactions in a safe place under the guidance of experts. Grounding nursing simulations in caring allows faculty to create an environment in which the uniqueness of the human person and the fullness of nursing practice can be understood (Eggenberger & Keller, 2008). Likewise, in the online course environment, faculty members must ensure the wholeness of patients and families is preserved. Integrating knowledge from multiple sources is a skill necessary for quality care, so less emphasis on textbooks and more emphasis on professional literature early and repeatedly is wise. Finally, ensuring caring competency through formative and summative evaluation helps prepare professional nurses "to be" as well as "to do" nursing.

Diener and Hobbs (2012) postulate that the increasing reliance on simulated learning may isolate caring from task acquisition in nursing. They state:

> Forming caring relationships, enacting caring presence, and employing transpersonal caring requires reciprocity that is not developed between students and simulated patients. In an age of avatars, Webkinz, and virtual environments, simulation technology becomes just another venue of gaming. Relationships are contrived and patients are plastic. If patients live, students have won "the game." Tears shed when simulation patients die may be more about performance stress and "losing" a game than losing a human being. Twenty-first century nursing is situated in a landscape where care and skill are needed in equal measure. Technology does not negate caring; indeed, the isolation it fosters makes the significance of transpersonal caring all the more important. As educators in a domain of humanistic science, the charge is to guide twenty-first century nursing education within a caring curriculum using technology wisely and appropriately. We are called to create a new paradigm for nursing education that merges Nightingale's vision with technology's promise. Facilitating development of caring behaviors in nursing students must move beyond simulation labs to engage live patients and cultivate caring behaviors modeled by nurse educators. Caring begins in school. Students who have never experienced a caring education are unlikely to recognize the healing aspect care brings to practice environments. In a similar fashion,

unless time is spent with human beings in even the earliest stages of nursing education, transpersonal caring relationships do not have space to develop. Learning, crafting, and maturation of caring behaviors becomes a serendipitous event or, more concerning, is no longer perceived as an essential characteristic of nursing. (p. 37)

Wow, what a poignant quote! As educators, these authors are concerned about the fashionable and sometimes sole use of technology—as learning aids to health professions students' understanding and development of caring relationships, particularly those with patients and families.

Nursing educators will need to be savvy about integrating technology with real clinical experiences in order to meet the demands of health systems for value. The pedagogical challenge for faculty is to help students find meaning in their nursing, connecting it with values that affirm caring relationships as central to clinical practice. Consistent dialogue with relevant affirmations, clinical practice, and reflection is crucial.

To effectively build caring relationships, students and teachers must learn how "to be" in relationship with each other and, in a sense, co-learn. Through the relationship, the two become aligned in the learning process and new information is tossed about, questioned, and grasped as pertinent or not pertinent to clinical practice. In this manner, caring nurse educators transform the learning environment from a passive acquisition of facts to an active relational investigation of new ideas and partnership, much like clinical practice!

Facilitating the development of new knowledge about caring relationships through advanced inquiry is also a faculty responsibility that requires faculty mentors who understand its nature and who are involved with the science themselves. Research mentoring is crucial to building a future group of nurse scientists who can translate caring relationships into practice.

ADVANCING THE SCIENCE OF CARING RELATIONSHIPS

Evaluating how caring relationships impact patient outcomes (safety and quality in particular), how to improve and widely disseminate them as the basis for care, and sustaining longer term caring relationships is demanding; yet, as a central construct of professional practice, knowledge about this core process is necessary to improve and accelerate its translation into practice. Moreover, it provides needed feedback to health professionals about their practice, which is so often lacking in specialized departments. To extend the understanding and strengthen the evidence pertaining to caring relationships (specifically nurse caring) as a significant variable in the healthcare process, much more evaluation is necessary. However, there is a relative lack of data on the quality of nursing care and inconsistencies exist among the evaluation tools used to measure care quality. These inconsistencies exist even among data-collection initiatives focused on nursing performance, such as the National Database of Nursing Quality Indicators (NDNQI) and the California Nursing Outcomes Coalition Database (CalNOC) Project. For example, despite the National Quality Forum's (NQF) Voluntary Consensus Standards for Nursing-Sensitive Care (The Joint Commission, 2010), nursing performance databases are not inclusive of them. Efforts to align these initiatives with NQF standards are ongoing. Furthermore, patient characteristics (such as acuity) are not used to adjust for differences in nursing performance. Lastly, the new payment rules on reimbursement for adverse outcomes also leave a great deal open to interpretation.

Outcomes measures that reflect nursing's benefits may better showcase the value of nursing. Although the NDNQI indicators have been instrumental in generating awareness of and improving important nursing-sensitive indicators, there are numerous, more positive metrics that may better reflect the performance of nursing. For example, hospitalized older adults frequently leave the hospital with poorer physical function than when admitted. This is a national problem with significant cost and clinical burden, not to mention the personal burden it places on patients and families. Measuring and reporting the difference in functional status from admission to discharge for older adults would showcase how nursing's attention to mobility during hospitalization saves both clinical burden and actual dollars (and might enhance the patient's experience). Those with chronic illnesses, such as heart failure, cancer, and chronic obstructive pulmonary disease (COPD), often are readmitted within 30 days of discharge, financially draining the U.S. health system. This burden may be lessened if nurses worked, through caring relationships, to engage patients in their care prior to discharge. Patient engagement is a positive outcomes indicator that is measurable at hospital discharge, has been associated with decreased readmissions in certain patients (Peters & Keeley, 2017), reflects the relational aspect of nursing care, and could potentially raise positive regard for nursing.

Other, more positive indicators such as comfort (vs. pain), knowledge (vs. knowledge-deficit), dignity, health-related quality of life (HRQOL), optimistic mood (vs. depression), feeling "cared for," recovery time, adherence (vs. nonadherence), contentment (vs. anxiety), continence (vs. incontinence), self-caring, cognition (vs. cognitive impairment), empowerment, health-seeking behaviors, mobility (vs. functional decline), symptom control, and skin integrity (vs. pressure ulcers) are examples of affirming outcomes measures that could be used to report the outcomes of nursing care. Many of these indicators have well-documented instruments that would easily translate to the clinical environment, rendering measurement and reporting feasible. And findings might provide some much-needed encouragement to nurses!

To extend the understanding and strengthen the evidence of caring (specifically nurse caring) as a significant variable influencing health outcomes, more research must be conducted and disseminated. Although studies of nurse caring over the last 3 years are few, studies of the benefits of patient-centered care are emerging (see Chapter 4) as are those related to enhancing health professionals' self-awareness (a dimension of self-caring). In a systematic review, Papastavrou et al. (2012) found important differences between patients' and nurses' perceptions of caring and caring behaviors in the 23 quantitative studies reviewed. Results have important implications for clinical practice and education. In a Saudi Arabian study, the frequency of caring relationships attended to by nurses in teaching/learning and helping/trust behavior subcategories was rated lower than in other caring subcategories. The authors posit that such differences were most likely the result of cultural and language differences between patients and nurses in Saudi Arabia (Suliman, Welmann, Omer, & Thomas, 2009). In this global world with multicultural nurses, it is important that the host country's norms and values are appreciated and used in the delivery of care. This is important to consider in the United States as well—many patients, particularly hospitalized older adults, have conveyed to this author their anxieties about health professionals who do not speak the primary language, and the unease it creates in health situations.

Continuing to build on the foundation of existing caring knowledge using multiple methods will provide the evidence needed to justify the radical transformation driving health system change. Refining existing measures of caring using appropriate conceptual definitions and adequate psychometric properties, with particular emphasis on the patient's view, will allow for correlational studies and multisite comparisons. In-depth studies of outliers (those organizations and health professionals who successfully embrace quality caring principles), examination of how to improve relational competencies in organizations, the influence of culture on caring relationships, how caring relationships with self can be fostered amid the complexities of the health system, and leveraging information technology to enhance caring relationships and patient-centered care are all important questions for further study. Continuing to study the link between caring relationships and specific nursing-sensitive patient outcomes, such as comfort, functional status, and increased knowledge will strengthen the evidence base regarding the importance of caring relationships in clinical practice. And linking caring relationships to reimbursable outcomes, such as patient experiences, readmission rates, and adverse outcomes, may significantly impact hospitals' bottom line. Likewise, educational studies that examine the acquisition of deeper levels of caring and/or professionalism over the course of a program are necessary. Nursing administration studies that identify the contribution of health professionals' characteristics to the delivery of patient-centered care and how well relationship-centered leadership adds to organizational relational capacity will also be valuable to the scientific base.

Developing caring-based interventions for testing is necessary to provide high levels of evidence for caring-based professional practice and to validate caring theory. Caring-based interventions are complicated to design because little has been done in this area, and practical limitations for testing can be challenging. Nevertheless, caring-based interventions must be studied through research investigations to better understand how they contribute to healthcare outcomes. Using empirical data and a caring-based conceptual framework to support the intervention, a detailed description organized to meet the needs of the population under study is paramount. Developing a protocol describing the content, strength, and frequency of the intervention allows for replication. Using probability sampling and longitudinal studies, questions such as "What is the effect of the intervention on specific outcomes of care?" can be answered. Integrating cost-effectiveness components will add to the understanding of the intervention's worth.

Using strategies such as interprofessional teams, applying tools where data are pooled from multiple sites, and integrating biological, behavioral, and cost-effectiveness methods will eventually enable us to make predictions about how health professionals with certain characteristics perform the caring factors, the proper "dose" of caring for particular patient populations, the most effective ways to learn caring, and the relative worth of caring practices.

Relevant manuscripts and doctoral dissertations published in high-quality journals will expose others to caring research. Likewise, presentations at meetings of professional organizations and use of the results of caring studies to create or revise existing policy add to the science. Through the daily application of evidence-based practice, nurses at all levels who critically appraise caring research to judge the trustworthiness of study findings and to translate credible results to the bedside will strengthen the work of nursing. Applying new knowledge in the appropriate setting may help to transform the work environment for nurses such that they find meaning in the important work they do. Finally, drawing conclusions from research about caring theory helps to validate and refine it. Explicitly stating the caring theory that undergirds research studies adds valuable knowledge for the profession and provides the basis for future nursing care (Fawcett, 2007), supplies rationale for practice improvements, exposes the significant role of professional nurses in healing, and helps validate or reject existing theory. Professional nurses have a social responsibility to study, mentor, and facilitate scientific inquiry related to caring relationships, the cornerstone of their clinical practice.

THE PROMISE OF A VALUABLE HEALTH SYSTEM

Now what?

Evolving health care payment options, accelerations in technology, evidence-based practice, and expert clinical workforces are going to continue dominating the national discourse. Well-qualified and questioning nurses are needed more than ever; now is the time to double down on our work. There is no time for delays since the world is moving all around us. Real leadership is needed to advance nursing's focus on improving health and healthcare for individuals and communities. And the type of leadership needed is the human-to-human, caring, uplifting type that reminds us of our likenesses, common needs, and shared experiences.

Far from the noise and bluster of Washington, DC, we all are likely to benefit by focusing our attention on serving real communities whose voices don't easily break through in these contentious times and by coming together to achieve the quadruple aim (Bodenheimer & Sinsky, 2014). The quadruple aim can be succinctly summarized as better health for populations, better care for patients, engaging patients and employees, and lower costs of healthcare. It's a simple yet powerful concept, and it is frequently used as the measuring stick for improving the quality and affordability of health and healthcare.

Working together—community groups and health systems, universities and health systems, patients and providers, health providers and law enforcement, schools and primary care centers—in caring partnerships will generate strong, coherent groups of individuals who respond to health problem–rich communities. Characteristics such as flexibility, resilience, reliability, durability, self-monitoring, and self-repair are necessary. There is no room on this list of adjectives for self-doubt, mistrust, disregard, roughness, violence, inattention, or despair. Rather the former characteristics are born of confidence, being connected, feeling safe, and optimistic—all consequences of "feeling cared for."

In response to the 2017 natural disasters (Hurricanes Harvey, Irma, & Maria) that devastated large geographic areas, individuals, families, and communities, swarms of dedicated health professionals brought lifesaving interventions, connection, and hope to many suffering individuals. Although the suffering victims were described as resilient, the enthusiastic, moving, risky, and patriotic choice that dedicated health professionals made to purposely work together brought some healing to suffering communities. In other words, they cared enough for others, even with scant resources, to try novel approaches and work together for "what really matters."

Health professionals and health systems have a real opportunity to radically reform and provide value through the generation of new ways of doing clinical work, advancing their professions, themselves, and communities in the process. Thinking long term while simultaneously managing the present allows goals to become reality. And *productive* dreaming (brainstorming) in caring environments sustains long-term thinking, enabling emerging new ideas and strategies for achieving them. Health professionals and health systems need to acknowledge that the past may not always provide the right lessons; in other words, reshuffling roles or adding new activities to existing ones is not radical reform. Healthcare reform with its focus on technology, increased access, and modified reimbursement, by itself, is not enough—caring human relationships among health professionals and patients are essential.

Taken together, these principles have guided the evolution of the QCM such that it incorporates a longer term, holistic, and integrated set of relationships from which to guide professional practice. Although originally intended to blend the human caring aspect of patient care with the evidence base needed for quality outcomes, more recently, the model has focused on enhancing the *quality of caring relationships* in an effort to meet the demand for high value (and self-advancing health systems) amid the intricacies of a multicultural, patient-driven, and chronically ill population. It is within this dynamic paradigm that attending to the quality of caring relationships is a global health priority!

A s significant as caring is to the profession of nursing, it is now being extended to the health system level. Enabling caring relationships to flourish
by acknowledging the good work health professionals do, deriving meaning in
that work, performing the caring factors, and continuously improving clinical
practice offers health professionals and health systems a new way to demonstrate
their significance to society. Displacing the disease, illness, negative outcomes
paradigm with one that focuses on well-being, wholeness, and positive outcomes
transforms the future outlook to one of possibility, hope, and advancement.

Healthcare as we know is transitioning to a model not seen before.
Although health professionals have stretched to meet the demands for
health services in recent years, it is the anchoring foundation of caring that
must be stretched, providing energy (and renewal) for further enriching
those caring relationships so necessary for high-quality outcomes. This
takes hard work—showing up day after day, searching for "what matters"
to others, authentic collaboration, multiple small innovations, discipline,
genuine concern, openness and acceptance. Today's workforce has the
tools—but must take responsibility for creating value.

R eal, long-term teams of health professionals developed and led for the
purpose of providing expert care to patients and families, that acknowledge the need to do better, where continuous learning is the norm, and
real-time patient data prevail are beginning to transform health systems to
ones "set up for patients." Health systems and health professionals must
decide whether to sit on the sidelines and watch this unfold *or* risk organizing around the caring needs of patients and families.

Turmoil and instability sometimes prevent consideration of what really
matters—in this case, professional nursing's primary function, caring relationships. But it is precisely at this time that the essence of nursing (Watson,
1979, 1985) may provide the strength necessary to carry out dramatic change.
Refocusing skill acquisition and tasks/procedures to caring relationships
and teamwork, building relational capacity, and measuring "feeling cared
for" and other patient-defined positive outcomes extend nursing's relational
core to other health professionals and health systems. Taking advantage

of this time in history to enhance value is nursing's gift to health systems. It is time for nursing to find its place—and "choose how to be" (Wheatley, 2017), *use* its oftentimes hidden power, and *lead*. Self-advancing patients, health professionals, and health systems need them!

SUMMARY

Reflections about the future were presented. Particular attention was paid to healthcare, including a new values-based model and the challenges of patient-centered health systems. The growing, sophisticated nursing workforce that practices from a caring stance is already transforming health systems. Several outliers are mentioned with current examples, and clinical practice, leadership, and educational challenges are presented. In particular, reducing adverse outcomes attributed to nursing, redesigning clinical workflow to be patient centered, sustaining professionalism, and creating teams of first-rate front-line managers are reviewed. In education, using caring relationships as the basis for learning and evaluation, experiential learning with additional clinical time, and partnering with service are advocated. Evaluating and researching how caring relationships impact selected outcomes and widely disseminating findings are significant. However, using patient-derived feedback and more positive indicators might benefit health professionals. The revised QCM provides a framework for modern clinical practice that offers hope for future generations. Rethinking how clinical work is organized to add value is paramount. Finally, nurses who are experts in caring relationships can lead health systems to embrace caring relationships as the basis for practice-enabling self-advancing systems that will make a profound impact on patient outcomes.

Call to Action

Relationships, specifically caring relationships, as the basis for actions and decision making are necessary to remake valuable health systems. Highly developed, inclusive, and interdependent professional nurses who understand the significance of the whole and whose practice is based on caring relationships are the critical mass that can lead the health system toward a sustainable future. **Choose** to believe (caring intention) in the power of caring relationships—they drive actions. **Assume** that others

(continued)

(continued)

care—look for the positive—it changes the dynamic of relationships. **Walk the talk**—it establishes your credibility. **Identify** the caring leaders you can turn to for guidance. **Discover and imitate** the caring experts in your health system. **Create** transparency, **clarify** expectations, **keep** commitments. A mindful, engaged, and relational professional workforce that remains true to its caring roots will help shift the biomedical, task-oriented, shift-focused approach of today to an interactive, whole system, theory-based practice that invigorates the healthcare system. Regularly **participate** in self-awareness practices and research. Nursing educators who value caring relationships as essential to health will further the development of caring knowledge. **Internalize** the significance of caring relationships to health. Rethinking the task-focused work of clinical practice is a national priority. The nonlinear and multiple relationships so common to healthcare work require a completely different focus of attention—one that is driven by the patient and embraces little structure and form but allows for relationships to generate ideas and conditions for innovation. The goal of the leader is to enable the healthcare system to emerge and self-advance by increasing the number and quality of interactions, developing caring–healing–protective environments and being mindful of the unfolding world in which they function. **Generate** new ways of thinking about nursing work. Demonstrating a return on investment for the caring behaviors of professional nurses will be a leadership responsibility. **Offer** some practical evidence of nursing's value to your organization. Reflective analysis of the future work of professional nursing, including the identification of role dimensions, will require difficult decisions about how that work will be accomplished. **Think about** the meaning in patient encounters, including the technical skill required. Expecting caring relationships in all interactions minimally demands civil discourse. No tolerance for verbal or other abuse in the workplace starts with relationship-centered leadership that continuously focuses on what's best for patients and families. **Role model** caring relationships. How front-line nurse managers are prepared, hired, evaluated, rewarded, and retained for a work environment focused on caring relationships requires in-depth analysis and crucial decision making. **Challenge** front-line nurse managers to **embrace** caring professional practice models. Weaving the caring core of nursing with positive, patient-derived feedback about the process strengthens and forms new connections that influence the future. **Engender** hope and possibility.

REFLECTIVE QUESTIONS/APPLICATIONS

. . . for Students

1. Discuss professional nursing practice in 2050. What will the work environment look like? What actions will make up the majority of nursing time?
2. In preparing to be tomorrow's professional nurse, what do you consider are the top five needs? What can you glean from the pioneers in nursing that may help this transition?
3. What do we need to do as a profession to better prepare nurses of the future for the challenges that await them?
4. What attitudes need to change?
5. What do we want to conserve about nursing?
6. Explain how the caring factors assist in patient-centered care? Be specific.
7. React to the two case studies presented in the chapter related to nurses in clinical practice.

. . . for Professional Nurses in Clinical Practice

1. How can professional nurses extend caring to health team members? Be specific.
2. Explain how you have learned some life lessons from relating to patients and families.
3. Create a future scenario (50 years from now) of a patient situation from your area of expertise. What is different about professional nursing, and what remains the same?
4. Remember a time when you chose caring over some other response to a patient's needs. How did it feel?
5. Can you identify leaders in your health system who regularly use caring relationships as the basis for their practice? How are they different from others? Does their behavior impact others? How?

. . . for Professional Nurses in Educational Practice

1. Describe how a sophomore nursing clinical course could be enhanced through caring relationships with patients. What would be required of faculty and of students? How would the course be evaluated?

2. What are the necessary thinking patterns that will have to occur in graduate students in order to meet the challenges of relationship-centered caring?
3. Create a future clinical nursing scenario either for the simulation lab or for use as a case study. Evaluate it with real students and revise as necessary.
4. Design a leadership course introducing the QCM. Include objectives and an evaluation mechanism. How would you know if the students could apply the model to their practice?
5. Choose a proposition from the revised QCM. Using a population of interest, present a research question that could test this proposition. Include relevant variables and hypotheses. What instruments might be used to test your hypotheses?
6. Evaluate the necessity of more clinical time for undergraduate nursing students. What would need to happen?
7. Discuss with fellow faculty members the redesign and testing of one undergraduate and one graduate course using a caring-based approach. What would the objectives look like? Who would teach it? How would the students and faculty be evaluated?

. . . for Professional Nurses in Leadership Practice

1. Record the methodology you would use to justify increased RN staffing for a nursing unit with the majority population older than 65 years.
2. Create a plan for dramatically altering RN work at your organization to enable *real* patient-centeredness. Who would be involved? What methodology would be used? How long would it take? What implications for RN staffing and scheduling would occur? How would you ensure that all opinions and ideas were heard? How would you evaluate it?
3. What critical knowledge and skills concerning caring relationships has the nursing leadership team in your organization acquired? What caring knowledge and skills do they lack? Create a plan for attaining the requisite knowledge and skills for relationship-centered caring.
4. How do *you* help nurses stay focused on caring relationships in their day-to-day practice?

5. What nursing-sensitive indicators do you track? How could they be more patient centered? What suggestions do you have to focus more on "positive" outcomes indicators?
6. What will your legacy be? What will you leave the next generation of nurses and patients?

REFERENCES

Bodenheimer, T., & Sinsky, C. (2014). From triple to quadruple aim: Care of the patient requires care of the provider. *The Annals of Family Medicine, 12*(6), 573–576. doi:10.1370/afm.1713

Centers for Medicare and Medicaid Services. (2017a). Accountable Care Organizations (ACO). Retrieved from https://www.cms.gov/Medicare/Medicare-Fee-for-Service-Payment/ACO

Centers for Medicare and Medicaid Services. (2017b). *National health expenditure data.* Office of the Actuary, National Health Statistics Group. Retrieved from https://www.cms.gov/research-statistics-data-and-systems/statistics-trends -and-reports/nationalhealthexpenddata/nhe-fact-sheet.html

Centers for Medicare and Medicaid Services. (2018). Our innovation models. Retrieved from https://innovation.cms.gov

Chazal, R. A. (2017). Recognizing inevitable change and responding responsibly. *Journal of the American College of Cardiology, 69*(12), 1637–1639. doi:10.1016/ j.jacc.2017.02.019

Diener, E., & Hobbs, N. (2012). Simulating care: Technology-mediated learning in twenty-first century nursing education. *Nursing Forum, 47*(1), 34–38. doi:10.1111/j.1744-6198.2011.00250.x

Duffy, J. (2009). *Quality caring in nursing and health systems: Applying theory to clinical practice, education, and leadership.* New York, NY: Springer Publishing.

Edmonson, C. (2010). Moral courage and the nurse leader. *OJIN: The On-line Journal of Issues in Nursing, 15*(3), Manuscript 5. doi:10.3912/OJIN. Vol15No03Man05

Eggenberger, T., & Keller, K. (2008). Grounding nursing simulations in caring: An innovative approach. *International Journal for Human Caring, 12*(2), 42–46.

Fawcett, J. (2007). Nursing qua nursing: The connection between nursing knowledge and nursing shortages. *Journal of Advanced Nursing, 59*(1), 97–99. doi:10.1111/j.1365-2648.2007.04325.x

Fry, R. (2015). Millennials surpass Gen Xers as the largest generation in U.S. labor force. *Pew Research Center.* Retrieved from http://www.pewresearch.org/fact-tank/2015/05/11/ millennials-surpass-gen-xers-as-the-largest-generation-in-u-s-labor-force

Grundy, Q., & Malone, R. E. (2017). The "as-if" world of nursing practice: Nurses, marketing, and decision making *Advances in Nursing Science, 40*(2), E28–E43. doi:10.1097/ANS.0000000000000143

The Joint Commission. (2010). National Quality Forum (NQF) endorsed nursing-sensitive care performance measures. Retrieved from http://www .jointcommission.org/national_quality_forum_nqf_endorsed_nursing -sensitive_care_performance_measures

Kalisch, B., Tschannen, D., Lee, H., & Friese, C. R. (2011). Hospital variation in missed nursing care. *American Journal of Medical Quality, 26*(4), 291–299. doi:10.1177/1062860610395929

Kantarjian, H. M. (2017). The Affordable Care Act, or Obamacare, 3 years later: A reality check. *Cancer, 123*(1), 25–28. doi:10.1002/cncr.30384

Lack, D. M. (2011). Presenteeism revisited. A complete review. *American Association of Occupational Health Nurses, 59*(2), 77–89. doi:10.3928/08910162-20110126-01

LaSala, C. A., & Bjarnason, D. (2010). Creating workplace environments that support moral courage. *OJIN: The Online Journal of Issues in Nursing, 15*(3), Manuscript 4. doi:10.3912/OJIN.Vol15No03Man04

Letvak, S., Ruhm, C., & Gupta, S. (2012). Nurses' presenteeism and its effect on self-reported quality of care and costs. *American Journal of Nursing, 112*(2), 30–38. doi:10.1097/01.NAJ.0000411176.15696.f9

Lucero, R. J., Lake, E. T., & Aiken, L. H. (2010). Nursing care quality and adverse events in US hospitals. *Journal of Clinical Nursing, 19*, 2185–2195. doi:10.1111/j.1365-2702.2010.03250.x

Massachusetts Department of Health and Human Services. (2017). National TeleNursing Center. Retrieved from http://www.mass.gov/eohhs/gov/ departments/dph/programs/community-health/dvip/violence/sane/ telenursing

Oppel, E. M., & Young, G. J. (2017), Nurse staffing patterns and patient experience of care: An empirical analysis of U.S. hospitals. *Health Services Research.* ePub ahead of print. doi:10.1111/1475-6773.12756

Papastavrou, E., Efstathiou, G., Tsangari, H., Suhonen, R., Leino-Kilpi, H., Patiraki, H., . . . Merkouris, A. (2012). Patients' and nurses' perceptions of respect and human presence through caring behaviours: A comparative study. *Nursing Ethics, 19*, 369–379. doi:10.1177/0969733011436027

Peters, A. E., & Keeley, E. C. (2017). Patient engagement following acute myocardial infarction and its influence on outcomes. *The American Journal of Cardiology, 120*(9), 1467–1471. doi:10.1016/j.amjcard.2017.07.037

Price Waterhouse Coopers. (2017). Millennials at work Reshaping the workplace. Retrieved from https://www.pwc.com/gx/en/managing-tomorrows-people/ future-of-work/assets/reshaping-the-workplace.pdf

Rhodes, S. M., & Collins, S. K. (2014). The organizational impact of presenteeism. *Radiology Management, 37*(5), 27–32.

Shirey, M. R., McDaniel, A. M., Ebright, P. R., Fisher, M. L., & Doebbling, B. N. (2010). Understanding nurse manager stress and work complexity: Factors that make a difference. *Journal of Nursing Administration, 40*(2), 82–91. doi:10.1097/ NNA.0b013e3181cb9f88

Stalpers, D., de Brouwer, B.J.M., Kaljouw, M.J., & Schuurmans, M.J. (2015). Associations between characteristics of the nurse work environment and five nurse-sensitive patient outcomes in hospitals: A systematic review of literature. *International Journal of Nursing Studies, 52*(4), 817–835. doi:10.1016/ j.ijnurstu.2015.01.005

Steelman, G. M., & Westman, E. C. (Eds.). (2016). *Obesity: Evaluation and treatment essentials*. Boca Raton, FL: CRC Press.

Suliman, W. A., Welmann, E., Omer, T., & Thomas, L. (2009). Applying Watson's nursing theory to assess patient perceptions of being cared for in a multicultural environment. *Journal of Nursing Research, 17*(4), 293–297. doi:10.1097/ JNR.0b013e3181c122a3

Swanson, K. (2008). *Living caring*. Presentation delivered at the International Association for Human Caring Conference, Chapel Hill, NC.

Watson, J. (1979). *Nursing: The philosophy and science of caring*. Boston, MA: Little, Brown and Company.

Watson, J. (1985). *Nursing: Human science and human care*. Norwalk, CT: Appleton-Century-Crofts.

Weirich, B. (2017). A Millennial leader's views on the Millennial workforce. *Nurse Leader, 15*(2), 137–139. doi:10.1016/j.mnl.2016.12.003

Wheatley, M. (2017). *Who do we choose to be: Facing reality, claiming leadership, restoring sanity*. Oakland, CA: Berritt-Koehler.

Appendices

Appendix A

Quality and Caring Resources on the Internet

Affordable Care Act (www.healthcare.gov/law/full/index.html)

Agency for Healthcare Research and Quality (www.ahrq.gov)

American Association of Colleges of Nursing (www.aacnnursing.org)

American Council on Education (www.acenet.edu/pages/default.aspx)

American Health Care Act of 2017 (www.govtrack.us/congress/bills/115/hr1628)

American Organization of Nurse Executives (www.aone.org)

Association of American Medical Colleges (www.aamc.org)

The Berkana Institute (www.berkana.org)

Bureau of Health Professions of the Health Resources and Services Agency (bhpr.hrsa.gov)

Centers for Disease Control and Prevention (www.cdc.gov)

Centers for Medicare & Medicaid Services (www.cms.gov)

The Commonwealth Fund (www.commonwealthfund.org)

The Daisy Foundation (www.daisyfoundation.org)

Hahn School of Nursing and Health Science (www.sandiego.edu/nursing/research/nursing-theory-research.php)

Institute for Healthcare Improvement (www.ihi.org/Pages/default.aspx)

Institute of Medicine (www.ihi.org/resources/Pages/OtherWebsites/TheInstituteofMedicine.aspx)

International Association for Human Caring (www.humancaring.org)

The Joint Commission (www.jointcommission.org)

National Association for Healthcare Quality (www.nahq.org)

National Database of Nursing Quality Indicators (www.pressganey.com/solutions/clinical-quality/nursing-quality)

National Institute for Nursing Research (www.ninr.nih.gov)

National League for Nursing (www.nln.org)

Nursing Theory Link Page (www.clayton.edu/health/nursing/nursingtheory)

Patient-Centered Outcomes Research Institute (www.pcori.org)

Picker Institute (pickerinstitute.org)

Plexus Institute (www.plexusinstitute.org)

Quality and Safety Education for Nurses (www.qsen.org)

Relational Coordination Research Collaborative (rcrc.brandeis.edu/about-us/index.html)

Relationship Centered Health Care (www.rchcweb.com)

Appendix B

Example Health Systems Using the Quality-Caring Model© as the Foundation for Professional Practice

Association of Women's Health, Obstetric and Neonatal Nurses, Washington, District of Columbia
Children's Mercy Hospital and Clinics, Kansas City, Missouri
Hannibal Medical Center, Hannibal, Missouri
Holy Cross Hospital, Silver Spring, Maryland
International Association of Forensic Nurses, Elkridge, Maryland
Johns Hopkins Bayview, Baltimore, Maryland
Lakeland Regional Medical Center, Lakeland, Florida
Lowell General Hospital, Lowell, Massachusetts
McLaren Northern Michigan Medical Center, Petoskey, Michigan
MD Anderson Medical Center, Houston, Texas
Methodist Hospital, Henderson, Kentucky
Moffitt Cancer Center, Tampa, Florida
Novant Health Forsythe Medical Center, Winston-Salem, North Carolina
Novant Health Presbyterian Medical Center, Charlotte, North Carolina
Novant Health Prince William Hospital, Manassas, Virginia
St. Joseph's Medical Center, Towson, Maryland
Swedish American Hospital, Rockford, Illinois
Texas Health Resources, Arlington, Texas (multiple hospitals)
Torrance Memorial Hospital, Torrance, California
University of California at San Diego Medical Center, San Diego, California
UMC Health System, Lubbock, Texas
West Virginia University Hospitals, Morgantown, West Virginia

RECENT ADDITIONS

Banner Gateway Medical Center, Gilbert Arizona

Massachusetts Department of Health and Human Services National TeleNursing Center, Boston, Massachusetts

Miriam Hospital, Providence, Rhode Island

Montefiore Health, New York, New York

St Barnabas Health System, Livingston, New Jersey

University of Colorado Anschutz Medical Campus, Aurora, Colorado

Winchester Medical Center, Winchester, Virginia

Appendix C

Nursing Implications of the Quality-Caring Model©

NURSES IN CLINICAL PRACTICE

Know the state of nursing quality in your organization
Accept responsibility for your own professionalism
Use nursing theory to guide your practice
Learn and practice the caring factors
Focus on caring relationships as the primary aspect of nursing work
Use the caring factors to effectively collaborate with health team members
Remind yourself often of the important work you do
Listen to patients and families—they are the best source of information and life lessons
Practice caring for yourself
Balance "being" and "doing"
Understand your role on the health team
Evaluate your caring intention
Use communication that conveys caring
Engage in ongoing practice improvement

NURSES IN EDUCATIONAL PRACTICE

Set the tone for student success
Increase clinical learning experiences
Familiarize yourself with PCORI
Test the Quality-Caring Model
Center learning around patients and families versus disease and geographic areas

Teach enduring nursing concepts in depth
Sustain caring relationships with students
Use caring as a pedagogy
Mentor emerging relational scientists
Evaluate caring capacity of students
Care for yourself, patients and families, health team members, and the community
served

NURSES IN LEADERSHIP PRACTICE

Evaluate and redesign nursing work; organize it for effective patient–provider
relationships
Build professional practice models and design patient care delivery systems that
embrace caring relationships as the foundation for nursing practice
Revise roles and responsibilities of first-line nurse leaders to focus on caring
relationships
Understand how the context influences caring relationships
Appreciate and preserve the important work nurses do
Partner with those in academia
Recognize, reward, and incentivize nurses for their caring practice
Make tough decisions in the best interests of patients and families
Practice caring for yourself, your staff, your patients, health team members, and
the community served
Focus on the fundamental work of the health system—high-quality patient care
Lead from within
Use principles of relationship-centered leadership

Appendix D

Using the Caring Factors to Keep Patients Safe

- Help patients and families understand the threats to their safety
- Listen to patients' concerns
- Clarify questions
- Routinely check in, offering assistance with basic human needs
- Anticipate patient and family needs
- Ensure availability
- Call patients and families by preferred name
- Allow patients to choose when and where they receive care
- Remove noxious stimuli—lights, noise, and so on
- Position and reposition often
- Know what is important to patients
- Relieve muscle tension through range of motion massage, exercises, and relaxation techniques
- Provide fast and effective pain relief and then evaluate its effectiveness
- Assist patients with food, sleeping arrangements, and elimination
- Maintain privacy and confidentiality
- Protect patient information
- Be alert for environmental variables that represent risks to safety
- Provide gentle, sensitive, physical care
- Provide anticipatory guidance
- Engage family members in patient's care and decision making
- Communicate (including shift report and other handoffs) at the bedside, including the patient in the discussion
- Use consistent, caring verbal and nonverbal behaviors
- Show patients they can depend on you by walking the talk
- Help patients understand their illnesses
- Accept feedback from patients and families
- Look for and praise safe behaviors
- Allow family members to stay and engage them in safe practices

Appendix E

Using the Caring Factors to Advance Quality Health Outcomes

Listen attentively to patients' health and illness stories.
Provide information about specific illnesses to patients and families.
Use multiple formats to present information.
Allow patients and families to ask questions about living with their illnesses.
Ask patients to teach *you* about living with their illnesses.
Encourage forward thinking.
Recognize patients' rights.
Praise attainment of intermediate goals.
Allow expression of both positive and negative feelings.
Follow up often.
Set up transitional activities.
Know what is important to patients and families.
Avoid assumptions.
Routinely assess patients' perceptions of "feeling cared for."
Understand the patient's frame of reference.

Appendix F

Assessment of Professional Work Environments for Quality-Caring Practice

Directions: To answer the question "Where are caring relationships evidenced at your institution?" evaluate the following for the presence and/or links to the caring behaviors. Next, evaluate how well they were represented on a scale from 1 (poor) to 5 (extremely well). (Note: Higher scores reflect better representation of caring professional practice.)

Admission

The admission process 1 2 3 4 5
Admission database—Is it holistic? 1 2 3 4 5
Care plans—Are they nurse-, system-, or patient-driven? 1 2 3 4 5
Documentation system—How are caring behaviors recorded and monitored? 1 2 3 4 5

Daily processes

Shift report/handoffs 1 2 3 4 5
Delegation of responsibilities to patient care assistants 1 2 3 4 5
Hygiene and mobility care 1 2 3 4 5
Transfers and "road trips" 1 2 3 4 5
Preventative management 1 2 3 4 5
Patient education materials 1 2 3 4 5
Discharge planning processes 1 2 3 4 5
Decision making at unit level 1 2 3 4 5
Family visitation 1 2 3 4 5

Physical environment

Family waiting areas 1 2 3 4 5
Bulletin boards 1 2 3 4 5
Meeting areas and learning resources for staff 1 2 3 4 5
Staff meetings 1 2 3 4 5

Scheduling/staffing 1 2 3 4 5
Assignments 1 2 3 4 5

Team caring

Rounds/physician visits 1 2 3 4 5
Engagement in practice improvement 1 2 3 4 5
Team meetings 1 2 3 4 5

Patient outcomes

Routine measurements of nursing-sensitive outcomes 1 2 3 4 5
Routine measurements of shared outcomes 1 2 3 4 5
Routine measurements of "feeling cared for" 1 2 3 4 5
Feedback mechanism for outcomes reporting 1 2 3 4 5

Policies

Policy and procedure manuals 1 2 3 4 5
Protocols 1 2 3 4 5
Practice guidelines 1 2 3 4 5

Appendix G

Potential Research Questions

- How do caring relationships contribute to specific nursing-sensitive outcomes?
- What are the characteristics of environments and communities that are perceived by patients to be caring?
- How does nurse caring influence patient outcomes in multiple settings or patient populations (e.g., long-term care, schools, home healthcare)?
- What contextual factors influence nurse-caring capacity?
- How effective are caring-based interventions on health promotion, quality of life, self-caring, patient experiences of care, decreased adverse outcomes, illness knowledge, and hospital readmission rates?
- What is the relationship between nurse-caring capacity and collective relationship capacity?
- Does patient feedback in real time influence the delivery of patient-centered care?
- What is the relationship between nursing leadership and nurse-caring capacity?
- What are the psychometric properties of caring tools for specialized patient populations?
- How do professional nurses differ in terms of nurse caring capacity?
- What improvements in nursing-sensitive patient outcomes are linked to nurse caring?
- What is the nature of the student–teacher relationship? Explain with reference to undergraduate and graduate students.
- What is the relationship between faculty caring and student learning?
- How does caring practice affect system outcomes (e.g., length of stay, readmission rates, costs)?
- What is the best approach to mentor nursing students in relationship-centered research?
- How are caring relationships with healthcare providers best sustained over time?
- How do outcomes of care differ between those sites that use caring professional practice models and those that don't?
- Does relationship-centered leadership improve organizational relational capacity?
- What hiring and orientation practices influence relational capacity?

Appendix H

Reflections on Practice

- Think about someone you have experienced as a caring leader. Identify his or her key attributes. How do these attributes correspond to the caring factors? Or do they?
- Reflect on an experience in your professional career in which a patient or family member taught you something about life. How did you use these lessons in your own life? Or did you?
- Reflect on a time your practice was truly "professional." What were you doing? What did it feel like?
- Think about the last time you worked. How did you connect with the health team? What did you do? What did you learn?
- In your last patient interaction, what nonverbal behaviors did you convey? How do you know?
- Remember the last time you cared for yourself. What did you do? How did it feel? When will you do it again?
- What reminders in the practice environment would help you to stay focused on relationships? List them.
- Do your patients/employees "feel cared for"? How do you know?
- Are you creating value in your health system? Describe how. What indicators are you using to evaluate it?

Appendix I

Quality-Caring Organizational Self-Assessment Tool

Domain	Item	Low = 1	2	3	4	High = 5	Comments
Leadership	Clear statements of commitment to QCM exist						
	Explicit expectations, accountabilities, and measurements related to QCM exist						
	QCM included in nursing philosophy, policies and procedures, guideline development						
	Nurse leaders set clear expectations for professional practice (consistent with the QCM)						
	Nurse leaders understand and can inform others about all components of the QCM						
	Nurse leaders assume accountability for ongoing support and development of the QCM						

(continued)

(*continued*)

Domain	Item	Low = 1	2	3	4	High = 5	Comments
	Clinical nurse leaders champion the QCM						
	Nurse leaders facilitate research and evidence-based practice						
	There is an established succession plan to ensure sustained professional practice						
Performance Improvement	QCM informs nursing strategic plan, QI plans, performance metrics						
	QCM evaluation data are used in future planning						
Personnel	QCM informs hires, RN job descriptions, and clinical advancement						
	Overall employee norms of behavior reflect the QCM						
	Nurses and other employees can articulate elements of the QCM						
	RNs provide care that best utilizes their full scope of practice						
Environment	RNs assume accountability for exemplary professional practice						
	The QCM is perceived by RNs as compatible with RN work						
	Employees are comfortable expressing their opinions and report "feeling heard"						

(*continued*)

(*continued*)

Domain	Item	Low = 1	2	3	4	High = 5	Comments
Professional Development	Web portals provide specific resources for QCM						
	Orientation contains information and expectations related to QCM						
	Multiple sources of continuing education are available for the QCM						
	Educators understand and embrace the QCM						
Documentation	There is evidence of QCM language in the medical record						
Care Processes	Families participate in discussions, rounds, change of shift report						
	Family presence assured 24/7						
	Patients engage in collaborative goal setting with care team						
	Patients express feeling listened to, respected, treated as partner in care						
	Patients actively involved in planning and care transitions						
	Patient discomfort is respectively managed in partnership with patients and families						
	Patients report feeling safe with dignity maintained						

(*continued*)

(*continued*)

Domain	Item	Low = 1	2	3	4	High = 5	Comments
	Patient information is held confidentially						
	Patients' basic human needs are attended to consistently and in a timely fashion						
	Patients' understanding about their illness is achieved through tailored educational approaches						
	Patients are routinely monitored for changes in condition						

QCM, Quality-Caring Model©; QI, quality improvment.

IMPROVEMENT PLAN

_____

_____

_____

_____

_____

_____

_____

_____

_____

_____

Index

Printed in the United States
By Bookmasters